Pharmacy Practice

Third edition

Patricia Stone

BPharm, MRPharmS, MCPP

Independent Pharmaceutical Consultant
Essex, UK

Stephen J Curtis

BPharm, MSc, MIPharmM, FRPharmS, MCPP

Director
Unit for Health Services Development
School of Pharmacy
London, UK

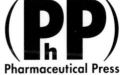

London • Chicago **Pharmaceutical Press**

Published by the Pharmaceutical Press
Publications division of the Royal Pharmaceutical Society of Great Britain

1 Lambeth High Street, London SE1 7JN, UK
100 South Atkinson Road, Suite 206, Grayslake, IL 60030-7820, USA

© Pharmaceutical Press 2002

First edition (1989) and second edition (1995) published by
Farrand Press
Third edition 2002

Text design by Barker/Hilsdon, Lyme Regis, Dorset
Typeset by Type Study, Scarborough, North Yorkshire
Printed in Great Britain by TJ International, Padstow, Cornwall

ISBN 0 85369 482 6

Contents

Preface   *ix*
Acknowledgements   *xi*
About the authors   *xii*
Abbreviations   *xiii*

Part One: Medicines and the patient   1

1   **Prescribers and patients**   3
Access to health services in the community   3
Medical and dental services in primary care   5
Nurses in primary care   10
Secondary referral   15
Patients' rights   19
References   21

2   **The manufacture and marketing of pharmaceuticals**   23
Suppliers of pharmaceuticals   24
Government control of pharmaceuticals   27
Marketing pharmaceuticals   34
New drugs   37
Clinical trials: the role of the pharmacy   40
Postmarketing studies   42
References   45

3   **Primary care pharmacy**   49
Prescribing support in the primary care setting   49
National Prescribing Centre   51
Collaborative National Medicines Management Services Programme   52
Pharmacy Community Care Liaison Group (PCCLG)   53
Pharmaceutical support in practice   54
Pharmaceutical services to private health care providers   58
References   65

4   Pharmacy in the community   69

The extended role: the way forward   69
Services provided by community pharmacists   74
Organisation of a community pharmacy   83
Administration of a community pharmacy   85
Supply and control of medicines   86
Financial controls   90
References   91

5   Dispensing prescriptions   95

Receiving the prescription   96
Reading and checking prescriptions   98
Potential prescription problems   98
Operating a safe system of work   105
Dealing with a dispensing error   108
Dispensing extemporaneous preparations   110
Concordance: a more liberal approach to taking medicines   114
Older people   119
Infants and children   121
Services for drug addicts   124
Wound management products   127
Surgical equipment, appliances and reagents   127
Medical gases   128
References   132

6   Hospital pharmaceutical services   137

Ward and department stock drugs   138
Controlled Drugs   142
Storage of pharmaceuticals on wards   144
Midwifery services   147
Hospital inpatients   148
Hospital outpatients   156
Hospital staff as patients   162
Private patients in NHS hospitals   162
Intermediate care   163
Community services   164
Emergency procedures   166
Ward and clinical pharmacy   169
References   175

7   Specialised hospital pharmaceutical services   179

UK Medicines Information Service   179
Medicines information: wider aspects   187
Pharmaceutical production in hospitals   190

Quality assurance in hospitals   201
References   208

8   The pharmacist as a health care professional   213
Introduction: the profession of pharmacy   213
Professional indemnity insurance   213
Relationships with other professions   214
Professional practice standards   219
Procedures for maintaining safety standards   221
Poisoning   229
References   230

Part Two: Management of resources, quality and audit   233

9   Human resource management   235
Employment law   235
Staff recruitment and training   242
Staff development   246
Education and training   249
Departmental management   253
References   256

10   Quality management in health care   257
Quality standards imposed by government   258
Accreditation by independent bodies   270
Quality from within the organisation   273
References   276

11   Finance, information and procurement   279
National Health Service (NHS) funding   279
Health authority finance   280
Control of finance within NHS trusts   283
Computing and information technology   286
Procurement of medicines   293
Management of stock and assets   298
References   299

Part Three: Health care organisation   303

12   Health care organisation in the UK   305
Accountability   305
Structural change in the NHS   306
Government policy documents   307

Current NHS structure and organisation   309
NHS management   310
Contracting for health care   315
Family health services in primary and community care   316
Hospital organisation and administration   325
Pharmacy organisation at trust level   326
Medical staff grading structure   330
Medical staff organisation   332
Nursing staff organisation   333
Other staff groups   337
Management and administration   337
References   340

Index   343

Preface

As a student, my teacher and mentor (no tutors in those days!) was Frank Allen, then Chief Pharmacist at Whipps Cross Hospital, who taught me a great deal about the practice of pharmacy, and also encouraged me to write. Two of the most significant facts he imparted were first, he told me: 'it doesn't matter so much what you know, as long as you know where to look it up', and second, that he introduced me to a book called *The Handbook of the Royal Naval Sick Berth Attendant*, of which he had an ancient copy. Now this book intrigued me, as it was intended to be a complete guide for someone who was isolated from professional advice, and yet who needed to find out quickly how to deal with problems as they occurred. Remote from pharmacy though some of the advice in this book was – how to organise a burial at sea, or where to dig the latrines if landing on an island, for example – it made me realise that our profession needed a similar reference source, and as a young preregistration student and later, as an inexperienced pharmacist, I longed for a similar book to help me. It was this memory that has provided an inspiration for this book, reinforced by the experience gained while Stephen Curtis and I have been organising preregistration student training in our district.

We have realised that students have to acquire a wealth of information to supplement their practical experience which cannot be found in the standard range of reference works. We have planned this book to provide most of this information in one convenient source, giving at the same time an insight into all the main areas of practice. Thus, it is intended mainly for preregistration students, but will be valuable for undergraduates learning about practice, and for pharmacists during their first few years on the register, or when changing their branch of the profession. Those studying for the examination for Practitioner Membership of the College of Pharmacy Practice will also find material which is relevant.

Since the first edition of this book was published in 1989, the National Health Service has undergone continuous management re-organisation, which will not be completed for at least another 2 or 3 years, if then. The main emphasis is directed towards the needs of the patient. Much importance is now attached to quality aspects of patient care, and since the second edition the concept of clinical governance – both encompassing and adding to previous quality initiatives – has become the main driving force to raise clinical standards. With the advent of primary care groups and trusts, there has also been a shift of management emphasis from the centre to a more locally managed service tailored to the needs of the local population. To reflect this change, we have added a chapter on primary care pharmacy. The remaining chapters have been completely revised to discuss the effects of important new legislation and current developments in practice and standards.

We see this book as an introduction to advanced pharmacy practice, and therefore have given an extensive reference list of further reading, drawing upon a wide range of sources, some familiar and some less so – the latter deliberately to illustrate that one must range widely in search of further education, drawing on the wisdom of other professions.

Patricia Stone
Stephen J Curtis
June 2002

Acknowledgements

The authors wish to thank their many colleagues for their help and suggestions during the preparation of this book. In particular, we appreciate the contributions of the following pharmacists: Robert Adamson, Brian Baker, Victor Irvine, Brian Miller and Marion Walker.

About the authors

Patricia Stone BPharm, MRPharmS, MCPP followed a career in hospital pharmacy, being mostly based at Whipps Cross Hospital, in East London, where at various times she managed the full range of clinical services and pharmacy support services. Seconded to several management projects, she also conducted a year-long study of community pharmacies for the Redbridge and Waltham Forest Family Practitioner Committee. Always interested in supporting and advancing the profession of pharmacy, she has been active in the College of Pharmacy Practice from its foundation, being (with her co-author) one of the first group of associates to achieve College membership by examination. She later worked as an associate examiner and as an examiner for College examinations in pharmacy practice and pharmacy law and ethics modules. Following retirement from full-time National Health Service (NHS) work, she has undertaken consultancy work.

Stephen J Curtis BPharm, MSc, MIPharmM, FRPharmS, MCPP pursued a career as a hospital pharmacist, working at a number of hospitals until becoming Area/District Pharmaceutical Officer at the then Redbridge and Waltham Forest Health Authority, with, latterly, general management responsibilities. Subsequently he became Regional Pharmaceutical Officer for the North-East Thames region, and Secretary to the Committee of Regional Pharmaceutical Officers. After a secondment to the Scottish Office, he left the NHS to set up the Unit for Health Services development at the School of Pharmacy, London University, of which he is currently the Director. He is the Chief Executive Officer of Curtis Buckley, a management consultancy undertaking work for the pharmaceutical industry.

Abbreviations

A&E	accident and emergency
ABPI	Association of the British Pharmaceutical Industry
ADR	adverse drug reaction
ADROIT	Adverse Drug Reactions On-line Information Tracking
AIDS	acquired immunodeficiency syndrome
API	Association of Parallel Importers
ATO	assistant technical officer
BACS	Banking Automated Clearing System
BAN	British Approved Name
BAPEN	British Association for Parenteral and Enteral Nutrition
BASICS	British Association for Immediate Care
BMA	British Medical Association
BNF	*British National Formulary*
BOPA	British Oncology Pharmacy Association
BPC	British Pharmaceutical Conference
BS	British Standard
BTEC	Business and Technicians' Education Council
CBS	Common Basic Specification
CD	Controlled Drug
CEPOD	Confidential Enquiry into Perioperative Deaths
CHC	community health council
CHI	Commission for Health Improvement
CI	clinical indicator
CIVA	centralised intravenous additive
CIVAS	central intravenous additive service
CNMMP	Collaborative National Medicines Management Project
CNPS	centralised NHS pharmaceutical store
COSHH	Control of Substances Hazardous to Health
CPD	continuing professional development
CPMP	Committee for Proprietary Medicinal Products
CPP	College of Pharmacy Practice
CPPE	Centre for Pharmacy Postgraduate Education
CPR	cardiopulmonary resuscitation

CRD	Centre for Reviews and Dissemination
CSM	Committee on Safety of Medicines
CSSD	central sterile supply department
CTX	clinical trial exemption
CV	curriculum vitae
CVMP	Committee for Veterinary Medicinal Products
DDX	Doctors' and Dentists' Exemption scheme
DGH	district general hospital
DHA	district health authority
DHSS	Department of Health and Social Security
DIAL	Drug Information Advisory Line
DMS	Diploma in Management Studies
DoH	Department of Health
DSS	Department of Social Security
DUMP	disposal of unwanted medicines
EAN	European article numbering
EBM	evidence-based medicine
EDI	electronic data interchange
EHC	emergency hormonal contraception
EHR	electronic health record
EMEA	European Medicines Evaluation Agency
ENB	English National Board
EPA	Environmental Protection Act
EPoS	electronic point of sales
EPR	electronic patient record
EU	European Union
FDA	Food and Drug Administration
FHSA	family health services authority
FHSAA	Family Health Services Appeals Authority
FPC	family practitioner committee
FRCS	Fellow of the Royal College of Surgeons
GP	general practitioner
GPFH	general practitioner fundholder
HA	health authority
HAZ	health action zone
HCHS	hospital and community health services
HDA	Health Development Agency
HImP	health improvement programme
HIV	human immunodeficiency virus
HLPI	high-level performance indicator
HPC	Health Professions Council

HTA	health technology assessment
HTM	health technical memorandum
INN	International Non-proprietary Name
IPPR	Itemised Prescription Payment Report
IRMER	Ionising Regulations (Medical Exposure) Regulations
ISO	International Organization for Standardization
IT	information technology
IV	intravenous
JCAHO	Joint Commission for the Accreditation of Health Organizations
LMC	local medical committee
LPC	local pharmaceutical committee
LPS	local pharmaceutical services
MAA	marketing authorisation application
MBA	Master of Business Administration
MCA	Medicines Control Agency
MCPP	Member of the College of Pharmacy Practice
MDA	Medical Devices Agency
MDS	monitored dosage system
MEP	*Medicines, Ethics and Practice*
MI	medicines information
MRCGP	Member of the Royal College of General Practitioners
MRCP	Member of the Royal College of Physicians
MS	Master of Surgery
MSc	Master of Science
MTO	medical technical officer
NAO	National Audit Office
NBM	nil by mouth
NCSC	National Care Standards Commission
NHS	National Health Service
NHSC	National Horizon Scanning Centre
NHSME	National Health Service Management Executive
NHSSA	NHS Supplies Authority
NICE	National Institute for Clinical Excellence
NMC	Nursing and Midwifery Council
NPA	National Pharmaceutical Association
NPC	National Prescribing Centre
NPSG	National Pharmaceutical Supply Group
NRT	nicotine replacement therapy
NSAIDs	non-steroidal antiinflammatory drugs
NVQ	National Vocational Qualification

O/D	overdose
OTC	over-the-counter
P	pharmacy medicine
PAC	Public Accounts Committee
PACT	Prescribing Analysis and Cost
PAGB	Proprietary Association of Great Britain
PAS	Patient administration system
PASA	Procurement and Supply Agency
PAYE	pay-as-you-earn
PCCLG	Primary Community Care Liaison Group
PCG	primary care group
PCT	primary care trust
PDG	pharmacy development group
PEC	postgraduate education committee
PFI	Private Finance Initiative
PGD	patient group direction
PGEU	Pharmaceutical Group of the European Union
PIANA	Pharmacy in a New Age
PICTF	Pharmaceutical Industry Competitiveness Task Force
PIL	patient information leaflet
PL[PI]	parallel importing product licence
PMCPA	Prescription Medicines Code of Practice Authority
PMR	patient medication record
PMS	personal medical services
PMS	postmarketing surveillance
POM	Prescription Only Medicine
PPA	Prescription Pricing Authority
PPM	planned preventive maintenance
PPP	public private partnerships
PPRS	Pharmaceutical Price Regulation Scheme
PSD	patient services department
PSNC	Pharmaceutical Services Negotiating Committee
QA	quality assurance
RAWP	Resource Allocation Working Party
RHA	regional health authority
RIDDOR	Reporting of Injuries, Diseases and Dangerous Occurrences Regulations
RPSGB	Royal Pharmaceutical Society of Great Britain
SAMM	safety assessment of marketed medicines
SATO	senior assistant technical officer
SCOPE	Standing Committee for Pharmacy Postgraduate Education

SHA	special health authority
SO	standing order
SOPs	standard operating procedures
SPAC	Standing Pharmacy Advisory Committee
SPM	senior pharmacy manager
SQP	suitably qualified person
SSP	Statutory Sick Pay
StHA	strategic health authority
SVQ	Scottish Vocational Qualification
TDM	therapeutic drug monitoring
TPN	total parenteral nutrition
TTA/O	to take away/out
UKCC	UK Central Council
UKMIPG	UK Medicines Information Pharmacists Group
VAT	Value Added Tax
WDA	waste disposal authority

Part One

Medicines and the patient

1

Prescribers and patients

Access to health services in the community

Primary care

The term 'primary care' is used to describe the first contact that a patient has with health care personnel to diagnose or treat his/her complaint. It includes measures to prevent disease, such as immunisation and, in its broadest sense, health education. If the patient is then referred to hospital, this is termed 'referral to secondary care', and should this hospital then seek further diagnosis or treatment from a specialist centre, this would be 'referral to a tertiary centre'. In a 1986 paper, the government stated[1] that over 90% of the contacts that people in primary care make with the health service are with either the family practitioner services (family doctors, dentists, community pharmacists and opticians), or the community health services (community nurses, midwives, health visitors and other professions allied to medicine). General practitioners (GPs), prescribing on form FP10 (in Scotland, GP10), generate most of the prescriptions which are dispensed by community pharmacists.

Care in the community

Apart from the normal everyday primary health care contacts, there are significant groups of individuals with long-term needs for access to health care. Many of these individuals were previously maintained in institutions such as the large mental illness hospitals. Although successive governments and health and social care organisations have shown considerable concern for the concept of caring for these people with long-term health problems outside institutions, in reality until 1987 no serious attempts were made to identify and meet the needs of these clients and their carers. A hotchpotch of services grew up, partly provided by health authorities, partly by family practitioner services, and partly by social services departments. Budgetary issues were always paramount, with, for example, the National Health Service (NHS) trying to discharge patients into the community so that the cost of care could be lost to the local authority social services department. In addition, it is believed that there are up to six million voluntary carers – family, neighbours and friends – that is, almost one in eight of the population. These people save the NHS and welfare services considerable cash – estimated at about £24 billion per year – often without receiving any support or respite. This is being addressed by voluntary organisations such as Carers UK (similar to Carers Scotland), who have their own support schemes as well as putting pressure on government to support carers.[2]

In the NHS and Community Care Act of 1990, the first serious attempts were made to rationalise and improve the care in the community of defined groups of clients – the aged, the mentally ill and physically ill, and those with learning disabilities. Its key objectives were to promote care at home ('domiciliary care') and holidays for carers ('respite care') to enable people to live in their own homes, to ensure practical support for carers, to make a proper assessment of care needs and to promote good care management. It also encouraged the development of the independent (private) sector, clarified the responsibilities of the various agencies to make each more accountable for its actions and sought to obtain good value for money. There were a number of ways in which pharmacists became involved in the new models of care which evolved in response to the new legislation. These ranged from entering into contracts to provide services to nursing homes to contracting to visit certain clients at home to provide counselling services or medication review. Aspects of this are now core to practice, with elements such as 'advice to care homes' and 'patient medication records' incorporated in the terms of service in the *Drug Tariff*.[3] Training packages are available for pharmacists wishing to provide these services from the National Pharmaceutical Association and from the Centre for Pharmacy Postgraduate Education, and the Royal Pharmaceutical Society of Great Britain (RPSGB) includes statements on related issues in its yearly publication *Medicines, Ethics and Practice*.[4] Much work has been done, and continues to be done, by pharmacists in both the managed services and in the community, to further these aims. (See also Chapter 3.) Many innovative schemes have been set up to encourage liaison and to provide so-called 'seamless care', but much still remains to be done. It is also recognised by workers in the field that many of the same problems occur with patient groups that fall outside the legislation. Thus, the growth of day surgery, 'hospital at home' schemes and the growth of home intravenous (IV) therapy for oncology and human immunodeficiency virus (HIV) patients all provide a challenge for the pharmaceutical services. A report of a conference in 2001 reviews the broad spectrum of pharmacy issues which are being addressed.[5]

Further government action was initiated by the publication of a White Paper *The New NHS: Modern, Dependable* in December 1997.[6] This introduced a broad range of evolutionary changes for the NHS, with diverse implications for all sectors. The NHS was required to 'take a big step forward and become a modern, dependable service' with improved quality, national standards of care and easier, swifter access for patients based on need. A system of integrated care, founded on partnership and driven by performance, was to be developed to replace the internal market in health care.

Medical and dental services in primary care

General medical practitioners

GPs are mainly independent contractors in much the same way as community pharmacists, although increasingly doctors are salaried as part of personal medical services (PMS) run by health authorities (to be succeeded by primary care trusts). Each contractor practitioner is registered with the health authority or, in future, the local primary care organisation, and undertakes to provide basic medical care to the patients on his/her list, including home visits if the patient cannot attend the surgery. The health authority maintains a list of GPs, and also performs some administrative functions for them, e.g. stocking and issuing supplies of official stationery such as prescription forms and medical certificates, notifying them if necessary about drug recalls, and sending them copies of relevant Department of Health (DoH) circulars.

Having first been proposed in the 1997 Act,[7] PMS pilots are becoming more widespread at the time of writing (2002). In these pilots, GP practices or organisations bid to be part of a scheme of innovative and experimental contracting models. Most parts of the country have at least one or two PMS pilots that are, in effect, allowed to contract for services outside the standard GP terms of service and other regulations. GPs in such pilots are normally salaried. Local pharmacy service pilots are also being developed,[8] and a consideration of the relevance of existing medical and dental schemes was published in the *Pharmaceutical Journal*.[9] (See also Chapter 12.)

General practitioners: training and continuing education

Doctors who want to take charge, i.e. become principals, of practices have to complete a formal vocational training scheme to bridge the gap between their hospital-based early training and the very different problems and style of general practice. Doctors who were already practising when these regulations were introduced were allowed to continue. These schemes are usually centred on a district general hospital and general practices in its vicinity. Over a period of several years, the GP trainees rotate through several 6-month senior house officer posts in particularly relevant specialities, such as accident and emergency (A&E), gynaecology, paediatrics, ear, nose and throat and the care of the elderly. Interspersed are attachments to GP training practices where they work under the supervision of an approved experienced GP, and a programme of lectures and seminars.

The Royal College of General Practitioners was founded in 1952, with the aims of encouraging, fostering and maintaining the highest possible standards in general medical practice. It encourages and assists in postgraduate training and continuing education for GPs, and conducts and promotes research into clinical and operational aspects of primary care through its four research units. An examination for the Membership of the Royal College of General Practitioners (MRCGP) has been established, in line with higher medical qualifications in other fields such as surgery. It is acknowledged that the College has had a very strong influence in shaping the improvement in standards of general medical practice which have been seen to have taken place since its inception. This is of considerable interest to pharmacists, since our own College of Pharmacy Practice was instituted along broadly similar lines, and with aims which are comparable.

Private practice

There are GPs working in the private sector. Some of these work in private health centres which offer a range of facilities similar in scope to NHS health centres. All drugs must be prescribed on a non-NHS basis and dispensed as private prescriptions.

Group practices

Traditionally, GPs worked alone or with a junior assistant. In recent years, the trend has been towards group practices. This has obvious advantages for the doctors in that they can share duties at unsociable hours and cover each other's leave without the use of locums unfamiliar with the practice and its patients. It also avoids the professional isolation which has been seen to be a problem with single-handed practitioners (and which may also afflict pharmacists who work in small businesses if they do not seek outside professional contacts). Patients are still registered with a given doctor, but may on occasion be seen by one of the others in the practice. The practice premises housing groups of doctors is often, but not invariably, termed a 'health centre'. Some of these are owned and administered by health authorities which lease the accommodation and certain facilities to the doctors; some health centres are owned by the doctors themselves. Economies of scale make it easier to employ other workers in the practice, e.g. nurses, secretarial staff and receptionists. Many employ a practice manager who is responsible for the day-to-day administrative and personnel management aspects of the practice. Some clinics may be run by nurses, e.g. ear syringing, immunisations and dressings. In some cases social workers may be attached to the practice. The group practice was particularly active in the development of GP fundholding and subsequently primary care groups, where the scale of operation can allow robust management arrangements.

Health centres

The original concept of a health centre was that of a 'health care shop' with a team all contributing to decisions on patient care. Health centres were to include pharmacies, and indeed some do. In some cases, these have been set up by allowing existing pharmacy contractors nearby the opportunity to participate in a consortium running the business. In some cases, health centre premises have not been designed to accommodate a pharmacy and therefore that has proved impossible. The concept of health centres has not proved to be as successful and as popular as it might have been, but it is reawakening with the development of integrated schemes to meet the new NHS structures, e.g. primary care groups, walk-in centres and PMS pilots.

Dispensing doctors

Some doctors provide dispensing services to their own patients, a right continued since the inception of the NHS which has caused considerable conflict between the medical and pharmaceutical professions. The current legislation states that, in rural areas, patients who live more than 1 mile (approx. 1.5 km) from a pharmacy, or who because of distance or difficulty have problems in getting to a pharmacy, may apply to be included in a doctor's list of patients for whom he/she may dispense. Frequent disputes have arisen when pharmacists attempted to open new businesses in rural areas, or doctors tried to extend their dispensing lists.

Medical receptionists and prescribing

Pharmacists are likely to have many contacts with medical receptionists, and so should be aware of their training and functions. Although formal qualifications are not mandatory, many will have obtained the Certificate in Medical Reception of the Association of Medical Secretaries, Practice Managers, Administrators and Receptionists.[10] Medical receptionists make the patients' surgery appointments and take details of house calls and other requests to the doctor, as well as typing correspondence and generally performing secretarial duties. Most practices have computerised their records and repeat prescription monitoring. To facilitate this, a computer-compatible version of form FP10 was introduced in 1981. In most practices, the receptionist writes or prints repeat prescriptions, which are then checked and signed by the doctor. Computer-generated FP10 prescription forms provide the patient with a counterfoil giving details of medications prescribed, and these may be used to request repeats by patients who are on long-term medication, rather than making an appointment to see the doctor. Alternatively, patients may be issued with a written medication record card.

Out-of-hours services

There are various ways in which GPs can arrange for their patients to obtain emergency medical cover out of surgery hours, and particularly at evenings and weekends, and at the same time have some time off themselves. In a group practice a rota can be arranged, or alternatively a rota can be set up between several doctors practising nearby. Another way is to use a commercial deputising service, which intercepts the calls to the surgery and usually sends a doctor employed by the service to see the patient. Deputising services provide the doctors with drugs for emergency use; these are bought either from a wholesaler or a pharmacy. Pads of prescription forms FP10 are issued by the health authority to the deputising service, and issued by them to the participating doctors. These pads are stamped with the address of the service, not the individual doctors, and, in the event of a query, the only way to contact the prescriber is by telephoning the deputising service office, which will then contact the doctor and ask him/her to telephone the pharmacy.

General practice out-of-hours co-operatives

With the twin objectives of reducing requests to GPs for home visits when surgeries are closed and inappropriate attendances at A&E departments, in many areas out-of-hours GP units have been established, often adjacent to a local A&E department. Patients who telephone their GP's surgery when it is closed may be directed to attend such a unit. There they will be seen by a GP, but not necessarily their own, since a rota of the participating GPs covers the unit. In some cases emergency supplies of medicines may be made using prepacks prepared by the hospital pharmacy, or an FP10 prescription may be written. Details of the visit and any treatment given or prescribed will be relayed to the patient's GP, often by fax.

Dentists

Like other primary care professionals, all general practice dentists undertaking NHS work are listed on the Dental List maintained by each health authority. Patients register with a dentist in the same way as they do with a doctor. Since the introduction of the current contract, however, a significant proportion of dentists solely undertake private work, and this has led to difficulties for patients in some areas in being unable to obtain NHS dental treatment. In addition, some forms of treatment are not allowed by the NHS. Dentists are now obliged by their terms of service to provide out-of-hours cover, or to participate in a rota offering emergency treatment. A patient with an acute dental problem, such as a severe haemorrhage following an extraction, requiring emergency treatment, and who cannot contact his/her dentist, will require referral to his/her own doctor or a hospital A&E department.

Dentists have a special pale yellow NHS prescription form, FP14 (in Scotland, GP14). On this they may prescribe only items listed in Part XVII of the *Drug Tariff*;[3] these items are also detailed in the *Dental Practitioners' Formulary*, further reproduced in the *British National Formulary*.[11] On private prescriptions they are not so limited, and can prescribe any Prescription Only Medicine (POM). Drugs and other items such as dental filling materials which are administered or used in the surgery are purchased by the dentist from a wholesaler or pharmacy.

Dentists may refer patients either to dental hospitals or, more commonly, to the oral surgery departments of district general hospitals for specialised treatment. These patients receive their drugs in exactly the same way as other hospital patients; any outpatient prescribing is either for in-house dispensing or on form FP10(HP). There are no restrictions on the items which may be prescribed other than those which apply to doctors. In fact, many hospital oral surgeons are medically and surgically qualified as well.

Some dentists are employed in the community dental service, which serves primarily schoolchildren, especially those attending special schools for the physically handicapped, those with learning disabilities, pregnant women and adults in long-term residential care. Such dentists may work in community health service clinics and health centres; they are salaried as opposed to being independent contractors, and are managed within the hospital service, usually as part of a surgical care group or clinical directorate. They are able to prescribe on form FP14 as above, following the guidance of a Department of Health and Social Security (DHSS) circular.[12] Pharmaceuticals and other items used in the clinics are usually supplied by the hospital pharmaceutical service.

Nurses in primary care

NHS Direct and walk-in centres

To promote effective use of GPs' time and to minimise inappropriate attendances at A&E departments, the government has established a national telephone helpline for patients, known as NHS Direct. Callers speak first to a 'call taker' who can divert the call to a nurse adviser or the emergency services (999). Describing the facilities on trial in a pilot in Essex, Pandya[13] reported that medication queries could be diverted to the regional medicines information unit or poisons unit. For symptom-based queries, the nurse adviser worked through a computerised Clinical Decision Support System. The outcome might be for the client to contact his/her GP, to attend a local A&E department or be given self-help advice. According to the NHS Direct website,[14] callers may expect to receive sensible advice on general health queries, such as 'why have I been given this medicine?' and may also get health information such as the location of the nearest late-night pharmacist. The early pilot schemes showed that there is a need for a 24-hour dispensing service, and in at least one pilot scheme, this has been met by contracting with a local NHS trust, which has a pharmacy residency scheme.[15]

In a second initiative to improve access to medical advice, the government is establishing a chain of NHS walk-in centres located in high streets or, in some cases, near existing hospital A&E departments. Nurse-led, the centres offer advice and treatment for minor illnesses and injuries. Centres are able to supply medicines under the authority of patient group directions (PGDs), or, if the nurses hold appropriate qualifications, they may prescribe items listed in the *Nurse Prescribers' Formulary*. Mason[16] describes the operation of two pilot walk-in centres, and discusses the implications for community pharmacy.

Macmillan nurses

Macmillan nurses are nurse practitioners specialising in cancer and palliative care.[17] There are more than 2000 nurses in the UK: some are based in hospitals and outreach services and others are based in the community. All are registered nurses with a minimum of 5 years' experience, including at least 2 years in cancer or palliative care. The Macmillan Cancer Fund is a charity that funds the nurses during their first 3 years in post; thereafter, the NHS takes over.

Patient group directions

In March 1997, a group to review the prescribing, supply and administration of drugs was set up under the chairmanship of Dr June Crown. Two reports were published, the first dealing with the supply and administration aspects, and the second with nurse prescribing. The first Crown Report[18] made recommendations about the supply and administration of drugs on group protocols, the legal term for which is now patient group directions (PGDs). Similar documents had been used in hospitals for many years, mainly to authorise specified nurses to administer drugs from ward stocks to inpatients. Since the advent of limited nurse prescribing, there had been considerable pressure from nurses to extend the use of group protocols to permit nurse prescribing and even supply in certain circumstances not covered by the prescribing regulations, e.g. in family planning clinics and vaccination clinics. While stating that the majority of prescribing should be on an individual patient-specific basis, the Crown Report recognised that there would be a continuing need for supply and administration on the authority of group protocols in certain cases, and recommended that the law should be amended to permit this. In 2000 the relevant Medicines Act Regulations were amended and the DoH issued detailed guidance on the use of PGDs.[19–21] The DoH circular confirmed that PGDs 'should be reserved for those limited situations where the PGD offers an advantage for patient care (without compromising patient safety), and where it is consistent with appropriate professional relationships and accountability'.

Under the new amending orders, a PGD is defined as a written direction, signed by a doctor or a dentist and by a pharmacist, relating to the supply and administration, or administration only, of a POM or a pharmacy medicine to persons generally, subject to any exclusions that may be set out in the direction. The *Medicines, Ethics and Practice*[4] guide identifies three main types of PGD:

- The first category allows authorised health care professionals to supply medicines on behalf of an NHS body (e.g. an NHS trust).
- The second type is to assist a doctor or dentist providing primary care NHS services.
- The third type is where an NHS body (e.g. a health authority, primary care group or trust) authorises a PGD for the supply of a POM by a named person lawfully conducting a retail pharmacy business (i.e. the owner of a pharmacy).

The responsibilities of pharmacists involved in writing and/or approving PGDs are set out in Section 23 of the Code of Ethics and Standards.[4] Pharmacists working with doctors and other health care professionals to draft PGDs must read the above references and also the RPSGB Professional Standards Directorate resource pack for pharmacists on the subject of PGDs, which can be downloaded from their website,[22] to get the full details of the requirements, of which only an outline is given below. There is also a website[23] that has been designed as a database of approved group protocols for the supply and administration of medicines; it is managed from the pharmacy at the Hope Hospital, Salford.[24] Each PGD has been approved for use in a specific locality by practitioners employed there.

Although the Crown Report recommended that the new regulations should apply to both the NHS and the private and voluntary sectors, at the time of writing (March 2002), further law changes are required to bring this about, and PGDs are not permitted outside the NHS. Details of the consultation process initiated by the Medicines Control Agency which, when concluded, will lead to amendments in the regulations permitting the use of PGDs in private, charitable and voluntary sector hospitals, and to prisons, police custody suites and defence medical services, have been reported.[25] The health professionals who will then be able to sell, supply or administer medicines under the authority of a PGD will be the same as those listed for the NHS.

A senior doctor/dentist and a senior pharmacist, both of whom should have been involved in developing the direction, must sign PGDs. In the case of PGDs intended to assist doctors or dentists in providing

Table 1.1 Registered health professionals who may supply or administer medicines under a patient group direction *as named individuals*

Ambulance paramedics	Optometrists
Chiropodists	Orthoptists
Health visitors	Pharmacists
Midwives	Physiotherapists
Nurses	Radiographers

Table 1.2 Information to be contained in a patient group direction (PGD)

The name of the business or National Health Service organisation to which the direction applies

The date it comes into force and the date it expires (guidance has indicated that a PGD should be reviewed every 2 years)

A description of the medicine(s) to which it applies

Details of appropriate dosage and maximum total dosage, quantity, pharmaceutical form and strength

Route and frequency of administration, and minimum/maximum period over which the medicine should be administered

Class of health professional who may supply or administer the medicine

Signature of a senior doctor/dentist as appropriate, and a senior pharmacist

The clinical condition or situation to which the direction applies

Description of those patients excluded from treatment under the direction

Details of the circumstances in which further advice should be sought from a doctor/dentist, and arrangements for referral

Relevant warnings, including potential adverse reactions

Details of any necessary follow-up action and the circumstances

A statement of the records to be kept for audit purposes

primary care NHS services, the PGD must also be signed by the relevant health authority, i.e. health authority or primary care group or trust. Health professionals who may supply or administer medicines under a PGD are listed in Table 1.1.

There are specific details that must be included in a PGD. These are listed in Table 1.2.

The circular directs that there must be comprehensive arrangements for security, storage and labelling of all medicines, which should preferably be in prepacks prepared by a pharmacist. An audit trail must be created showing who treated which patient, and when. The records should allow incoming and outgoing stocks to be reconciled. Medicines should normally be ordered only in accordance with the Summary of

Product Characteristics, although the guidance acknowledges that there may be exceptional circumstances where this cannot be followed. There are special warnings about including antimicrobials in PGDs; at the time of writing, all Controlled Drugs and radiopharmaceuticals, covered by additional legislation, are specifically excluded, although a possible law change might permit the inclusion of Schedule 4 and 5 Controlled Drugs in future.

Nurse prescribing

At the time of writing, prescribing by nurses is limited to community and practice nurses who are identified as nurse prescribers in the Nursing and Midwifery Council (NMC; formerly the UK Central Council) register. Full details of the implementation of nurse prescribing and the regulations surrounding it were given in a briefing document for pharmacists;[26] although this was written in the early phase of the implementation of nurse prescribing, only a few details have changed subsequently to date. Pharmacists can check whether a particular nurse is qualified to prescribe by telephoning the NMC. Only items listed in the *Nurse Prescribers' Formulary*, which is further reproduced in the *British National Formulary*,[11] may be prescribed. At the time of writing, there are no provisions for nurses working in hospitals or other practice settings to prescribe on their own authority.

The Health Minister announced a new policy in May 2001.[27, 28] With immediate effect, existing nurse prescribers can prescribe nicotine replacement products. During 2002, further nurse prescribers will be trained and will have the authority to prescribe on the NHS all non-Black-listed Pharmacy and General Sale List medicines. Palliative care nurses and nurses treating patients with chronic conditions, e.g. asthma and coronary heart disease, will be able to prescribe a broader range of medicines. In addition, 'supplementary prescribing' for nurses is to be introduced by provisions of Health and Social Care Act 2001. After amendments to the relevant Medicines Act and NHS legislation have been passed, nurses will be able to prescribe for a further range of conditions after initial assessment by a doctor. An extended formulary for nurse prescribers has been drafted; it includes a number of POMs, but no oral antibiotics, and will come into force during 2002.

Nurses working as community nurses, i.e. employed by community NHS trusts, prescribe using form FP10(CN) in England and Wales. Practice nurses use form FP10(PN). In Scotland, nurse prescribers use form GP10(N), and in Northern Ireland, form HS21(N). In order to act as a nurse prescriber, the nurse has to complete the specific training for prescribing successfully, and to hold an appropriate post. Each nurse prescriber retains a personal prescription pad, with his/her details printed in a box at the foot. Community nurses must enter the GP practice code.

Currently, to qualify as a prescriber, the nurse already practising must:

- hold a district nurse or health visitor qualification;
- complete an English National Board (ENB) open learning pack on nurse prescribing;
- attend a taught course at an ENB-accredited nurses' education provider for specialist practitioner courses in district, i.e. community nursing and/or health visiting;
- pass a written examination.

Nurses undertaking specialist training in these fields have had the prescribing training included in their qualification since 1999. With the expansion of nurse prescribing discussed above, there are plans to extend nurse prescriber training to add a further 10 000 prescribers to the 20 000 already qualified.

Nurse prescribers will require ongoing information and support from pharmacists. This has been recognised by the National Prescribing Centre (NPC), which has produced *Prescribing Nurse Bulletins* and a series of Powerpoint presentations for nurse training, which can be downloaded from their website.[29] These currently cover:

- wound management;
- scabies and threadworms, with a patient information leaflet on applying treatment for scabies;
- management of head lice, also with a companion patient leaflet;
- urinary incontinence;
- constipation.

Nurse prescribers will also need access to medicines information services, and ideally will establish good working relationships with their local community pharmacists.

Secondary referral

A general medical or dental practitioner often wishes to refer the patient to a consultant (or 'specialist') for advice in diagnosis or treatment. Patients may opt for referral to an NHS hospital, or, particularly if they have private health insurance, referral to a consultant privately.

NHS consultant outpatient clinics

The patient is seen by appointment, the GP having asked the consultant by letter or telephone for a consultation. The patient is usually seen by the consultant in person on the first visit, but on follow-up visits may well see the registrar or senior house officer; this accounts for the oft-heard complaint that patients never see the same doctor twice. In England and Wales the doctor in the clinic may prescribe drugs, which will either be dispensed by the hospital pharmacy, or prescribed on form FP10(HP). It is normal hospital practice to prescribe not by number of doses to be supplied, but by length of time – traditionally to last until the next appointment. Latterly, many hospitals have tried to contain their drug budgets by supplying prescriptions for only a minimal length of time, and then attempting to pass responsibility for prescribing long-term supplies to the GP. Whilst this may cause no problems where familiar drugs are involved, GPs rightly object to being expected to prescribe drugs which require specialised knowledge and possibly hospital monitoring. (See Chapter 3 for a discussion of prescribing at the primary/secondary care interface.)

In some cases, shared-care protocols are developed which define the responsibilities of each party and ensure that the GP receives all the information necessary to prescribe for the patient in good time to ensure continuity of supply. If necessary, there should be liaison between hospital and community pharmacists. In the event of a query, hospital pharmacists can check the case notes for details of therapy. They will need either the patient's unit (or hospital) number – usually to be found on the appointment card – or name and address, or date of recent outpatient appointment, in order to trace the case notes. Age or date of birth is also helpful since there are often several registered patients with the same names living at the same address. Consultants often visit several hospitals, holding clinics at the same day and time each week in each location; if prescription queries arise on the day following the appointment, it is better to telephone the consultant's secretary in the first instance, to find out where he/she may be found.

There have been many initiatives to promote seamless pharmaceutical care. Leach[30] identified a number of potential obstacles and some solutions, including the need for hospital and community pharmacists to be aware of each other's problems. He identified several needs of community pharmacists, including receiving copies of the local hospital formulary and any prescribing bulletins. Lord[31] also considered the problems that can arise at the interface, including in her assessment those facing the hospital pharmacist when patients are admitted with an incomplete or inaccurate medication history. She points out that the community pharmacist's patient medication record can be a valuable source of information. At her hospital, discharge information is communicated direct to community pharmacists in certain cases. The documents used are based on checklists drawn up by the RPSGB in conjunction with the Hospital Pharmacists' Group in 1993;[32] however, these have not become widely used. Choo and Cook[33] describe a system initiated in their locality, where discharge information was provided to community pharmacists by fax. They concluded that faxed discharge information can offer a better level of communication and cooperation between hospital and community pharmacists, and can provide an opportunity to resolve potential medication problems rapidly.

Some GPs have made arrangements for consultants to hold outreach clinics at the practice premises. This is useful both because it saves patients having to travel to distant hospitals, and also because it improves communications between GPs and consultants.

Domiciliary visits

If patients are too infirm to travel to hospital, on very rare occasions the GP may arrange for a consultant to visit them at home. Medical etiquette dictates that the GP should be present at the consultation and prescribe any drugs required. In practice, this does not always occur and the consultant may have to write an FP10(HP) form.

Hospital admission

Planned admissions ('cold admissions' in hospital parlance), often for non-emergency surgery or for diagnostic procedures, are usually arranged at an outpatient consultation. Immediately prior to admission, the patient's GP is asked to complete a questionnaire detailing current drug therapy. Patients are often asked to bring their current medication with them as an aid to identification. If still valid, this may possibly be used for their own treatment during their stay or may be returned home. On discharge, the patient is usually given at least an initial supply of medicines to last until repeat supplies can be prescribed by the GP. The take-home medicines will be dispensed by the hospital pharmacy; form FP10(HP) may not be used for this purpose. During the inpatient stay, medicines are often deleted from the pre-admission regimen. Lord[31] observes that, unfortunately, such changes are not always recorded accurately at the surgery, and at times deleted items may be prescribed.

Accident and emergency departments

Patients may attend A&E departments without being referred by their GP, for genuine accidents and acute medical emergencies; unfortunately there are many abuses of the system by people who attend for non-urgent and trivial conditions – and also for non-medical social reasons. Persons having a serious accident, or being taken acutely ill at home may summon an ambulance by making a 999 call – also a possibility for people urgently requiring medical attention in a pharmacy. The ambulance will take them to the nearest A&E department; if they telephone their GP and the GP summons the ambulance, he/she can specify to which hospital they are to be taken. Patients who the GP thinks require urgent hospital admission, but not necessarily needing an ambulance, will also be referred to the A&E department. Either way, they will be examined by a hospital doctor who may decide to admit them, or may initiate treatment and return them home. During normal working hours, prescriptions are usually dispensed by the hospital pharmacy, but out of hours, forms FP10(HP) are often used. Most hospital pharmacies also provide a range of commonly used drugs – usually antibiotics and prescription analgesics – as 'starter packs' packed and labelled ready for issue by A&E doctors or by A&E nurse practitioners under the authority of a PGD. A&E departments have no facilities for dispensing prescriptions written by GPs which cannot conveniently be supplied by a chemist contractor, or supplying oxygen cylinders, masks or other types of equipment.

Private consultations

Patients requiring referral to a consultant may opt for private treatment. Consultations may be held at a private hospital; many have their own pharmacies that dispense outpatient prescriptions. Failing this, or if the consultations are held at consulting rooms, patients will be given private prescriptions. If they are covered by medical insurance, this may cover the cost of drugs. Private patients are not eligible for NHS prescriptions, although it is not unknown for the GP to prescribe continuation treatment on form FP10. It is possible for consultants to hold private clinics in NHS hospitals. Prescriptions may be supplied by the hospital pharmacy for these patients, charging the patient. Since the passing of the Health and Medicines Act 1988, trusts may set their own charges.

Private patients may be admitted direct or transferred to NHS hospitals (see Chapter 6).

Patients' rights

NHS complaints procedure

Considering the number of people involved, complaints against practitioners providing NHS services are quite rare. When they do arise, it is often because of misunderstandings, and a little time spent discussing or anticipating potential problems with patients would prevent much of the anxiety and misunderstandings which may lead patients to believe that they have cause for complaint. Thus, patients may believe that they have been given the wrong tablets when the brand or appearance changes, or may believe that their doctors are incompetent when one doctor refers to the diagnosis as a 'heart attack', the next as a 'myocardial infarction' and a third as 'a coronary' – a sequence which led to an actual complaint on one occasion, since the patient thought that the medical staff were unable to find out what was wrong. In hospitals, a regular cause of complaint is the loss or destruction of the patient's own tablets upon admission. If substantiated, there is no alternative but to provide replacements or financial recompense at the going rate (NHS prescription charges or reimbursement for private prescriptions), since the drugs are legally the patient's property.

In 1996, an Executive Letter[34] introduced a new statutory NHS complaints procedure. A companion book[35] setting out the new procedures in full was published at the same time. The procedure is set out on the NHS website.[36] In outline, the procedure requires:

- all NHS trusts, health authorities and primary care practitioners to formulate a complaints procedure;
- all NHS trusts, health authorities and primary care practitioners to nominate a person to act as complaints manager. This manager's role is to acknowledge receipt of the complaint, to set up an in-house investigation into the circumstances, and to report back to the complainant promptly (normally within 20 working days for hospital complaints, or within 10 working days for family health services providers);
- the chief executive of the trust or other body to respond to all written complaints;
- the complaints procedure to be separate from any disciplinary process.

Unlike the earlier procedure, the health authority has no formal role in dealing with the initial stages of complaints against primary care contractors; it is hoped that complaints will be resolved locally whenever possible. However, the health authority may nominate a person to act as conciliator between complainant and professional if necessary. The complaints process ceases if the complainant decides to take legal action.

If local resolution fails, within 28 days the complainant may request that the matter be referred to a review panel. Trusts and health authorities must appoint at least one person to act as convenor to consider requests from complainants for unresolved complaints to be referred to independent review panels. The convenor must obtain a written statement from the complainant which sets out the nature of outstanding grievances, and why the complainant is dissatisfied with the outcome of local resolution. The convenor will then consult an independent lay chairperson drawn from a list held by the regional office of the NHS Executive, and they will jointly decide whether further action can be taken locally, or whether it is necessary to convene a review panel. Should a complaint relate to professional judgement, an independent professional opinion will be sought.

When it is deemed necessary to convene a review panel, it is set up as a subcommittee of the health authority or trust, but is chaired by a person from outside the organisation. Also on the panel is the convenor and a third person whose choice is determined by the nature of the complaint. The panel, which sits in private, investigates the complaint as reported to them by the convenor, and may obtain further independent professional advice. It finally reports to the parties concerned. Finally, the chief executive reports back to the complainant, giving details of any actions taken after the panel's report, and also pointing out the complainant's right to refer the matter to the Ombudsman if they remain dissatisfied.

In pharmacies, it is likely that complaints may be received about alleged or actual dispensing errors. All pharmacies should have a written procedure to follow should this occur. This should be based on the relevant RPSGB Professional Standards Directorate Fact Sheet.[37]

Parliamentary and Health Service Commissioner (Ombudsman)

The Ombudsman investigates complaints about failures in NHS hospitals or community health services, about care and treatment and about local NHS family doctor, dental, pharmaceutical or optical services. Members of the public may complain directly to the Ombudsman, but the complaint will normally only be pursued if the NHS complaints procedure has been carried out first.[38] The complaint must reach the Ombudsman within a year of the event. If the Ombudsman is not satisfied with the response received after he/she has investigated a complaint, it is possible to arrange for the person involved to be summoned before a parliamentary select committee. In an editorial on the subject,[39] Clare Dyer, a legal correspondent, commented that this committee could impose no sanctions: its chief weapon is embarrassment. Nevertheless, at that time no authority had failed to take action after this experience.

References

1. Command 9771: *Primary Health Care: An Agenda for Discussion*. London: Her Majesty's Stationery Office, 1986.
2. Carers UK website (2001). www.carersuk.demon.co.uk (accessed December 2001).
3. Department of Health and National Assembly for Wales. *Drug Tariff*, published monthly. London: Stationery Office.
4. Royal Pharmaceutical Society of Great Britain. *Medicines Ethics and Practice: A Guide for Pharmacists*, published yearly. London: Royal Pharmaceutical Society of Great Britain.
5. Report of a conference of the Primary Care and Community Pharmacy Network. Meeting the challenge of change. *Pharm J* 2001; 267: 654–655.
6. Department of Health. White Paper, *The New NHS: Modern, Dependable*. London: Department of Health, 1997.
7. Department of Health. *Personal Medical Services Pilots under the NHS (Primary Care) Act 1997 – A Comprehensive Guide*. London: Department of Health, 1997.
8. News item. First come, first served for LPS pilots? *Pharm J* 2002; 268: 3.
9. Russell R, Craig G. Local Pharmaceutical Services – what can we learn from doctors and dentists? *Pharm J* 2001; 267: 865–866.
10. Association of Medical Secretaries, Practice Managers, Administrators and Receptionists website (2002). www.amspar.co.uk (accessed January 2002).
11. Mehta D K, ed. *British National Formulary*, published twice-yearly. London: British Medical Association/Royal Pharmaceutical Society of Great Britain.
12. Department of Health and Social Security. *School and Priority Dental Services: Prescribing of Listed Drugs and Medicines*. HSC(IS)82/WHSC(IS)74.
13. Pandya A. Pharmacy's future role in NHS Direct. *Pharm J* 1999; 263: 983.
14. NHS Direct website home page (2001). www.doh.gov.uk/nhsexec/direct.htm (accessed 7 May 2001).
15. Conference report. Improving access to care: NHS Direct and pharmacy. *Pharm J* 2000; 265: 578.
16. Mason P. NHS walk-in centres: implications for pharmacy. *Pharm J* 2000; 265: 305–307.
17. Macmillan Cancer Fund website (2001). www.macmillan.org.uk (accessed 9 May 2001).

18.   Department of Health. *Report on the Supply and Administration of Medicines under Group Protocols*. HSC 1998/051.
19.   News item. New legislation paves the way for patient group directions. *Pharm J* 2000; 265: 219.
20.   News item. NHS issues guidance on PGDs. *Pharm J* 2000; 265: 255.
21.   Department of Health. *Patient Group Directions [England]*. HSC 2000/026.
22.   RPSGB Professional Standards Directorate (2001). Site map/Law and Ethics/Law/*Patient Group Directions, A Resource Pack for Pharmacists*. Website: www.rpsgb.org.uk (accessed 9 May 2001).
23.   Group protocols website (2001). www.groupprotocols.org.uk (accessed 9 May 2001).
24.   Untitled news item. *Hosp Pharm* 2000; 7: 87.
25.   News item. PGDs to be extended beyond the NHS. *Pharm J* 2002; 268: 46.
26.   The Pharmacy Community Care Liaison Group. Nurse prescribing: a briefing paper for pharmacists. *Pharm J* 1999; 262: 660–665.
27.   United Kingdom Central Council website (2001). *News*. www.ukcc.org.uk (accessed 8 May 2001).
28.   News item. More nurses to prescribe more. *Pharm J* 2001; 266: 636.
29.   National Prescribing Centre website (2001). *Nurse Prescribing*. www.npc.org.uk/ (accessed 8 May 2001).
30.   Leach R H. How can hospital and community pharmacists work together? *Hosp Pharm* 1997; 4: 218.
31.   Lord S. The interface – steps towards seamless care. *Hosp Pharm* 1999; 6: 83.
32.   News item. Checklists for admission and discharge. *Pharm J (Hospital suppl.* 13 March) 1993; 250: HS6.
33.   Choo G C C, Cook H. A community and hospital discharge liaison service by fax. *Pharm J* 1997; 259: 659–661.
34.   NHS Executive. *Implementation of New Complaints Procedure*. EL(96)19.
35.   NHS Executive. *Complaints: Listening . . . Acting*. 1996.
36.   NHS website (2001). *Patients' Voice*: www.nhs.uk/patientsvoice/how_to_complain.asp (accessed 7 May 2001).
37.   Royal Pharmaceutical Society of Great Britain Professional Standards Directorate. *Fact Sheet 11: Dealing with Dispensing Errors*. London: RPSGB Professional Standards Directorate, 2001.
38.   Parliamentary and Health Service Commissioner website (2001). www.ombudsman.org.uk (accessed 10 April 2001).
39.   Dyer, C. Called to account. *BMJ* 1987; 294: 663.

2

The manufacture and marketing of pharmaceuticals

The pharmaceutical industry plays an important role in the national economy. In 1999, the gross UK sales for pharmaceutical products and preparations were in the region of £8000 bn.[1] The value of UK pharmaceutical exports in 1998 totalled nearly £6 billion; the pharmaceutical industry is the UK's second biggest exporter after North Sea oil, creating a trade surplus in 1998 of nearly £2.5 bn.[2] There are two important trade associations which represent the interests of pharmaceutical manufacturers: the Association of the British Pharmaceutical Industry (ABPI) and the Proprietary Association of Great Britain (PAGB). Members of the former make prescription, and the latter non-prescription, medicines. In each case, the association protects the interests of member companies at home and abroad, represents their views to government departments and attempts to influence proposed legislation affecting the industry. Examples of ABPI papers and briefing documents may be seen on the website cited above.[2] Both organisations have a self-regulated code of practice, with which their members comply, that regulates certain activities such as advertising and promotional methods (see below). The ABPI code may be found in its *Compendium*,[3] which also gives details of the constitution and procedures of the ABPI Prescription Medicine Code of Practice Authority.

Most pharmaceuticals are purchased ready-made by pharmacies, and the dispensing operation is simply a matter of providing a quantity convenient for the patient's treatment and labelling it with directions for use. Since a major part of a pharmacist's work is concerned with the procurement of pharmaceuticals from various suppliers, it is necessary to be familiar with the types of product, their manufacturers and the service they offer.

Suppliers of pharmaceuticals

Branded products

Most modern drugs are developed by research in the laboratories of a multinational pharmaceutical company; this company will market the drug in countries where it has an established marketing organisation, or may sell the right to produce or sell it to another company in those countries where it has not. These products are assigned a brand name by the manufacturer and this name will be given prominence on the label and in promotional material. It will often be easier to remember than the non-proprietary name which, in the UK, the manufacturer is obliged by the Medicines Act also to include on the label. Since the implementation of Directive 92/27/EEC, the non-proprietary name used has to be the recommended International Non-proprietary Name (INN), i.e. recommended by the World Health Organization. This replaces the former rules, under which the British Approved Name (BAN) invented by the British Pharmacopoeia Commission could be used. During a transitional period, in the interests of safety, both names are given for certain drugs. Details will be found in the *British National Formulary*.[4] Until the expiry of the patent, usually only one brand is marketed in each country, but occasionally two brands of the same drug are launched simultaneously by different companies, both presumably having bought the right to make or market the drug from the patent holder. In an interesting review, Thompson[5] surveys the process of inventing and gaining approval for both generic and brand names.

Pharmaceutical manufacturers sometimes have to register different brand names for their product when sold in other countries, possibly because a similar name has already been allotted to another product. In fact, there may even be differences in formulation and presentation to comply with different drug regulatory bodies, although harmonisation of requirements has been achieved within the European Union (EU). Large companies have a registration department whose job it is to elucidate and deal with requirements worldwide. Problems may arise when dealing with patients newly arrived from overseas: most foreign brand names can be found in *Martindale*[6] or by consulting the Royal Pharmaceutical Society of Great Britain (RPSGB) information service. Not all branded drugs are sold in all countries, e.g. cefotetan disodium, a drug similar to cefoxitin, is available as Apatef (Lederle) in Australia and Darvilen (Schering) in Italy, but has never been marketed in the UK. In less developed countries, the range of drugs available is much less, and furthermore, drugs which have been withdrawn from sale by licensing authorities such as the Medicines Control Agency (MCA) or the American Food and Drug Administration (FDA) because of an unacceptably high incidence of adverse reactions may still be promoted. Intending travellers with chronic health problems such as diabetes may find themselves in difficulty, since some types of insulin and other drugs may not be available in Africa and many other countries. The pharmaceutical company's UK head office will provide information about availability in other countries, including the addresses of their local offices or distributors. Further complications may be introduced by religious and political extremism – in certain Middle Eastern countries, drugs of porcine origin may be restricted, and there may be difficulties in obtaining drugs made by companies with operations in Israel.

In addition to the range of 'ethical' medicines – that is, intended for doctors' prescription and only advertised to members of the medical and pharmaceutical professions – there is a wide range of over-the-counter (OTC) products which may be advertised to the public. Many large ethical companies have an OTC division with a different name and range of brands, although some of these may contain the same ingredients as the company's ethical brands. The distinction has been blurred since the government introduced legislation prohibiting certain hitherto 'ethical' products from National Health Service (NHS) prescription (the 'Black List'): some of these are now being advertised freely. Yet other divisions may sell cosmetics and toiletries, and adult and baby foods.

Generic products

This term usually, but not always, describes products where the patent of the brand leader has expired, making it possible for other manufacturers to make and sell the drug. These manufacturers sometimes themselves register brand names. Not all those companies that offer a product for sale are themselves manufacturers; some buy or import the drug either as a raw material or as a pharmaceutical formulation which they, or a subcontractor, then pack. The source of the material, or the subcontractor, may not be the same on each occasion, and this may lead to misgivings about bioequivalence. It must be remembered that, contrary to popular belief, this certainly does not apply to all suppliers of generics. All the major generic companies are divisions of multinational groups with substantial international generics business. Generic products tendered for inclusion in hospital contracts are tested and monitored by the hospital quality assurance service nationwide, but the capacity does not exist to extend this facility to purchasers outside the managed service. Unfortunately, it has become a feature of pharmaceutical marketing that sometimes the sales force of the brand leader will attempt to discredit the products of other suppliers to doctors to encourage brand loyalty. However, all products are subject to the same controls during the licensing procedure, and thus the granting of a marketing authorisation is a guarantee of a product at least as good as any similar authorised product of the same drug.

Another type of generic is the standard formulary pharmaceutical that has not been patented for many years, if ever. An example might be morphine sulphate injection or calamine lotion. Hospitals are the main purchasers and infusion and irrigation solutions are the largest part of the market. It should be noted that not all standard preparations in fact have got a marketing authorisation, even though they may comply with, and be labelled, e.g. 'BP'. The purchaser is responsible for quality assurance of such products.[7] The whole field of generics manufacture and marketing was discussed in an article by Kay,[8] who included interesting comparisons between European and UK practice. He makes the point that the UK practice of 'open prescribing' of generics, where the choice of supplier is left to the dispensing pharmacist, is almost unique in Europe. Kay reviewed the subject again 4 years later, discussing changes within the marketplace and also commenting on supply problems which had arisen when one manufacturer had to cease production during 1999, with a resultant loss of 10% of production capacity nationally.[9]

'Specials' and specialised dispensing services

Some manufacturers are additionally licensed under the Medicines Act to make products for doctors and pharmacists to special order. Details may be found in *Dale and Appelbe's Pharmacy Law and Ethics*.[10] The manufacturer holds no marketing authorisation, and responsibility for quality control rests with the purchaser. Hospitals are the main customers. In recent years, the service available has been extended to include the provision of total parenteral nutrition (TPN) and antibiotic infusion preparation both for hospital inpatients and for long-term patients in their own homes. The drugs may be ordered via a hospital pharmacy, or may be prescribed by the GP on form FP10. Another development has been the commercial provision of cytotoxics reconstitution; this would require serious consideration before large sums were invested in an in-house facility.

'Orphan drugs'

Both adults and children may be diagnosed with rare disorders for which drugs can be supplied only on a 'named-patient' basis since no drugs with a marketing authorisation exist. Since the process of obtaining a marketing authorisation is long and may cost up to £300m per product, and potential patients are few, there is little commercial incentive for pharmaceutical companies to license such drugs, for which the term 'orphan drugs' has been coined. The current plight of 'orphan drugs', which are not all for children's diseases, is discussed fully in an article by Karr.[11] He points out that many are for diseases found mainly in developing countries where there may be many potential patients, but scarce funds to purchase treatment. A solution to the problem, at least for drugs for rare diseases, is for governments to provide incentives to pharmaceutical companies to encourage them to develop and license 'orphan drugs'. This already happens in some countries, including the USA, Japan, Singapore and Australia. In the USA, incentives include tax and other financial benefits and 7 years' market exclusivity. This legislation has demonstrably speeded up the introduction of new drugs for rare conditions. The EU regulation on orphan medicinal products (no. 141/2000) is in the process of implementation in member countries, with similar aims. Rare diseases have been defined as those affecting fewer than 5 per 10 000 of population.

Government control of pharmaceuticals

Controls on suppliers: quality, safety and efficacy

Drug manufacturers

Although these happened many years ago, it is worth recounting two disastrous events which probably had the most influence in shaping the present laws and official recommendations governing pharmaceutical manufacture and the use of medicines in the UK. They illustrate how easy it is for harm to occur in the use of medicines, and how such events can result in the initiation of ongoing controls relating to the quality, safety and efficacy of medicines. In 1961, the capacity of thalidomide to cause fetal abnormalities was realised, and the Medicines Act 1968 evolved from recognition of this and knowledge of other adverse effects arising from inadequately researched drugs. This placed emphasis on the testing of new drugs for safety, the control of quality throughout the manufacturing process and proof of efficacy before licensing for use. Then, in 1972 came the Devonport Incident,[12] in which at least 4 patients died as a result of receiving contaminated infusion fluid. An official enquiry ensued, which resulted in the Clothier Report in 1972;[13] this was followed in 1973 by the Rosenheim Report with its recommendations on the prevention of microbial contamination.[14]

Under the provisions of the Medicines Act, manufacturing premises became subject to statutory inspection, and the Medicines Inspectorate came into being. At the time of implementation, hospitals were exempt from the effects of such legislation ('crown immunity'). Hospitals also carried out widespread and large-scale manufacturing operations; the authors remember working in a district general hospital in which all sterile water, intravenous infusions and most solutions for injection in ampoules were made on site! So as to ensure that standards of manufacture between hospital and industry were standardised, the government imposed the controls under the Medicines Act on the health service through the issue of a specific circular.[15] As a result of their findings during inspections of industrial premises and hospital departments, the inspectors realised that definitive guidelines were needed. After passing through three UK editions, standards in the UK are now based on the European guide to pharmaceutical manufacturing practice.[16] The manufacturing facilities of suppliers of imported drugs may be subject to inspection by UK inspectors prior to product licensing, since there is no reciprocity between the regulatory authorities in various countries, and indeed, standards and requirements vary considerably.

Wholesalers

Bad storekeeping practice at the wholesaler was one of the causative factors of the Devonport incident. It is not surprising, therefore, that the Medicines Act does not limit its influence to the site of drug manufacture, but requires wholesalers to comply with standards of good practice in order to be eligible for a Wholesale Dealer's Licence. Since most pharmacies buy the bulk of their drugs from wholesalers, it would be disastrous if their standards were inferior. There are around 12 full-line wholesalers in the UK, providing a comprehensive range of items, including specialised items for hospitals.[17] In addition, there are about 4000 so-called 'short-line' wholesalers, who can provide only a restricted range.[18]

Wholesalers' frequent deliveries make it possible for stocks to be reduced in pharmacies; most have streamlined ordering by using electronic transfer of stock data. Some of these work in real time so that the pharmacy is informed at the time of order if there is a problem with an out-of-stock item. Many drug companies minimise their distribution costs by using wholesalers to distribute their products even to buyers of large quantities like hospitals. Wholesalers compete for contracts and give discounts and, paradoxically, a given item may be cheaper bought in this way than directly from the maker.

Parallel importers

The importing (or reimporting) of branded drugs from Europe – so-called 'parallel importing' – emerged as an issue many years ago. At first it was unregulated, but now it is seen as part of legitimate business in the EU trading area. Products to be imported are controlled by the MCA through the issue of a parallel importing product licence (PL[PI]) which ensures minimum standards for the import. Certain wholesalers specialise in this activity; there is a parallel importers' association – the Association of Parallel Importers (API)[19] – otherwise known as the British Association of European Pharmaceutical Distributors. The financial advantage of importing stems from the fact that certain branded drugs are sold more cheaply in other EU countries than the same, or similar, products in the UK. However, the remuneration that the contractor receives for NHS prescriptions is at present based on the normal rate in the UK. This had led to concerns by manufacturers that their UK price is being undercut, and concerns by the government that pharmacists are making too large a profit by buying goods from overseas. The practice is quite legal, however, so there will undoubtedly be continued moves by both aggrieved parties to reduce their loss (whether perceived or actual).

Quite apart from fiscal concerns, there have been safety issues with the use of parallel imports. If inadequately controlled, the procedure can lead to the patient receiving an unsatisfactory product. In many cases, the foreign product and the UK brand differ, so substitution may expose the patient to variations in appearance, additives and even, in some cases, active ingredients. The foreign brand name often differs from that used in the UK. This, coupled with foreign-language instruction leaflets and calendar packs, may cause anxiety and problems in use for patients. Some pharmacists have reservations about using parallel imports because of these reasons. It must be remembered that the sale or supply of unlicensed products on prescription is illegal, and therefore the parallel import must be licensed and obtained from a reputable source.

Controls on suppliers: price

The government in the UK uses a whole range of measures to control expenditure on medicines in the NHS. One of the most important of these is the Pharmaceutical Price Regulation Scheme (PPRS). This is a voluntary scheme agreed between the pharmaceutical industry (through the ABPI) and the government. The ABPI publishes a useful briefing document on the scheme.[20]

The intention of the PPRS is to ensure that excessive prices are not charged to the NHS, but that price controls are not so rigorous that the industry's profitability, research and development capability and export potential are harmed. The methodology is to limit prices through control on the net profits of the industry. The net profit allowance is set by a complex formula linked to returns on capital, and is allowed to vary within bandings to allow for 'good' years (when, for example a new, successful product may be marketed) or 'bad' years. Within the agreed formula companies are restricted on some expenditure out of gross turnover. An example is a restriction on the percentage allowed to be spent on sales promotion. There are, however, no direct controls on how the money is spent within the allowance. One company might choose to spend a greater amount on its sales force than on direct advertising or on glossy literature. The scheme is agreed to last a set number of years (currently 5), and the negotiations are undertaken through high-level confidential discussions between the government and representatives of the industry through the ABPI. The most recent agreement was in October 1999, and in this the government tightened controls on the industry as part of measures to restrict NHS expenditure on medicines. The agreement included the imposition of an immediate cut in the price of medicines.

The high political interest in the pharmaceutical industry and the price of medicines was emphasised soon after the agreement of the 1999 PPRS. The government set up a high-level cabinet committee to address the position of the pharmaceutical industry, its research contribution to the country and its profitability.[21] This group, the Pharmaceutical Industry Competitiveness Task Force (PICTF) was set up to 'identify all the criteria for maintaining and developing the competitiveness of the UK as a successful and effective base for an innovative pharmaceutical industry in a global market' and 'to report to the Prime Minister on any action needed to retain and strengthen the competitiveness of the UK business environment'. The final report[22] indicated that the pharmaceutical industry was worth between £2bn and £4bn a year to the UK economy.

It also published a comparison of how new medicines are licensed and assessed in different countries, and a set of indicators to assess how the UK pharmaceutical industry is performing in comparison with other countries.[23]

Controls on prescribing

Drug Tariff

Although perhaps not the easiest of books to assimilate, the *Drug Tariff*[24] (separate editions are published for Scotland and Northern Ireland) is essential reading for all pharmacists. One important section lists the price that will be used in the calculation of ingredient costs of prescriptions for non-branded drugs by the Prescription Pricing Authority. Also of concern to hospital pharmacists are the sections listing which dressings, appliances and reagents are permitted to be prescribed under the NHS, since only items listed in the *Drug Tariff* may be prescribed on either FP10 or FP10(HP) for dispensing by a community pharmacy. Other important sections deal with oxygen, elastic hosiery and prescription charges for composite prescriptions and packs. The book also includes specifications for certain items. The *Drug Tariff* is published every month, and is distributed to chemist contractors by health authorities, and to hospital pharmacies via trusts.

Generics

For many years a cornerstone of government policy on prescribing has been to encourage the use of generic medicines. In the hospital service generics are substituted for branded medicines, where available, under the authority of the Drugs and Therapeutics Committee. In the community substitution is illegal, so pressure is put on prescribers to write their prescription using the generic name. The Department of Health (DoH) has set a target for 72% of prescriptions to be written generically by March 2002, and this will no doubt be a rolling programme. In this way, price is controlled through competition between manufacturers of generic medicines, and reflected in the price allowed by the *Drug Tariff*. This market economy had worked well until 1999 when a shortage of some generic medicines caused rapid rises in prices. The causes for this were varied, including the closure of a large manufacturer, and the government acted swiftly to reduce the effect of the price rises on the prescribing budget. A House of Commons Select Committee reported on the issue, and the implications of this are discussed in an article by Kay and Baines.[25] Subsequently the DoH issued a consultation paper on long-term measures to control the generics market.[26] The tension between the imperative to reduce costs by better use of generics and the need to maintain a viable branded industry is reflected in the need for the strategic discussions such as PICTF, referred to above.

Medicines not prescribable on the NHS

Although the basic prices of ethical medicines are controlled through the PPRS, the government has always looked at wider issues in its attempts to control drug costs. As early as April 1985 action was taken to limit the availability of prescribable items which were deemed to be ineffective, in duplication of cheaper medicines, or were expensive proprietary medicines with alternative therapy available. The NHS Regulations were amended to limit the range of preparations available in particular therapeutic groups, listed in Table 2.1. This list has been maintained and is included in the *Drug Tariff* as 'Drugs and other substances not to be prescribed under the NHS pharmaceutical services'.

The selection of drugs within these groups was made by the Advisory Committee on NHS Drugs. Popular parlance soon coined the name 'Black List' for the prohibited items, which are identified by symbols in both the *British National Formulary*[4] and the *Monthly Index of Medical Specialities* (MIMS),[27] and 'White List' for those still available on NHS prescription. A series of DoH circulars followed which elucidated various ambiguities and extended the new regulations to cover hospital prescribing as well as general practice. In public the medical profession was strongly opposed to the new restrictions, which were

Table 2.1 Categories of medicines included in original 'Limited List'

Analgesics for mild or moderate pain
Antacids
Benzodiazepine tranquillisers
Bitters and tonics
Cough and cold remedies, including cough suppressants, expectorants and
    demulcents, etc
Inhalations
Laxatives
Mucolytics
Nasal decongestants
Vitamins

Table 2.2 Additional categories of medicines to be considered by the Advisory Committee on National Health Service Drugs

Antidiarrhoeal drugs	Drugs for allergic disorders
Appetite suppressants	Drugs for vaginal/vulval conditions
Contraceptives	Drugs used in anaemia
Drugs acting on the ear and nose	Hypnotics and anxiolytics
Drugs acting on the skin	Topical antirheumatics

seen as a limitation on clinical freedom. If a patient really wants a 'black-listed' Prescription Only Medicine, to the extent of being prepared to pay for it, the doctor may write a private prescription. In practice, this seems to happen rarely. A review body has been set up to consider appeals against the prohibition of certain items, and as a result, some of the original 'Black-listed' items have been reinstated.

As well as limiting prescribing in the above categories, by the same amendments, the opportunity was taken to remove the right to prescribe a list of obsolete and obscure preparations, some of which had never had, or had no great likelihood of ever obtaining, a product licence. The position of a number of borderline preparations was also clarified (see below).

By 1992, the DoH was referring to the 'Selected List' rather then the 'Limited List', and the terms of reference of the Advisory Committee had been changed to allow further groups of drugs to be included in the scheme. These are listed in Table 2.2.

In addition to those medicines not prescribable on the NHS, there is also a list of medicines whose prescribing is controlled by limitation to certain medical conditions. Early examples, such as acetylcysteine for use in cystic fibrosis, were fairly non-contentious, but other examples, such as listing restrictions on the use of sildenafil for erectile dysfunction, caused much public debate. The latest list will be found in the *Drug Tariff* as 'Drugs to be prescribed in certain circumstances under the NHS pharmaceutical services'.

Borderline substances

Certain preparations have been known for many years as 'Borderline Substances', i.e. it was not clear whether they were to be regarded as drugs, or as foods and cosmetics, the latter never having been available on NHS prescription. Doctors who unwittingly prescribed them were liable to have their prescriptions disallowed, and to have to pay for the items themselves. Confusion is liable to arise since in some cases the items are likely to be recommended to the general practitioner by a hospital consultant, who is free to prescribe within the institution. The unfairness of this was eventually recognised by the establishment of the Advisory Committee on Borderline Substances which has drawn up a list of approved medical conditions for which the prescription of these items should be allowed. A list of the medical conditions and the preparations prescribable may be seen in the *Drug Tariff* as 'Borderline Substances' both as a list of conditions and as a list of products.

Post-licensing evaluation

In addition to the methods described above, there is internationally a move to evaluate the cost-effectiveness of medicines and to restrict public reimbursement of medicines which are deemed not to meet strict criteria set by the government. In England and Wales this function is carried out by the National Institute for Clinical Excellence (NICE; see Chapter 10). In December 2001, the DoH updated its guidance on prescribing to make the implementation of NICE guidance mandatory on health authorities and primary care trusts.[28]

Marketing pharmaceuticals

Association of the British Pharmaceutical Industry

The ABPI is a trade organisation set up to represent pharmaceutical companies. Although the majority of its members are ethical companies, generic manufacturers may be members, and indeed some are. Member companies are committed to observe the Code of Practice for the Pharmaceutical Industry. Drawn up in consultation with the DoH, the MCA and the British Medical Association (BMA), this lays down standards of conduct to be followed in the marketing of medicines intended for use under medical supervision. In 1993, the ABPI set up the Prescription Medicines Code of Practice Authority (PMCPA) to operate the Code on its behalf. It operates independently, and copies of the Code of Practice itself and a quarterly review of cases which it has considered can be obtained from the PCMPA.[29] Complaints against companies by practitioners are investigated by the ABPI Code of Practice Committee, and, if upheld, an undertaking is obtained from the company that the undesirable practice will be discontinued. So that justice may be seen to be done, an account of the complaints considered by the committee is published from time to time in the *Pharmaceutical Journal*. The Code has sections covering all aspects of drug promotion and the conduct of medical representatives, including sampling, gifts, inducements and hospitality. There is also a section on market research. Hospital pharmacists should be aware that additionally, as purchasing officers of a public authority, their actions are governed by the Standing Financial Instructions of their health authority or trust, with which they should be familiar, and by the confidentiality aspects of regional and national drug contracts.

Medical representatives

Like anyone else working in sales, drug company representatives are trained in marketing psychology and techniques as well as being taught the salient facts about their products. The representative is at the lowest level in the hierarchy of the company's marketing department, and this is likely to be his/her first job in this industry, although he/she will have a science or paramedical qualification (rarely pharmaceutical) and may well have selling experience in another field. Thus he/she may have little understanding at first of the niceties of trading in a professional medical setting; this may cause problems, particularly in hospitals. Of course, many talented representatives never put a foot wrong and it is a pleasure to see them; such people are soon likely to be promoted to greater responsibilities as divisional/regional sales managers.

Although, of course, drug sales staff call on pharmacists, there can be little doubt that the mainstay of their activities is the visit to the doctor, during which they will promote whatever products are the subject of the current sales drive. Wide use is made of 'detail aids' – hand-held visual aids for use during the sales talk. If the company has no new products, it will push old ones, sometimes by bringing forward new information. The representative will be keen for the doctor to start using his/her drug at all costs, and so will be anxious to provide samples. Some doctors do not realise that the relatively flimsy sample packaging may not afford the same shelf-life or protection against possibly adverse storage conditions as the conventional commercial pack. In hospitals, a rule that all samples must be handed to the pharmacy minimises potential problems – without this, at 5 p.m. on Friday, one is liable to get a request for a non-stock drug for a patient part-way through a course. On the credit side, representatives are keen to deal with queries, act as public relations agents and generally to serve as an information link with head office.

Other promotional activities

Subsidised conferences in exotic locations to which doctors are invited to read papers favourable to a newly launched product have received much adverse media publicity. It is less well known that some companies, in the interest of good customer relationships, sponsor conferences – more often than not in university accommodation – for other health service professionals, including pharmacists, and sessions are devoted to subjects which have no bearing on the company's products at all. It is DoH policy, set out in a guide issued in 2000,[30] *Commercial Sponsorship; Ethical Standards for the NHS*, that pharmacists and other NHS personnel should not accept offers of free luxury accommodation, and they should pay their own travelling expenses. Examples of activities approved and disallowed are included in this guide. A further circular[31] gave guidance on the need for declaration of interest in this area.

The ABPI Code does not permit firms to send out unsolicited reprints of papers from medical journals; however, they are pleased to supply them on request, usually via the representative. Drug companies sometimes sponsor special editions of journals devoted entirely to their drug – often these contain reports of papers delivered at a subsidised conference. The papers so published are quite likely not to have been submitted to the adjudication procedures which are the norm in scientific journals for papers submitted in the ordinary way.

A promotional activity which has caused much aggravation to hospital pharmacists is the so-called clinical trial/clinical assessment of an established drug, usually one which is not in general use in that hospital. This is quite distinct from real trials of unlicensed drugs, and is merely a way of starting the habit of prescribing the drug, which the sales representative hopes will then continue after the 'trial' is over. Doctors may even be charmed into believing that they are performing worthwhile research and indeed they may reap direct or indirect financial benefits, as the firm may pay for the completion of patient records, or supply equipment. From the drug company's point of view, this is a particularly elegant way of sampling – an added refinement being that often the free drug supplied (if any) is enough for only a few patients, and to complete the 'trial' the hospital will have to buy the rest. It is to counteract this kind of activity that hospitals have established rigid 'new drugs' policies, which usually allow only consultants to order new items, after discussion with the pharmacist, or possibly making a case to the Drug and Therapeutics Committee. Drug formularies are also seen as a way of limiting the range of drugs available, and ensuring that those selected are as cost-effective as possible.

In 1986, Bayer UK Ltd was suspended from the ABPI for allowing its representatives to organise 'trials' of this type for its drug Adalat Retard, as this contravened the ABPI Code of Practice.[32] The question of the relationships between doctors and drug companies has been explored by the Royal College of Physicians. Their report was summarised in the *Pharmaceutical Journal*.[33] On the subject of promotional 'clinical trials', it concluded that: 'Such trials threaten to undermine the trust of patients and the respect of the public'. Postmarketing surveillance (PMS) guidelines have now been agreed between the ABPI, the BMA and the Royal College of General Practitioners. They state several features which are essential in the design of company-sponsored PMS, e.g.: 'there should be a valid medical reason; design and methods used must permit the achievement of the stated scientific and medical objectives; the study must not be designed for, or conducted as, a promotional exercise'. Appropriate fees for doctors participating in studies have been agreed with the BMA, as a recompense for record-keeping and other extra work involved.

New drugs

In 2001, about £6.5m per day was spent on research and development by the UK pharmaceutical industry.[34] The drug development process is so costly because of a number of factors. These include the high drop-out rate of new chemical entities, which fail to live up to early promise during the testing stages and are discarded, and the complexity of the testing procedures required before marketing authorisation is achieved.

Registration of medicinal products

In developed countries, medicines have to be registered and authorised for sale by a national regulatory authority such as the MCA in the UK and the FDA in the USA. There is often no reciprocity between national agencies, with the result that companies have to apply for product registration through a full licensing procedure, and may have to conform to differing requirements. Within the EU, however, a mutual recognition procedure has been agreed. A marketing authorisation application (MAA) will be assessed by the regulatory authority of one member state and, when successful, the applicant can then request that the initial EU member state should apply for approval of the authorisation in other member states. This process is described more fully in an article by Harman,[35] which forms part of a series – The drug development process – published in the *Pharmaceutical Journal*. For mutual recognition to be permitted, the MAA submitted to subsequent member states must be identical with that submitted in the original member state. If the mutual recognition application occurs after postmarketing clinical experience has added knowledge to the drug profile, the MAA will have to be updated with the agreement of both the original and the subsequent member states.

In some cases, instead of following the mutual recognition procedure, the MAA can be handled by a centralised agency, the European Medicines Evaluation Agency (EMEA), whose headquarters is in London. In an organisation comparable to that of the MCA, which evaluates medicinal products through the Committee on Safety of Medicines (CSM), the EMEA works through two committees, the Committee for Proprietary Medicinal Products (CPMP) for human medicinal products, and the Committee for Veterinary Medicinal Products (CVMP) for animal medicines. For certain products, i.e. those derived from biotechnology processes such as proteins, enzymes, antibodies, genetic materials and other naturally occurring substances, within the EU, MAAs must be handled by the EMEA. More information will be found in Harman's paper.[35] The centralised procedure is available to manufacturers as an option for other substances that are deemed innovative, i.e. entirely new chemical entities, new delivery systems, a new indication for an existing product or a product whose action is based on the presence of a radioisotope.

Stages leading to marketing authorisation

A period of 8–12 years may elapse between the isolation and patenting of a new drug to its marketing authorisation, and during this period no profits are made. Figure 2.1 gives an outline of the pathway from new chemical entity to marketed product.

Once a promising molecule has been synthesised and patented – a process that may take several years – the preclinical testing programme is launched. This will determine the pharmacological profile, and also assess toxicity, using both animal and, where feasible, *in vitro* testing methods. The information accumulated will be submitted at the first stage of the MAA. In another article in his series, Harman[36] gives background and details of the legislation at each stage; he sets out the structure of the application, and gives insight into the scale and complexity of the data needed before any trials on human subjects can be undertaken. The reader seeking fuller information is advised to read further articles in Harman's series.[37–39]

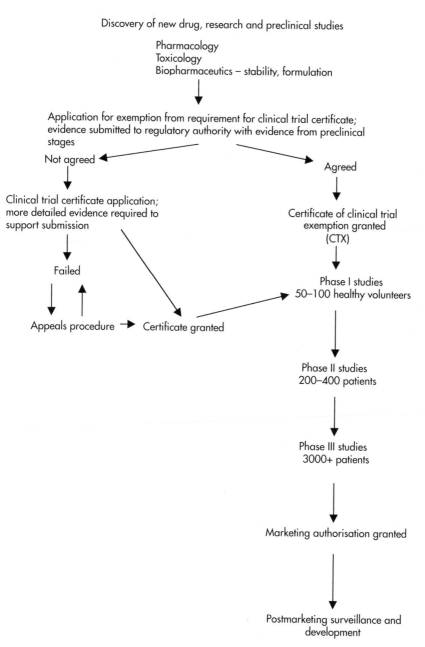

Figure 2.1 Stages in the development of a new drug.

Once the preliminary stages have been completed, the next stage is the application to the local regulatory authority – in the UK the MCA – for a clinical trial certificate or a clinical trial exemption (CTX) certificate, which permits the holder to start clinical trials on humans. The CTX scheme, which avoids the need to apply for a full clinical trial certificate, was started in response to complaints that the original full licensing procedure took so long to complete that the useful patent life of the product had expired before marketing was possible. Data are submitted to the MCA in a summarised form, and must be signed by a medical practitioner who declares that it is reasonable for the trial to take place. Under the existing regulations, if there are no objections, a CTX can be granted within 35 days. (However, this is to be extended to 60 days under the provisions of the European Directive on clinical trials.) Further details may be found on the MCA website[40] and in an article by Wiffen.[41]

A new European Directive (2001/20/EEC) on clinical trials was published in 2001.[42] Once its provisions have been enacted in the UK, it will have far-reaching effects on the conduct of clinical trials, both in manufacturers' facilities and within hospitals. The major changes are summarised in the article cited. The implications for both manufacturers and hospitals were discussed at a symposium held by the Joint Pharmaceutical Analysis Group, reported in the *Pharmaceutical Journal*.[43]

Clinical trials: the role of the pharmacy

Phase I studies using healthy volunteers are undertaken to confirm the previous pharmacological and toxicological studies, and normally take place in specialist units. Currently not included in UK clinical trials regulations, volunteer studies will be covered under the new EU directive. Only when these studies have been completed satisfactorily is it possible to move on to phase II and III studies, involving at first small numbers of patients, normally in a hospital, and then, finally, larger studies at several centres, or possibly in the community.

Planning for a clinical trial

Pharmacists expecting to be involved with clinical trials must familiarise themselves with the section 'On dealing with clinical trials' in the practice advice section of the *Medicines, Ethics and Practice* guide,[44] which includes practical guidance on the role of the clinical trials pharmacist and references to relevant guidance and legislation. There is now a specialist clinical trials qualification for pharmacists and pharmacy technicians. Launched jointly by the Liverpool School of Pharmacy and the Association of Clinical Research for the Pharmaceutical Industry, the clinical trials module can form part of studies for a Certificate of Professional Development or a Postgraduate Diploma in Clinical Research.[45]

It cannot be emphasised too strongly that the preparation and planning stages of clinical trials are pivotal in ensuring that they run smoothly and produce valid results. Plans will be formulated by collaboration between the clinical trials/medical department of the pharmaceutical company and the hospital consultant assuming responsibility for the patients, and ideally should include clinical support services as appropriate. At each hospital the trial protocol has to be submitted to the local research and ethics committee. This will include consultants not involved in the trial, lay members and nurses, and exists to consider the ethics of the proposals. However, should the trial design not conform to recommended professional standards, the committee should be so advised and should reject it or require modifications to the protocol. Under the terms of the CTX, any refusal of a trial by an ethical committee has to be reported to the MCA by the pharmaceutical company.

Running clinical trials

The pharmaceutical company often does the dispensing into patient packs. In such cases, it may be necessary for the local pharmacy to add hospital name-and-address labels. This will be important should the patient be admitted to another hospital; few drug companies' medical departments will be able to provide an Accident and Emergency doctor with details promptly in the middle of the night, but an on-call pharmacist can. Cautionary and advisory labels, e.g. 'Keep out of the reach of children' should be added or requested as appropriate. Under the new European Directive, there will be mandatory guidance about the labelling of clinical trial supplies. The company should be asked to use child-resistant packaging at the planning stage. Some trials involve a comparison with an established drug, and the shelf-life of both the trial agents and any other drugs used must be recorded. Most trials take much longer to complete than originally envisaged and it is easy to overlook the impending expiry of the drugs. The batch numbers should also be recorded for use in a recall.

Before the trial starts, the clinical trials pharmacist should draw up a procedure detailing exactly what is to be done at each outpatient attendance by dispensary staff, or by clinical pharmacists on the wards. A log book should be kept to record events; the facts to be noted will vary according to the requirements of the trial design, but should always include names, addresses and telephone numbers of patients for emergency use. If returned tablet counts are to be done to monitor compliance, this is the place to record them. Should patients fail to collect their treatment, this should be followed up and the investigator informed. In 'blind' trials, the pharmacy usually holds the key to the randomisation code, which is opened and read only at the end of the trial, or in the case of an individual patient, if some medical emergency arises. At the end of the trial, continuation supplies of drugs deemed effective should be made available for continuing treatment; such supplies are usually made free of charge by the company. This may mean supplying from the hospital pharmacy, with no prospect of referral to the general practitioner, for long periods if marketing authorisation is delayed.

Pharmacies handling significant numbers of clinical trials may find that the best way to handle the data storage and retrieval problem is by using a database. O'Hare et al. describe the design and use of such a database at the Belfast Royal Hospitals.[46]

Postmarketing studies

The total number of subjects exposed to the drug during the trial stages may not be enough for rare adverse drug reactions (ADRs) to become apparent, and so assessment is continued after marketing. The main ways in which this is achieved are illustrated in Figure 2.2.

Postmarketing safety assessment schemes

In 1993, agreement was reached between the MCA, CSM, the Royal College of General Practitioners, the BMA and the ABPI, which led to the publication of guidelines for company-sponsored safety assessment of marketed medicines (SAMM Guidelines).[47] They were formulated at a time when there was growing disquiet because some so-called assessments were in fact marketing schemes with incentives for doctors to prescribe new products. In some cases, the reporting of identified ADRs was delayed until the end of the study. For the purpose of the guidelines, SAMM is defined as 'a formal investigation conducted for the purpose of assessing the clinical safety of marketed medicine(s) in clinical practice'. The guidelines, which are reproduced in the ABPI Compendium,[3] would not normally apply to formal trials in which the company

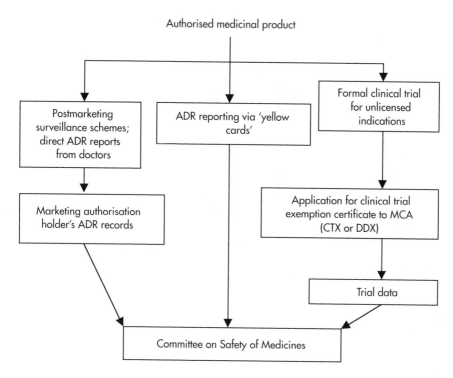

Figure 2.2 Postmarketing studies. ADR, adverse drug reaction; MCA, Medicines Control Agency; CTX, clinical trial exemption; DDX, Doctors' and Dentists' Exemption scheme.

provides the medicines (phase IV studies), for which there are separate guidelines.

Adverse drug reaction reporting: the 'Yellow Card' scheme

The monitoring of ADRs is a function of the Pharmacovigilance Section of the CSM. Marketing authorisation holders have to report any ADRs reported to them to this section, which maintains the UK Adverse Drug Reactions On-line Information Tracking (ADROIT) database. To facilitate ADR reporting, and to receive information from ADROIT, there is a 24-hour 'hot-line' whose number is listed in the *British National Formulary*.[4]

In addition, the CSM asks doctors and pharmacists to complete yellow report cards giving details of any diagnosed or suspected ADRs. Since 1999, community pharmacists have been included in the Yellow

Card scheme. At the time they were requested to focus their reporting particularly in those areas where they have specialist knowledge and where there is limited reporting by doctors – OTC medicines and licensed and unlicensed herbal medicines.[48] Reports sent in by community pharmacists will be acknowledged, and a copy of the report will be sent to the patient's general practitioner. Since 2000, patients' names are not required, but health professionals using the cards are requested to code them in a way which would enable subsequent retrieval of case notes, e.g. practice or hospital number, and to file a copy of the yellow card details in the notes. To encourage reporting, the *British National Formulary*[4] includes 'yellow cards' and information on reporting. Newer drugs are marked with the symbol ▼ and doctors are asked to be particularly vigilant in reporting ADRs suspected with these drugs.

Feedback from the ADR reporting schemes is provided either in response to individual queries addressed to the CSM, or via the bulletin, *Current Problems in Pharmacovigilance*, that is circulated to doctors and pharmacists. When a serious problem is identified, a product withdrawal may ensue and the marketing authorisation is usually revoked to prevent further marketing. Residual stocks of such drugs are usually returned to the makers for disposal; prescriptions received after the withdrawal should be referred back to the prescriber.

Unlicensed indications

Manufacturers may promote a drug for only those indications listed in the marketing authorisation. At times, prescribers may wish to investigate the drug's effects for novel indications, or by using a dose form by an unconventional route, e.g. inhalation of an injection solution or vice versa, or in a dosage regimen different from that recommended. A doctor may prescribe an unlicensed product for an individual named patient, provided that the doctor is aware of what he/she is doing and accepts responsibility for the outcome, but if he/she embarks on an organised investigation in a series of patients, this constitutes a clinical trial and may require an application for a clinical trial certificate. In most cases, a full clinical trial certificate application procedure will be waived by the MCA under the Doctors' and Dentists' Exemption (DDX) scheme. Full details of the application procedure will be found on the MCA website,[40] and the scheme is also described in the article by Wiffen.[41] At the time of writing (March 2002), two guidance booklets produced by the MCA[49, 50] are under revision.

References

1. National Statistics. *Monthly Digest of Statistics*, no. 661. London: Stationery Office, 2001.
2. Association of the British Pharmaceutical Industry website (2001). *Pharmaceutical Facts and Statistics*: www. abpi.org.uk (accessed 30 April 2001).
3. Association of the British Pharmaceutical Industry. *Medicines Compendium*. London: Pharmaceutical Press/DataPharm Communications, 2002.
4. Mehta D K, ed. *British National Formulary*, published twice-yearly. London: British Medical Association/Royal Pharmaceutical Society of Great Britain.
5. Thompson F. Where do generic and brand names come from? *Pharm J* 2001; 267: 223–224.
6. Sweetman S, ed. *Martindale: The complete drug reference*, 33rd edn. London: Pharmaceutical Press, 2002.
7. Law and ethics bulletin. Unlicensed products for dispensing. *Pharm J* 2001; 266: 279.
8. Kay A. Generic medicines. *Pharm J* 1997; 258: 554–559.
9. Kay A. Four years of ups and downs in the generics marketplace. *Pharm J* 2001; 266: 788–791.
10. Appelbe G E, Wingfield J. *Dale and Appelbe's Pharmacy Law and Ethics*, 7th edn. London: Pharmaceutical Press, 2001.
11. Karr A. Who wants to adopt an orphan? *Hosp Pharm* 2000; 7: 165–167.
12. Meers P D, Calder M W, Mazhar M M, Lawrie G M. Intravenous infusion of contaminated dextrose solution. The Devonport incident. *Lancet* 1973; 2: 1189–1192.
13. *Report of the Committee Appointed to Inquire into the Circumstances, Including the Production, which led to the Use of Contaminated Infusion Fluids in the Devonport Section of the Plymouth General Hospital*. London: Her Majesty's Stationery Office, 1972.
14. *Report on the Prevention of Microbial Contamination of Medicinal Products*. London: Her Majesty's Stationery Office, 1973.
15. Department of Health and Social Security. Application of the Medicines Act to health authorities. HSC(IS)128.
16. *Rules and Guidance for Pharmaceutical Manufacturers and Distributors (The Orange Guide)*. London: Stationery Office, 1997.
17. Mulholland D. Full-line wholesaling: regionals go national, nationals go European. *Pharm J* 2001; 268: 107–109.
18. Fawhan F. Short-line wholesalers: what part do they really play? *Pharm J* 2002; 268: 112–113.
19. Association of Parallel Importers website (2002). www.api.co.uk (accessed January 2002).
20. Association of the British Pharmaceutical Industry. *Understanding the PPRS*. Available at www.abpi.org.uk (accessed 19 March 2002).
21. News item. Task force to strengthen industry. *Pharm J* 2000; 264: 598.
22. Association of the British Pharmaceutical Industry and the Department of Health. *The Pharmaceutical Industry Competitiveness Task Force. Final Report. March 2001*. www.doh.gov.uk/pictf (accessed January 2002).
23. News item. Pharmaceutical industry worth extra £2–£4bn to United Kingdom. *Pharm J* 2002; 268: 6.

24. Department of Health and National Assembly for Wales. *Drug Tariff*, published monthly. London: Stationery Office.

25. Kay A, Baines D. The House of Commons Health Select Committee's report on generic prices – implications for primary care prescribing. *Pharm J* 2000; 265: 689–691.

26. News report. Fixed prices or competitive tendering: latest options for generic medicines. *Pharm J* 2001; 267: 109.

27. *Monthly Index of Medical Specialities*. London: Haymarket Medical.

28. Department of Health (2002). PCG/PCT prescribing and budget setting 2002/2003. www.doh.gov.uk/prescribingbudgets/index.htm (accessed January 2002).

29. Prescription Medicines Code of Practice Authority website (2002). www.abpi.org.uk/links/assoc/pmpca (accessed January 2002).

30. Department of Health. *Commercial Sponsorship; Ethical Standards for the NHS*. London: Department of Health, 2000.

31. Department of Health. *Standards of Business Conduct: Declarations of Interest*. EL(96)12.

32. ABPI Code of Practice Committee Report. Bayer UK Ltd suspended over actions by representatives. *Pharm J* 1986; 237: 821.

33. News report. Advice on relationships with physicians. *Pharm J* 1986; 237: 431.

34. Association of the British Pharmaceutical Industry website (2001). *Pharmaceutical Facts and Statistics*: www. abpi.org.uk (accessed 30 April 2001).

35. Harman R J. The drug development process: (2) administrative processes and options for registration of medicines. *Pharm J* 1999; 262: 928–931.

36. Harman R J. The drug development process: (1) introduction and overview. *Pharm J* 1999; 262: 334–337.

37. Harman R J. The drug development process: (3) quality issues (I). *Pharm J* 1999; 263: 394–398.

38. Harman R J. The drug development process: (4) quality issues (II). *Pharm J* 2000; 265: 206–208.

39. Harman R J. The drug development process: (5) pharmacotoxicological studies (I). *Pharm J* 2001; 266: 155–159.

40. Medicines Control Agency website (2001). www.opengov.uk/mca/mcahome.htm (accessed 10 March 2001).

41. Wiffen P J. A guide to the licensing system. *Hosp Pharm* 1995; 2: 15–16.

42. News item. New directive for clinical research will have huge impact on pharmacists. *Pharm J* 2001; 267: 7.

43. Phillips G, Secretary, Joint Pharmaceutical Analysis Group. Implications of the new clinical trial directive. *Pharm J* 2001; 267: 26–27.

44. Royal Pharmaceutical Society of Great Britain. *Medicines, Ethics and Practice: A Guide for Pharmacists*, published yearly. London: Royal Pharmaceutical Society of Great Britain.

45. News item. Clinical trials qualification for pharmacists launched. *Pharm J* 2000; 264: 85.

46. O'Hare M C B, McFarland M, O'Hare J D G. The development of a clinical trials database. *Pharm J* 1997; 259: 226–227.

47. *SAMM Guidelines: Guidelines for Company Sponsored Safety Assessment of Marketed Medicines*. London: Medicines Control Agency, 1993.
48. Medicines Control Agency, Committee on Safety of Medicines. *Community Pharmacists can now Report Suspected Adverse Drug Reactions via the Yellow Card Scheme*. London: CSM, MCA, 1999.
49. Medicines Control Agency. *A Guide to the Provisions Affecting Doctors and Dentists (MAL 30)*. Revised June 97. London: MCA, 1997.
50. Department of Health and Social Security. *Clinical Trials Using Marketed Products (MAL 32)*. London: Her Majesty's Stationery Office, 1974.

3

Primary care pharmacy

During most of the history of the profession, little pharmacy was practised in the primary care or community setting outside the confines of the localities' community pharmacies. The National Health Service (NHS) payment system, which was centred on the supply of prescriptions and with no means of paying for professional pharmaceutical advice, did nothing to encourage innovative practice. In recent years, this has begun to change. From small beginnings, e.g. the provision of services to residential homes, pharmacists have moved outwards into the community and are becoming integrated with the other providers of primary care as members of the team. This trend will be accelerated by the proposals for the future of pharmacy set out in the recent government plan.[1] These include the introduction of new legislation to allow a new form of agreement leading to the establishment of 'local pharmaceutical services', i.e. arrangements tailored to local circumstances. This could lead to new ways of contracting for pharmacy services such as medicines management and health promotion schemes, not necessarily provided by traditional pharmacy contractors. This chapter sets the scene for the developments now occurring and discusses the current initiatives in this changing field of practice.

Prescribing support in the primary care setting

Before and during the 1980s, there was little incentive for general practitioners (GPs) to rationalise prescribing by introducing practice formularies, by prescribing generically or otherwise try to save money on their prescribing, because the drugs budget was not apportioned to individual general practices and was open-ended, i.e. not cash-limited. The bill for both the ingredients component and pharmacists' professional fees was the responsibility of the Family Health Services Authority (FHSA: the forerunner of the present health authority (HA)) in whose area the prescription was dispensed. By contrast, hospital drugs budgets were cash-limited. This period was marked by repeated attempts by hospitals to cut their drugs expenditure by transferring responsibility for long-term prescribing of expensive drugs to the GP by curtailing outpatient prescribing and by reducing quantities of drugs issued on discharge. The writing of outpatient prescriptions on form FP10(HP) does not fall into this category, since the costs revert to the issuing hospital or trust. This practice not only upset the FHSAs, which objected to funding part of the hospitals' drugs expenditure, but it also led to problems about determining who was clinically responsible for therapy, and often soured relationships between GPs and hospital doctors. An NHS Management Executive letter[2] gave guidance on prescribing at the interface between hospitals and general practice. Based on the recommendations of a multidisciplinary working party, the letter stated that there should be liaison between hospital doctors and GPs to decide who should be responsible for prescribing. It was no longer appropriate for hospitals to refuse to supply long-term medication to avoid paying for expensive drugs. The letter established the principle that drugs should be prescribed by the clinician who retains clinical responsibility for the patient. GPs should not be expected to prescribe unfamiliar drugs, and shared-care protocols should be agreed between hospital consultants and GPs. When a drug is involved which is not normally dispensed in the community, the hospital pharmacy should liaise with the community pharmacy to ensure continuity of supply. Shared-care arrangements with agreed protocols for prescribing are now the norm in managing many long-term conditions. In addition, in most HAs, area prescribing committees have now been established; these consider issues such as the introduction of new drugs, hospital discharge policies and resolving potential conflicts at the primary–secondary care interface.

In 1991, in a move towards improving the cost-effectiveness and quality of general practice prescribing, indicative prescribing budgets (i.e. budgets to which the practice was supposed to adhere, but not actually cash-limited) were assigned to practices by FHSAs,[3] and monitoring began of prescribing performance by using Prescribing Analysis and Cost (PACT) reports provided by the Prescription Pricing Authority (PPA). An enhanced version of PACT is now available to HAs online as EPACT Net. This enables data sets to be manipulated to provide comparisons between individual or groups of GP practices, e.g. in a primary care group (PCG). Further information is contained in the Itemised Prescription Payment Report (IPPR) which is sent each month to HAs.

In 1989, the concept of fundholding was introduced in a government White Paper.[4] Thereafter, some GP practices became fundholders, one result being that their drugs budgets were genuinely cash-limited. In 1993[5] and 1994[6] the National Audit Office had undertaken studies of general practice prescribing, which revealed that GP prescribing accounted for 10% of the total NHS budget at that time, and this gave the government a powerful incentive to try to curb expenditure. GPs were encouraged to obtain pharmaceutical advice on controlling their expenditure by methods including generic substitution and proper controls of repeat prescribing. The 1999 Health Act abolished GP fundholding, and introduced PCGs, in which GP practices serving a population of around 100 000 patients were grouped together to serve as a commissioning unit. From April 2000, these have been able to apply for primary care trust (PCT) status, with an enhanced role in planning, providing and commissioning services, taking on some of the roles previously carried out by the HAs. (See Chapter 12.) The financial allocation to PCGs and PCTs for all forms of care, including prescribing, is cash-limited. By 1999, GP prescribing accounted for one-third of the primary care budget – over 500 million prescriptions were dispensed annually, costing more than £4.5bn.[7]

From the initiatives discussed above, the concept of 'pharmaceutical support' of prescribing has emerged. Jackson[8] defined this as the use of additional professional input into one or more elements involved in the prescribing process, with the objectives of promoting high-quality medicine use and of improving the pharmaceutical care of patients.

National Prescribing Centre

In 1996, the NHS Executive set up the National Prescribing Centre (NPC) following a review of centrally funded support for prescribing and medicine use. According to its website,[9] its current aim is 'to facilitate the promotion of high quality, cost effective prescribing through a co-ordinated and prioritised programme of activities aimed at supporting all relevant professionals and senior managers working in the NHS'. Since the NHS management structure is constantly changing in the light of government reviews and plans, the work of the Centre has to adapt to this process. An outline of its work is summarised in Table 3.1.

Pharmacists will be familiar with some of the publications listed in the table, such as the *MeReC Bulletin*. *GP Prescribing Support: A Resource document and guide for the new NHS*, reported by Jackson, was published by the NPC following a national conference held during 1997.[8] The purpose of the guide is to bring to the attention of those interested in prescribing the wide range of services available. As far as pharmacists are concerned, it is intended for those directly concerned in providing prescribing support, and also for others who may be planning

Table 3.1 Examples of work produced by the National Prescribing Centre

Information on medicines	*MeRec Bulletins* and *Briefings*
	Connect newsletters
	Information resource documents
	New Drugs in Clinical Development bulletins
	New Medicines in the Market bulletins
Training and education	Targeted therapeutic workshops, day seminars and conferences for advisers and other relevant professionals
Dissemination of good practice	*Prescribing initiative* database
	Medicines and the NHS: A Guide for Directors publication
	GP Prescribing Support: A Resource Document and Guide for the New NHS
Information technology	Helping in the development of information systems related to prescribing
Informing research and initiatives	Keeping relevant NHS staff informed of key information

NHS, National Health Service.

services or commissioning them. Clive Jackson, the Director of the NPC, states that the guide categorises the types of prescribing support potentially available to GPs into three categories:

- clinical (involving issues usually based around individual patient care);
- prescribing policies, procedures and analyses (involving issues usually to be implemented at practice level);
- issues and policy at the interface between practices, PCGs and hospitals (involving issues usually best coordinated and facilitated across a locality).

Collaborative National Medicines Management Services Programme

As part of *The NHS Plan*[10] in the section 'Helping patients to get the best from their medicines', *Pharmacy in the Future*[1] included plans to provide funding for medicines management services to provide targeted support for patients. In 2001 these plans took shape when the Department of Health (DoH) launched a Collaborative National Medicines Management Project (CNMMP),[11] in which during 2001–02 £1.9m would be invested in 25 NHS schemes based in PCGs/PCTs. The project is a step in the establishment of a national Medicines Management

Services Programme, to be hosted by the NPC working in conjunction with the National Primary Care Development Team. During the first stage of the project, applications were invited for schemes in which local facilitators would work closely with GPs, pharmacists and primary health care teams to reshape local services to meet the needs of patients, and to ensure that money spent on medicines is used to best effect. The main aims for the programme, set out in the CNMMP publication,[11] are to achieve:

- improvements in health through improved medicines management, using accepted markers;
- a reduction in the wastage of medicines;
- a reduction in unmet, evidence-based pharmaceutical need in at least one priority therapeutic area;
- an improvement in medicines taking through the development of patient partnerships;
- a reduction in inappropriate clerical and professional time taken up with existing medicines management processes (e.g. repeat prescribing);
- improved patient satisfaction with medicines management services provided.

In July 2001, the successful bids were announced. The schemes that they proposed to implement were outlined in the *Pharmaceutical Journal*,[12] and included assessing the ability of certain patient groups to self-medicate; the referral of patients needing assistance with their medicines to a local pharmacist for assessment and advice; management of minor ailments by pharmacists; improving the quality of repeat dispensing and prescribing; and the monitoring of anticoagulant prescribing by community pharmacists. In the same report, it was announced that the NPC is to include a section about the medicines management scheme on its website (www.npc.co.uk).

Pharmacy Community Care Liaison Group (PCCLG)

The PCCLG, with representatives from England, Wales and Scotland, exists to advise on issues in primary and community care; its members are appointed from various backgrounds covering community, learning disabilities, mental health, universities, HAs, the NHS Executive, the Royal Pharmaceutical Society of Great Britain (RPSGB) and the DoH.

The remit of the PCCLG is to:

- identify important developments in community care which affect pharmaceutical services;
- promote and support best practice in community care pharmaceutical services and the use of medicines;
- produce information to facilitate greater involvement of pharmacists in national and local service developments within a multidisciplinary environment.

The PCCLG produces papers on various subjects that are circulated to interested organisations as appropriate. These mostly define standards of pharmaceutical support for specialised patient groups such as those with learning difficulties. The papers are sometimes published in the *Pharmaceutical Journal*, but may also be found on the PCCLG website (www.nmhc.co.uk/pcclg.htm).

Pharmaceutical support in practice

Health authority pharmaceutical advisers

The provision of pharmaceutical advice at a senior managerial level had become an established feature of hospital pharmacy during the 1970s and 1980s following the reorganisations that took place following the 1970 Noel Hall report.[13] Equivalent developments were slower to take effect in the community. However, this was to change in the wake of two reports – the 1986 Nuffield Report[14] and the Joint Working Party of the DoH and the Royal Pharmaceutical Society, which reported in 1992.[15] The second report stated 'we recommend that each Family Health Services Authority (FHSA) should employ a pharmaceutical adviser'. The Working Party alluded to the development of hospital prescribing formularies, and recommended that FHSA pharmaceutical advisers should work alongside medical advisers to promote similar developments in general practice, and also to encourage consistency between hospital, community and primary care staff.

Since then pharmaceutical advisers have been appointed to all HAs. Initially envisaged by the Working Party, it would seem, as general facilitators and providers of practice-level prescribing advice, their role has developed over the years and is now more strategic in nature, while much of the original practice-based work is now being undertaken by community pharmacists. Amongst a raft of other activities, the advisers assist in formulating prescribing policies, particularly at the hospital–community interface; advise on the pharmaceutical aspects of planning and commissioning health care for the local population; advise on commissioning pharmaceutical services locally; and generally provide pharmaceutical advice to the HAs' medical and nursing advisers. In addition, they have had an important role in assisting the medical adviser in the setting and monitoring of prescribing budgets and prescribing in general practice. This latter role is liable to change with the advent of the more autonomous PCTs, since they will take on some of the commissioning functions currently undertaken by HAs. Some of these changes are outlined by Leach.[16] Increasingly, it is to be expected that the advisers will be less involved with practice-level matters, and more with coordinating policies between secondary care providers, PCGs and PCTs.

The role of the HAs, and with it their pharmaceutical advisers, will change in the wake of the planned reduction from 99 to 30 HAs, which is taking place currently as part of the restructuring of NHS top-level management. The new HAs are to take over the strategic role which at present is undertaken by the NHS Executive regional offices, which are being abolished. The possible impact of the changes on HA pharmaceutical advisers was explored by Thompson.[17] Pharmaceutical advisers interviewed concluded that there would be a continuing role in the new structure, but the emphasis would shift towards the PCT/PCG level.

Primary care pharmacists

PCGs and PCTs have recognised the need for pharmaceutical support by appointing pharmaceutical advisers on a full- or part-time basis; alternatively, they may have entered a contract with either a hospital pharmacy or an independent contractor to provide advice. Thus, a new speciality has arisen – the primary care pharmacist. The need for standards for individuals and organisations working in this field has been recognised by the NPC which, together with the Pharmaceutical Advisers' Group has formulated a core competency framework for primary care pharmacists.[18] In addition, the National Primary Care Research and Development Centre and the NPC have collaborated to produce a quality guide for pharmacists. This book defines terms currently used and also explains how to assess quality in this field. There is also advice on methods used to improve prescribing practice.[19]

Primary care pharmacists provide pharmaceutical advice to the boards of PCGs and PCTs, most of which have no pharmacist board members. This will be on topics such as commissioning services with a pharmaceutical component, e.g. a respite care facility or a medication management programme. They also monitor prescribing budgets by using PACT and EPACT reports. The implementation of policies set by the HA, or by government priorities and initiatives such as national frameworks (see Chapter 10) may require pharmaceutical input to the development of local action plans by the PCG or PCT. The PCG/PCT pharmacist adviser will also manage and coordinate pharmacists working with GP practices. There may also be some educational/training component to the job, with, for example, seminars on various topics relevant to prescribing support being arranged. Curwain[20] summarises the various prescribing support initiatives that the PCGs/PCTs are likely to require.

Practice-level prescribing support

There are various models for the provision of prescribing support at GP practice level. Jesson and Wilson[21] set out the options and summarise the tasks that may be undertaken. These are listed in Table 3.2.

Table 3.2 Primary care pharmacist activities

Cost-effective prescribing	PACT analysis
	Formulary development
	Review repeat prescribing systems
	Review repeat requests
	Rationalising prescriptions
Medicines management	Clinics
	Meeting drug company representatives
	Storage of medicines
	Audit of 'brown bags'
	Drug treatment protocol development
	Medication review in nursing homes
	Medication review of high-risk groups
	Review of patients on multiple therapy
Education	Seminars on therapeutic issues
	Update sessions
	Drug information
Patient contact	Clinics
	Adherence (compliance) problems
	Hospital admission and discharge
	Domiciliary visits
	General query response

Reproduced with permission from Jesson J and Wilson K. Primary care pharmacists: a conceptual model. *Pharm J* 1999; 263: 62.
PACT, Prescribing Analysis and Cost.

Possibly the most usual scenario is for a PCG/PCT or a GP practice to fund a community pharmacist on a sessional basis to work on a specific project such as a review of repeat prescribing or the development of a practice formulary. There have been many pilot schemes, mostly aimed at improving cost-effectiveness rather than other aspects of prescribing, particularly since the DoH in 1995 commissioned 17 projects including different models for the provision of prescribing advice. An evaluation of the effect of community pharmacists on GP prescribing was undertaken by Geoghegan *et al.* in 1998.[22] Their paper is of great interest, since as well as reviewing previous work in the field, it details the results achieved over a 3-year period in various therapeutic groups, comparing them with control groups. The cost of providing the advice to 23 GP practices in St Helens and Knowsley over a 2-year period was calculated at £50 000. However, an estimate of the savings in just three therapeutic groups – ulcer-healing drugs, corticosteroid inhalers and non-steroidal antiinflammatory drugs – in eight practices in 2 years came to £89 000 when compared with controls. In 1999, Leach and Wakeman[23] evaluated the effectiveness of joint working between pharmacists and GPs, and concluded that 'interested pharmacists who have received special training are able to work well with GPs to improve the cost-effectiveness of prescribing'.

Training for prescribing support

Pharmacists planning to enter this field are advised to study the NPC book,[18] which sets out the competencies required. Providers of training are listed in an appendix to this book. As with any speciality, practitioners gain from interaction with others in the same field. There is now an organisation catering for primary care pharmacists – the Primary Care Pharmacists' Association. The RPSGB has launched a journal *Primary Care Pharmacy*, which may be received by pharmacists working within this speciality. In addition, there have been many initiatives in which shared learning between GPs and pharmacists has been organised. This has been valued by participants, who have found that their professional relationships with other health care professionals have been improved. A Scottish scheme for shared learning has been evaluated by Parr *et al.*[24] They conclude that the course participants experienced considerable benefits, but they warn that commissioning authorities will want to see that improvements in patient care can be achieved via this route.

Pharmaceutical services to private health care providers

Regulation and standards

Until recently, privately owned and voluntary sector residential homes and nursing homes have been licensed, regulated and inspected according to regulations made under the Registered Homes Act 1984, or the Nursing Homes Registration (Scotland) Act 1938 as amended. Residential care accommodation provided by the local authority was inspected but not licensed. Such accommodation has become progressively less common since the passing of the 1990 NHS and Community Care Act. The reasons for this are discussed by Hill.[25] The social services departments of local authorities were responsible for licensing and regulating residential homes, while HAs carry out similar functions for nursing homes. In both cases, the legislation covered a variety of matters, including registration and inspection, the fitness of the people running the home, record-keeping, services and facilities to be provided and criminal offences for breaching the regulations.[26] Compliance with the regulations has, up to now, been monitored by inspection units set up within social services departments and HAs. In practice, many homes have so-called dual registration as both nursing and residential homes. This has led to the formation of joint inspection units in some areas, to ensure uniformity of requirements and procedures. Local authority inspection units are also responsible for standards in other types of residential accommodation provided by the authority, e.g. community homes and children's homes with more than three children. As described later, pharmacists often have an input into inspection teams.

During the 1990s, there were a number of reports that highlighted deficiencies in the existing system. One of these, the 1995 *Moving Forwards* consultation document,[27] identified major deficiencies in the existing registration and inspection system. The main deficiency was that it was not comprehensive, since it failed to include many private health care providers, including domiciliary and day care which had become increasingly part of health care provision. There was also inconsistency in applying the regulations by the 150 local authorities in conjunction with about 100 HAs.

The Care Standards Act 2000 has been designed to meet these shortcomings.[28] As its regulations take effect, it will replace and extend existing legislation. Under its provisions, regulation and inspection will become the responsibility of a new body, the National Care Standards Commission (NCSC), established in April 2001; it took on its regulatory functions in April 2002. There will be about 80 area offices that will carry out the work of registration and inspection, to standards currently being developed. The Act will impose registration and inspection on private health care providers, some of whom are not currently regulated appropriately for their scale and range of services, and others which are not currently regulated at all:

- Independent hospitals, i.e. non-NHS hospitals (with the exception of Ministry of Defence hospitals, which are specifically excluded). Under the previous legislation, private hospitals were not distinguished from nursing homes, although the services they offered could be much more extensive. Some establishments were not subject to any form of regulation because they had a Royal Charter or had been established by a special Act of Parliament. The new Act has a specific category for hospitals regardless of their history, which includes all establishments providing: medical and surgical care; palliative care (including hospices but not a care home where a resident happened to require palliative care); psychiatric treatment for illness or mental disorder and for persons liable to be detained under the Mental Health Act 1983; treatment under all forms of anaesthesia (including Emla); private dental treatment under general anaesthesia; obstetric services, including maternity homes run by midwives; termination of pregnancy; cosmetic surgery and treatment using 'prescribed techniques or technologies'. The treatments to be so prescribed have not yet been fully defined. They will include class 3B and 4 lasers, that may be used to remove tattoos or in beauty parlours. The list may eventually include various other treatments when used outside hospitals, i.e. hyperbaric oxygen, pulsed light sources, endoscopy and dialysis.
- Intermediate care is envisaged as a 'whole-system approach' to a range of multidisciplinary, multiagency providers of services designed to reduce avoidable hospital admission, and to facilitate timely discharge from hospital with effective rehabilitation. It is expected that providers will plan new services in non-hospital environments, to minimise premature or long-term dependence on long-term care.
- Independent clinics: the Act will for the first time regulate private doctors and private dentists offering general anaesthesia. Registration and inspection will be required for practices ranging from Harley Street consulting rooms to walk-in private medical centres. Doctors practising from their own homes will also be included.

- Independent medical agencies: such doctors provide treatment or advice privately to patients, sometimes via a telephone, sometimes by making a house visit.

In addition, new statutory bodies will be formed: the General Social Care Council in England; the Scottish Social Services Council in Scotland; and the Care Council in Wales, taking over the functions of the existing Central Council for the Education and Training of Social Workers, which deals only with qualified staff. The new bodies will be responsible for the first time for the regulation of other key staff groups, in a manner similar to the Council for Professions Supplementary to Medicine. There may be some repercussions on the training of care staff in the use and handling of medicines (see below). Further details about the changes and other aspects of social services legislation to be amended by the Act will be found in Hill's book,[25] or from a summary of the Statutory Instrument, which may be viewed on the internet (at www.hmso.gov.uk/stat.htm).

The Registered Homes Act is also to be amended so that dentists' premises where wholly private dental treatment under general anaesthesia is undertaken will be subject to licensing and inspection under the provisions of the existing Act until its provisions are replaced by the requirements of the new Act.

According to the *Moving Forwards* consultation document,[27] 'regulation' means setting acceptable standards for services, and enforcing those standards by registering, issuing licences to or otherwise formally recognising service providers who meet them and taking action against those who do not. 'Inspection' means supporting the regulatory function by monitoring the initial and continued compliance by service providers with the standards set and identifying areas where the quality of care received by the user is inadequate.

The new inspection process will be based on the existing one, since it is intended to transfer staff from HA inspection units to the NCSC. Currently, when inspection teams identify failures, in the first instance advice is offered to the owner of the business. If this approach fails, and particularly if safety standards are compromised by legal violations, the owner may be prosecuted. If the closure of the care home is considered advisable, the local authority or HA may refer the matter to the Registered Homes Tribunal, established under the 1984 Act; the tribunal may recommend closure of the home. Such a case was described in 1992,[29] with some details of the infringements that led to prosecution, which included defective medicine administration procedures. It is expected that the new Act will have analogous procedures.

The Care Standards Act provides for the sharing of information between the Commission for Health Improvement (CHI; see Chapter 10) and the NCSC. A possible example cited in the implementation report is that of a CHI inspection team having concerns about the quality of care being provided by a private hospital to NHS patients; they could pass the information to the NCSC for action by their inspection team. It is also envisaged that staff may be seconded between the two commissions, to develop the inspection skills of the inspectors working for both organisations. The NCSC will have the power to utilise specialist staff such as pharmacists where they are not employed directly. It has formed a working group to identify the required competencies for inspectors. These are set out in a report of a study day[30] at which Hazel Somerville, a working group member, described her work. The competencies are to be incorporated into a national curriculum for NCSC inspectors currently being developed by the Open University. It is planned to develop a postgraduate diploma for all staff involved in inspection and registration.

Pharmaceutical requirements for registration

At the time of writing, the NCSC is developing national minimum care standards for all types of care accommodation due to be registered and inspected under the Care Standards Act 2000. These can be accessed from the NCSC website.[31] The national minimum standard for care homes for older people[32] contains a number of requirements about medicines management. These include having a medicines policy drawn up with pharmaceutical input and having policies and procedures for the receipt, recording, storage, handling, administration and disposal of medicines, which must comply with RPSGB guidelines as well as with current medicines legislation.[33]

There are many types of residential establishment that fall within the scope of this section. Some frequently met examples are listed in Table 3.3. Privately owned flats with a warden do not usually come into this category.

Table 3.3 Establishments that may require pharmaceutical services

Residential homes for the elderly	Children's homes
Nursing homes	Young offenders' institutions
Homes for persons with learning difficulties	Boarding schools
Homes for persons with physical difficulties	Hospices

Although the present law allows local authorities to develop their own sets of standards for registration, in practice agreements on standards across local authority boundaries have been made in some areas. Thus, in Greater London, common standards have been agreed between local authorities. The RPSGB has developed guidelines[34] for the administration and control of medicines in care homes for adults and children, and these define the standards that have been adopted by most local authorities. The guidelines set out the responsibilities of the home owner, which include, among other things:

- to enable medicines to be used appropriately for each patient;
- to enable safe, effective medicine administration and regular medication review;
- to enable self-administration of medicines by residents, where appropriate;
- to provide information and training for staff. It is recommended that those administering medicines should be trained to the level 3 of a National Vocational Qualification. Such training may be available from local colleges.

There is a long section on good practice procedures in the provision of medicines in care homes, and this is essential reading for anyone planning to work in this field. It is recommended that pharmaceutical advice should be available to all homes by a community pharmacist, irrespective of who supplies medicines to the home. (Some homes may obtain their medicines from a dispensing doctor.) In most cases, the pharmacist who regularly supplies the home will provide advice. The HA pays for and administers the contracts of pharmacists who provide advice to care homes on a formal basis, and may set local criteria for the services provided. This could include prescription review, staff training or the provision of drug information. A pharmacist could be employed by the HA specifically for this purpose, as in a scheme initiated in the Isle of Wight,[35] where it was believed that a more clinically oriented service could be provided by a specialist. Details of the NHS contract will be found in the *Drug Tariff*.[36]

HA inspection units usually have the benefit of pharmaceutical advice, whether from their own adviser, by purchasing the services of a pharmacist on a sessional basis from a local trust or by employing a part-time pharmacist. This is not necessarily the case with local authority inspection units. The PCCLG (see above) has published guidelines on the pharmacy inspection of nursing homes.[37]

Pharmaceutical services to care homes

Both standards and practice advice for services to residential and nursing homes have been drawn up by the RPSGB, and appear in the *Medicines, Ethics and Practice* (MEP) guide.[38] In addition to completing specific training (see below), pharmacists are recommended to draw upon the experience of others working in this field. In a review of pharmacy services to care homes, Sommerville[39] quotes work that demonstrates poor management of medicines, including inappropriate prescribing of psychoactive medicines. Also, she reports that many complaints about nurses to their governing body relate to inappropriate procedures concerning medicines in the private sector. It is clear that there is an important role for pharmacists in giving assistance in developing procedures, monitoring standards and training staff. In 1997, Corbett[40] studied repeat prescribing for 433 residents of care homes. She found that GPs were sometimes resistant to proposed changes for a variety of reasons, but in spite of this, she was able to show:

- use of less expensive therapeutic equivalents;
- increased use of generic medication;
- changes in the number of drugs per patient;
- reduced number of doses per patient per day;
- raised awareness of adverse drug reactions and drug interactions by the prescribers.

Hemmings *et al.*[41] describe services commissioned from community pharmacies for two community units set up to cater for mentally ill patients formerly cared for in a local psychiatric hospital; this could act as a model for other units. In fact, there was nothing about their proposals that was specific to a mental illness setting. Another group, Furniss *et al.*,[42] devised a system of documentation for use by pharmacists undertaking nursing home medication reviews. They recorded the following information about the pharmacist's activities:

- recommendations made to the GP regarding medication;
- reasons for the recommendations;
- whether the GP accepted the recommendations;
- whether the recommendations were acted upon;
- the outcome of any changes.

Pharmacists supplying care homes often agree to dispense medicines in monitored-dosage systems (MDSs). There are a number of systems on the market, e.g. the Nomad, which uses plastic cassettes holding 7 days' supply of medicines, and the Manrex, using plastic cards into which a foil-backed blister pack can be inserted. Some systems have associated software that generates patient administration records for use by home staff. NHS regulations do not list a payment for this service to the chemist contractor, who may be able to negotiate payment from the home owner. The MEP contains advice about the production facilities and procedures required for filling MDSs, including information about preparations that are not suitable for inclusion.

Hospices are currently regarded as a specialised type of nursing home providing palliative care for terminally ill adults and children. They are usually, but not always, run by charity or religious organisations outside the NHS; however, health purchasers are able to commission care for their patients in hospices. Hospices may contract with either hospital or community pharmacies to supply medicines. The rules for supplying nursing homes and hospices are complex, with important differences between those that are run by the NHS, voluntary organisations and charities and those which are privately operated for profit. Pharmacists new to this work are advised to consult the Professional Standards Directorate of the RPSGB.

Care homes are permitted to hold a stock of over-the-counter medicines or 'homely remedies' for administration without necessarily consulting a doctor. There are usually locally agreed guidelines about items which may be included in the list and conditions that may be treated. The list of ailments given in the RPSGB guidance[34] is indigestion, mild pains, cough, constipation, diarrhoea and mild skin conditions. There should be local agreement between HA, GP, pharmacist and home on the items to be supplied. The list may not include any Prescription Only Medicines. The home may purchase the medicines from a community pharmacy, preferably one which regularly supplies the home, or in some cases the GP may be able to prescribe a bulk supply.[36] Medicines labelled with the name of a resident may not be treated as a bulk supply and administered to other residents.

Training for work in care homes

This falls into two categories: training the pharmacist for undertaking this kind of work, and training the staff of the care home.

The minimum requirement for the pharmacist is to have successfully completed the *Home Away from Home* and the *Patient Medication Records* courses of the Centre for Pharmacy Postgraduate Education (CPPE). Several other CPPE courses will be helpful for those undertaking medication reviews for the elderly, and there is a course on palliative care. Further training, such as a clinical diploma or certificate, would benefit the pharmacist undertaking medication and repeat prescribing reviews.

In nursing homes, at least some of the carers will be registered nurses. They may benefit from refresher training or advice on an informal basis when the pharmacist visits the home. By contrast, people with no nursing qualifications usually run residential homes. Local authorities' standards for registration usually require managers to provide training for care staff. There are National Vocational Qualifications for this work. Pharmacists may have a contract to contribute to the training of care staff. There is a CPPE resource pack, *Take Good Care with Medicines,* for pharmacists undertaking this work, containing checklists and handouts, overhead projector slides and a video. Care staff who have completed the training will be able to:

- handle and administer medicines safely;
- support residents who are self-administering;
- use and maintain medication records.

The resource pack can be obtained from Centre for Pharmacy Postgraduate Education, School of Pharmacy, University of Manchester, Manchester M13 9HJ.

References

1. Department of Health. *Pharmacy in the Future – Implementing the NHS Plan.* London: Department of Health, 2000.
2. National Health Service Management Executive Letter (1991). EL(91)127.
3. Department of Health. *Improving Prescribing: Implementation of the GP Indicative Prescribing Scheme.* London: Department of Health, 1990.
4. Secretaries of State for Health, Wales, Northern Ireland, Scotland. *Working for Patients.* London: Her Majesty's Stationery Office, 1989.
5. National Audit Office. *Repeat Prescribing by General Practitioners in England.* London: Her Majesty's Stationery Office, 1993.
6. National Audit Office. *A Prescription for Improvement: Towards more Rational Prescribing in General Practice.* London: Her Majesty's Stationery Office, 1994.
7. News item. Community pharmacists and PCGs: which will be the most important areas? *Pharm J* 1999; 262: 169.
8. Jackson C. GP prescribing support: developing the professional opportunities. *Pharm J* 1998; 261: 422.
9. National Prescribing Centre website (2001). www.npc.gov.uk (accessed July 2001).
10. Department of Health. *The NHS Plan: A Plan for Investment, A Plan for Reform.* London: Department of Health, 2000.

11. Department of Health. *The Collaborative Medicines Management Project.* London: Department of Health, 2001.
12. News item. What will the successful medicines management sites be offering? *Pharm J* 2001; 267: 83.
13. *Report of the Working Party on the Hospital Pharmaceutical Service.* London: Her Majesty's Stationery Office, 1970.
14. Nuffield Foundation. *Pharmacy: The Report of the Committee of Inquiry Appointed by the Nuffield Foundation.* London: Nuffield Foundation, 1986.
15. Joint Working Party Report. *Pharmaceutical Care: The Future for Community Pharmacy.* London: Royal Pharmaceutical Society of Great Britain on behalf of the Department of Health and the pharmaceutical profession, 1992.
16. Leach R H. The impact of primary care groups and trusts. *Hosp Pharm* 1999; 6: 50–52.
17. Thompson M. What does the future hold for health authority pharmaceutical advisers? *Pharm J* 2001; 267: 117.
18. National Prescribing Centre. *Competencies for Pharmacists Working in Primary Care,* 1st edn. Liverpool: National Prescribing Centre and London: NHS Executive, April 2000.
19. National Primary Care Research and Development Centre and National Prescribing Centre. *Improving Quality in Primary Care: Supporting Pharmacists Working in Primary Care Groups and Trusts.* May be downloaded from National Prescribing Centre website www.npc.co.uk/publications/ ImprovingQuality/pharma.pdf (accessed 16 March 2002).
20. Curwain B. Provision of prescribing support for primary care groups. *Pharm J* 1999; 262: 338–339.
21. Jesson J, Wilson K. Primary care pharmacists: a conceptual model. *Pharm J* 1999; 263: 62–64.
22. Geoghegan M, Pilling M, Holden J, Wolfson W. A controlled evaluation of the effect of community pharmacists on general practitioner prescribing. *Pharm J* 1998; 261: 864–866.
23. Leach R H, Wakeman A. An evaluation of the effectiveness of community pharmacists working with GPs to increase the cost-effectiveness of prescribing. *Pharm J* 1999; 263: 206–209.
24. Parr R M, Bryson S, Ryan M. Shared learning – a collaborative education and training initiative for community pharmacists and general medical practitioners. *Pharm J* 2000; 264: 35–38.
25. Hill M, ed. *Local Authority Social Services: An Introduction.* Oxford: Blackwell, 2000.
26. Mandelstam M. *An A–Z of Community Care Law.* London: Jessica Kingsley, 1998.
27. Department of Health. *Moving Forwards: A Consultation Document on the Regulation and Inspection of Social Services.* London: Department of Health, 1995.
28. Department of Health. *National Care Standards Commission Implementation Project.* London: Department of Health, 2000.
29. News item. Nursing home owner convicted of medicines records offences. *Pharm J* 1992; 248: 279.

30. Joshua A. Study day report. Role for pharmacists in the National Care Standards Commission. *Pharm J* 2001; 266: 834.

31. National Care Standards Commission website (2001). www.doh.gov.uk/ncsc (accessed 12 August 2001).

32. National Care Standards Commission. *Care Homes for Older People: National Minimum Standards.* London: Stationery Office, 2001.

33. News item. Care homes must seek pharmacists' advice. *Pharm J* 2001; 266: 411.

34. Royal Pharmaceutical Society of Great Britain. *The Administration and Control of Medicines in Care Homes.* London: Royal Pharmaceutical Society of Great Britain, 2001.

35. News item. Isle of Wight Health Authority to appoint nursing homes pharmacist. *Pharm J* 2000; 264: 392.

36. Department of Health and National Assembly for Wales *Drug Tariff*, published monthly. London: Stationery Office.

37. *Pharmacy Inspection of Nursing Homes.* Pharmacy Community Care Liaison Group, 1997.

38. Royal Pharmaceutical Society of Great Britain. *Medicines, Ethics and Practice: A Guide for Pharmacists*, published yearly. London: Royal Pharmaceutical Society of Great Britain.

39. Sommerville H. Pharmacy services for the elderly in residential and nursing homes. *Pharm J* 1997; 259: 683–685.

40. Corbett J. Provision of prescribing advice for nursing and residential home patients. *Pharm J* 1997; 259: 422–424.

41. Hemmings E, Tompkins M, Curtis S J. Providing pharmaceutical services for two residential units for the mentally ill. *Pharm J* 1991; 246: 330–332.

42. Furniss L, Craig S K L, Scobie S *et al.* Medication reviews in nursing homes: documenting and classifying the activities of the pharmacist. *Pharm J* 1998; 261: 320–323.

4

Pharmacy in the community

The extended role: the way forward

Community pharmacists: extended role and Pharmacy in a New Age (PIANA)

The community pharmacist now has a wider role as a health care professional than ever before. Apart from dispensing prescriptions and all the established activities of the community pharmacy, he or she also increasingly works as part of the primary care team, and also has a role to play in health promotion, and advising health care colleagues in the safe and effective use of medicines. This chapter will describe some of these additional professional roles both currently and as they are expected to develop.

The expansion of the role of pharmacists was given impetus by several reports. In 1986 the Nuffield Report[1] stated: 'we believe that the service provided by the pharmacist (giving advice and treatment relating to minor ailments) could be more extensively used', but emphasised individuals' rights in choosing whether to ask the pharmacist or to go to their doctor. In 1992, a working party report[2] had amongst its recommendations that community pharmacists should be involved in promoting effective prescribing and in the selection of medicines; in the safe and effective use of medicines; in improving health; and in the provision of specialist services in community pharmacy. Over the intervening years many of these and other proposals have been enacted. In 1996, the Department of Health (DoH) changed the regulations for remunerating pharmacy contractors to make it possible to pay a professional allowance for specific services aimed at making better use of pharmacists' skills. Since then, a number of schemes have come into being, some of which will be described in the following sections.

In 1995–1996, the Royal Pharmaceutical Society of Great Britain (RPSGB) started a new initiative called Pharmacy in a New Age (PIANA). The first phase took the form of a consultation exercise in which the members of the Society were asked to provide their views on how pharmaceutical services should be developed to meet the needs of the public in the twenty-first century. The outcome was a document, *The New Horizon*.[3] It identified four major areas of activity crucial to the future of the profession:

- managing prescribed medicines – helping at every stage in the chain;
- managing chronic conditions – offering a better quality of life to patients with such conditions and helping to improve the outcomes of treatment;
- managing common ailments – giving patients reassurance and advice, with or without the use of non-prescribed medicines;
- promoting and supporting healthy lifestyles – helping people protect their own health.

At about the same time, a White Paper[4] was published that broadly made the same recommendations, but with the additional role of providing more advice on medicines to the rest of the primary health care team and others. The PIANA initiative is ongoing, and more recently has been promoted to the members by a nationwide tour of a roadshow entitled *Over to You*. This was designed to help pharmacists think about and work towards their professional future; presentations describing local initiatives were made by speakers from each area, covering a wide range of practice areas. These themes are supported and developed in the *Pharmacy in the Future* document,[5] which sets out a programme for the development of pharmacy in the National Health Service (NHS). This was published shortly after the government's plan for the whole NHS.[6]

Pharmacy development groups

Pharmacy development groups (PDGs) began to be set up as part of the PIANA initiative in England, to make it possible for pharmacists to network with others in their area, and to work jointly on projects to develop pharmacy services locally. In 1999, the RPSGB organised a meeting at which experiences of PDGs from different parts of the country were shared.[7] It emerged that PDGs have developed in various ways from local needs; some have been set up as subgroups of the local pharmaceutical committee (LPC); some had evolved from health authority (HA) and LPC working groups, and others have no allegiance to existing local groups. An earlier focus group of PDG members had identified nine objectives common to all, quoted from the report above (Table 4.1).

Table 4.1 Pharmacy development group objectives

Convincing others of the value of pharmacy
Influencing local strategic decisions
Identifying opportunities for local development
Developing new, sustainable models of practice
Disseminating details of successful initiatives
Meeting personal development needs of pharmacists
Attracting new resources for development work
Unifying the profession locally
Stimulating and mobilising the enthusiasm of pharmacists

The RPSGB has developed guidelines to assist pharmacists who wish to establish a PDG in their area. These are summarised by Mason.[8] Further information may be had from the Professional Development Directorate. Funds to support the activities of PDGs have to be identified locally; they may be available from government initiatives such as health improvement programmes; from primary care groups; and from pharmaceutical manufacturers. Additionally, the RPSGB has offered professional development awards to promote the development of pharmaceutical services locally. In 2000, there were two levels of award: the lower level, up to £500, to help to develop a PDG infrastructure locally – such awards might help with administration expenses; and the higher, up to £3000, to extend the contribution of pharmacy in a locality. The views of local primary care groups would be considered when applications are judged. A report[9] gave details of the successful bids made in 1999, and gives an outline of the types of project being undertaken by PDGs nationally. Some of the projects undertaken by PDGs have been entered for pharmaceutical care awards (see below).

Pharmaceutical care and medicines management

The term 'pharmaceutical care' originated in the USA but has been widely adopted in the UK. The preferred term for this process is now 'medicines management' according to the Society's President,[10] since 'medicines management' may be taken to imply a multidisciplinary team approach. However, the two terms have been used in parallel and, to a certain extent, interchangeably. Either way, it describes a concept of care that was first defined in 1990 by Heppler and Strand[11] as 'responsible provision of drug therapy for the purpose of achieving definite outcomes that improve a patient's quality of life'. However, this definition was later

Table 4.2 Minnesota project: the seven elements of pharmaceutical care

---

Review all active medication
Link each medication to an appropriate indication
Assess actual or potential drug therapy problems
Take action to resolve and/or prevent drug therapy problems
Establish a care plan with the patient to achieve desired therapeutic goals for each
  medical condition and drug therapy problem
Plan for follow-up evaluation
Document above elements in a readily retrievable, billable fashion

---

adapted by one of the authors to 'a practice in which the practitioner takes responsibility for a patient's drug related needs and holds him or herself accountable for meeting those needs'. A major community pharmacy trial of this model of pharmaceutical care is being undertaken by the University of Minnesota; two reports have appeared in the *Pharmaceutical Journal*.[12, 13] As part of the project, an assessment tool was developed by the Minnesota Pharmacists' Association, which set out the seven elements of pharmaceutical care. These are detailed in Table 4.2.

A further description of the philosophy, process of pharmaceutical care and management systems that underlie it will be found in the book by Cipolle *et al.*[14] Although the practice setting is the USA, the book includes information on record-keeping and personalised care plans for patients, which could be adapted for use in the UK.

The development of pharmaceutical care in the UK has been encouraged by the introduction, in 1992, of the annual Pharmaceutical Care Award Scheme, sponsored jointly by the *Pharmaceutical Journal* and Glaxo Wellcome UK Ltd. Each year a presentation ceremony has been reported with details of the prize-winning projects, which could provide inspiration for others to follow.[15-17] The awards are given in three categories: shared care, community care and hospital care. A theme common to many of the entries is teamwork, and many of them have been made by multidisciplinary teams. They cover a wide range of topics: medication review for elderly patients living at home; improving medicine use in nursing homes; community pharmacist supply of emergency hormonal contraception; an integrated head lice infection management programme; and a prescribing errors review, to name but a few.

Most of these schemes, whether undertaken for an award or not, involve an element of practice research. It is important to realise that for work to be valid and useful, researchers should have training in research

Table 4.3 National Health Service (NHS) research and development criteria

The work should be relevant to improving the health of the nation, or other legitimate business of the NHS
It should follow a clear, well-defined protocol
The protocol must withstand external peer review
The findings must be capable of being reported so they are open to critical examination, such as by publication
The findings should be generalisable

principles and techniques. Schools of pharmacy and some teaching hospitals have academic practice units, and advice and training may be available. An article by Cairns[18] documents the experience of the pharmacy academic practice unit at St George's Hospital, London. Amongst a wealth of information, which identifies problems and proposes strategies for overcoming them, the article lists the criteria for NHS research and development, reproduced here as Table 4.3.

Each year many practice research projects are presented as papers or posters at the British Pharmaceutical Conference (BPC), and these are published in a practice research supplement to the *Pharmaceutical Journal* each September. These give an excellent overview of the topics of interest of the day. In a helpful paper, Alexander[19] reviewed not only the subjects of the papers presented at the BPC 2000, but also commented on the methodology employed.

In 1991, *The Health of the Nation*[20] identified key areas to be addressed by the NHS. These key areas were causes of substantial morbidity – coronary heart disease, stroke, cancers and accidents; causes of substantial ill-health – mental health, diabetes and asthma; factors which contribute to mortality and ill-health; and finally, promoting healthy living – smoking cessation, diet and alcohol advice and physical exercise. It also named areas where there was scope for improvement and where there is potential for harm. Targets were set in some areas, e.g. by 2000, mortality from cardiovascular disease was to be reduced by 15%. Also particularly relevant to pharmacy were some areas named as being ones where there is scope for improvement or harm – the health of pregnant women; infants and children: human immunodeficiency virus (HIV)/acquired immunodeficiency syndrome (AIDS) and other communicable diseases.

To support pharmacists who plan to practise a system of pharmaceutical care, considerable information is now available, with the emphasis on the diseases and patient groups listed above. In recent years, there has been an occasional series in the *Pharmaceutical Journal* on various topics, e.g. sinusitis and otitis[21] and coronary heart disease,[22] and the RPSGB has developed guidelines for diabetes, mental health and asthma and chronic obstructive airways disease, available from the Practice Division or on the Society's website (www.rpsgb.org.uk). There is also a book, edited by Bond,[23] which describes the extended role of community pharmacists. It includes evidence that demonstrates the value of pharmacist involvement in areas such as disease management; this could be useful in supporting one's case when preparing bids for innovative schemes.

The Centre for Pharmacy Postgraduate education (CPPE), in collaboration with the Scottish Centre for Post Qualification Pharmaceutical Education, is now providing a pharmaceutical care training programme for community pharmacists. The course is designed to encourage community pharmacists to reflect on relevant local opportunities and to explore ways of developing systems for optimising medicines-related patient care.[24]

Services provided by community pharmacists

Prescribing in the pharmacy

For many years, people have expected to be able to get informed advice from a pharmacist on the treatment of minor ailments and on the response to the symptoms of illness, and this has been encouraged by the government in various ways. The Nuffield Report on pharmacy[1] also supported this role: 'we believe that the service provided by the pharmacist (giving advice and treatment relating to minor ailments) could be more extensively used', but emphasised individuals' rights to choose whether to ask the pharmacist or to go to their doctor. In recent years, people have been encouraged by DoH campaigns such as *Choose the Right Remedy* to visit their pharmacist rather than their general practitioner (GP) for advice, and NHS Direct now makes pharmacy referrals for some conditions. The reclassification of some medicines from Prescription Only Medicine (POM) to Pharmacy (P) status has made it possible for pharmacists to prescribe effectively for a wider range of conditions, and the *Pharmacy in the Future* plan[5] indicates that this trend seems set to continue. However, patients who are exempt from paying prescription charges have to pay for medicines prescribed by a pharmacist, and this acts as a powerful disincentive for poorer patients. Up to 9% of GP consultations have been shown to be for conditions for which a pharmacist might prescribe; in many cases patients visit their doctor simply to request a prescription, after receiving advice from a pharmacist.[25] A further barrier to seeking advice from a pharmacist may be the lack of privacy in some pharmacies. This must be overcome sensitively if patients are to present themselves for advice. Pharmacy layout should permit a secluded area where quiet discussion will not be overheard. Failing this, patients requesting advice may be drawn towards the dispensary – although pharmacists should be careful not to be alone with patients in possibly compromising circumstances.

Practice guidance has been developed by the RPSGB on prescribing in the pharmacy for self-limiting conditions and common conditions; this can be downloaded from the Society's website or obtained as a paper copy from the Practice Division. A high standard is achieved partly by good training, and partly by having written protocols to be followed by medicines counter assistants. Pharmacists should develop their own protocols, and update them in the light of new information or local circumstances. Two articles published in the *Pharmaceutical Journal* in 1994 when protocols were introduced will help those unfamiliar with developing written procedures.[26, 27] A special feature on the sale of medicines in pharmacies appeared in the *Pharmaceutical Journal* in 1997. It includes an overview of the factors governing the sales of medicines[28] and other papers on relevant topics.

Public confidence in the profession depends largely on the individual's performance in giving health care advice and prescribing. Over the years, several surveys carried out by *Which?* have generated adverse comment in the media, although recently they have conceded that the advice given by pharmacists to researchers was generally satisfactory, although that given by assistants often was not.[29]

There are two main facets to advising patients who come to the pharmacy for advice, both of which need the pharmacist to be informed and up-to-date. The first, and perhaps more important part of the pharmacist's role, is in the response to symptoms. It is essential for the pharmacist to be able to recognise those symptoms which may be indicators of serious disease needing medical attention, and to distinguish them from those of minor illness for which counter prescribing might be appropriate. Advice on eliciting a relevant history of the condition is given within the RPSGB guidance, and further information on this and treating diseases generally is published regularly in special features the *Pharmaceutical Journal*. There are also several books, some of which pharmacists should read and have available for reference. One such text is *Minor Illness or Major disease?*;[30] there is also a book by Li Wan Po and Li Wan Po[31] which acts as a ready reference source of common ailments and suitable over-the-counter (OTC) medications. Another reference source, describing minor illnesses frequently encountered in community pharmacy with suitable OTC medicine recommendations, is Nathan's book.[32] Nutrition and dietary advice may be found in a book by Mason.[33] The CPPE has several relevant distance learning packages; in particular their *Responding to Symptoms* should be completed (available from CPPE, School of Pharmacy, University of Manchester, Manchester M13 9HJ).

If the customer's consultation with the pharmacist results in a recommendation to seek medical advice, this may or may not be supplemented with the sale of a medicine. In either case, it is important that customers understand fully the reasons for referral. They should be firmly encouraged to go to their doctor without unduly worrying them, and the information given should enable them to give more useful information to their doctor.

The second important area is that of the pharmacist's response should the need for referral to a doctor have been eliminated. It is crucial to the professional standing of the pharmacist, and indeed to the future good will of his/her business, that medicines are sold only when clearly indicated, and that the customer is given a choice, including the least expensive alternative if appropriate. There will be occasions when the best advice does not require the provision of medication, and such instances must be recognised.

Wound management products and surgical appliances

The community pharmacist must supply on prescription any dressing or appliance included in the *Drug Tariff*.[34] In view of the wide range of items available, many pharmacists carry out this obligation by keeping only a small number in stock and obtaining others on demand from a wholesaler or manufacturer. The position of the community pharmacist as a stockist of routine dressings and appliances should not, however, be underestimated, and a reasonable range should be available for purchase. Some pharmacists have expanded this service by developing their expertise in, and keeping an expanded range of, surgical appliances, including disability aids and mobility aids such as wheelchairs.

The technology of dressings is, like drugs, continually changing, and it is important that the community pharmacist keeps up-to-date in this field. New products have been developed as a result of research into the wound-healing process, which has led to the realisation that some traditional methods actually retard wound healing by damaging regenerating tissue. This has led to the development of the concept of the 'environmental' type of dressing which, by maintaining a favourable temperature and humidity for epithelialisation, promotes wound healing. Since pharmacists may be asked to advise on the choice of dressings, knowledge of the various aspects of the subject is necessary, and a reference book should be available on this subject. There is a section on wound management products, and also on stoma care products, in the book by Harman.[35] The CPPE runs workshops on wound management, and also has a distance learning package on the subject (see above for address).

Health promotion and diagnostic services

In addition to the specific services mentioned above, the pharmacist has an extremely important part to play in health education and promotion. This role was emphasised in the Nuffield Report,[1] and has received considerable government support in recent years. One of the reasons for this is the fact that community pharmacists are virtually the only health care professionals to whom the public has unrestricted access, and whom the public often visit when they are not ill. Health educative advice may be far better accepted when individuals are feeling well rather than when they are apprehensively waiting to see their doctor or dentist. Some potential areas for pharmacy involvement in health promotion are listed in Table 4.4.

Health education may be promulgated by the use of visual aids, e.g. posters and leaflets, but it is just as important for the community pharmacist to disseminate health information by both words and deeds. This aspect is acknowledged in the Code of Ethics and Standards, which bans the sale of tobacco products and other products which may be injurious to health from pharmacies. Of equal importance is the need for pharmacists to keep informed of current advice on matters of public debate, such as the need for dietary fibre, and the role of fats in the prevention of heart disease.

Table 4.4 Pharmacy health promotion areas

Smoking cessation	Dealing with infestations
Dietary advice – infants and adults	Sun and skin protection
Peak flow measurements	

The RPSGB acknowledges the importance of the pharmacist in health promotion in several ways. There are sections on health care information and on diagnostic testing and health screening in the 'Service Specifications' section of the MEP, and the nationwide Pharmacy Healthcare Scheme is based at the Society's headquarters. Under the auspices of this DoH-funded scheme, free leaflets on health promotion topics are distributed to pharmacies, for them to display and use when counselling clients. The National Pharmaceutical Association (NPA) also publishes a range of leaflets on health advice topics. One of the criteria for receiving a payment for extra professional services under Part VIA of the *Drug Tariff*[34] is the display of up to a maximum of eight health promotion leaflets. In 1998, the RPSGB and the Pharmaceutical Division of the DoH jointly commissioned an investigation into pharmacy health promotion: one of the aims was to provide guidance for developing health promotion in community pharmacy. The report was summarised in the *Pharmaceutical Journal*.[36] It included recommendations about the features required in health-promoting pharmacies. Some key points are summarised below:

- a professional atmosphere and a consultation area;
- space for the display of health promotion information, which should be accessible, signposted and well maintained and updated regularly;
- links for referral with the primary health care team and, for example, self-help groups and drugs workers;
- product ranges that positively promote health, e.g. sugar-free weaning foods, sugar-free medicines;
- a wide range of mobility aids if appropriate for the client group;
- a health and safety policy and a no smoking policy;
- ramps for access and a suitable layout for disabled customers and pushchairs.

The Health Development Agency (HDA) has now superseded the Health Education Council, formerly the government agency responsible for directing policy. It has three main functions: commissioning research and evaluating evidence; advising on the setting and implementation of standards; and an advisory role on the training, development and resource needs of professionals. Some of the HDA's priority areas may have an impact on pharmacy – these include smoking cessation, inequality of health care provision and diet and nutrition.

There are some obstacles to overcome for pharmacists who wish to get involved in health promotion. One may be lack of specialised training and funding to cover attendance on courses during the day, or later to cover the time spent on health promotion activities. These have been addressed in pilot schemes run by some HAs, e.g. in Barnet and in Somerset. The Barnet scheme involved providing and funding training to supplement completion of distance learning, and subsequent evaluation of the effect on the pharmacists' performance in this field. It has been described by Anderson and Greene.[37] The Somerset scheme was outlined and evaluated in a paper by Ghalamkari *et al.*[38] Pharmacists unable to participate in formal schemes can complete the CPPE distance learning package *Improving the public's health through health promotion*, or may attend workshops run locally on relevant topics. There is also a textbook on the subject, edited by Harman.[39]

Smoking cessation

As part of an ongoing government initiative, including the publishing of a White Paper *Smoking Kills*, smoking cessation has been identified as a high priority in the *National Priorities Guidance* set for the next few years.[40] In 1999 a circular[41] announced that up to £60m of new money over the next 3 years would be made available for HAs to develop new smoking cessation services, initially in health action zones (HAZs). The circular refered to the evidence base for smoking cessation interventions,[42] and directed HAs and primary care groups to appoint staff to set up smoking cessation clinics; it emphasised the effectiveness of nicotine replacement therapy (NRT). At the time NRT products were not prescribable on form FP10, and initially provision was made for free supplies to be made to certain patients. HAs were reminded that any scheme set up to supply NRT, whether purchased privately or supplied free, must comply with the Medicines Act; they would need a Wholesale Dealer's Licence should they plan to distribute free supplies to pharmacies themselves. From early 2001, nicotine replacement products became prescribable on form FP10 and by nurse prescribers, and the free-supply scheme was phased out.

Pharmacists should familiarise themselves with the practice advice in the MEP guide,[43] which also lists resources available to supplement their own efforts. Each year there is a national 'No Smoking Day' with considerable publicity, and the *Pharmaceutical Journal* has included special features on the subject to enable pharmacists to prepare to participate.[44, 45]

Table 4.5 Pharmacy diagnostic services

Blood sugar measurement	Cholesterol testing
Blood pressure monitoring	Pregnancy testing

Diagnostic services

As a development of their role in health education, many pharmacists are introducing a range of additional services relating to health promotion or diagnosis. Diagnostic tests commonly performed in pharmacies are listed in Table 4.5. Standards for running these services are set out in the MEP[43] and, in some cases, e.g. diabetes screening guidance, may also be found on the RPSGB website (www.rpsgb.org.uk).

The provision of diagnostic services in pharmacies is very much in line with the government plan for pharmacy,[5] in which the pharmacist is expected to take an active role in helping patients get the most out of their medicines. Professor Moffat[46] believes that diagnostic testing could form a large part of the pharmacist's work in the future. In his article, he foresees that, in addition to the services which are already widespread, community pharmacists could be involved in asthma clinics, anticoagulant clinics, therapeutic drug monitoring and in screening for *Helicobacter pylori.*

Contraception and sexual health

One area in which the community pharmacist has always been involved is the provision of advice and the sale of requisites for family planning. In an interesting article, Anderson surveyed the role that community pharmacists have played in the sexual health of the nation.[47] This traditional role has perhaps been strengthened with the emphasis on the use of condoms within the government's education campaign against HIV. Further to the classical advice and sales involvement in family planning, many pharmacies have extended their role to running a pregnancy testing service.

Until recently, pharmacists were only able to supply without prescription spermicidal gels and condoms. In 1998, the first Crown Report[48] recommended law changes that would legalise the supply and administration of medicines by patient group directions (PGDs). In 2000, amendments were made to the relevant regulations made under the Medicines Act[49] and guidance about the use of PGDs was issued in a Health Service Circular.[50] Developing PGDs requires interprofessional teamwork, and more information about their drafting and use is found in Chapter 1. There are more potential applications for PGDs in hospitals and clinics than in community pharmacy, but at the time, their advent made feasible the supply of emergency hormonal contraception (EHC) by community pharmacies. There were a few pilot schemes in which community pharmacists who have successfully completed training have been funded by the HA to give contraceptive advice, and, when appropriate, to supply EHC.[51] Details of the planning of one scheme will be found in a paper by O'Brien and Gray.[52] Such schemes have been set up in HAZs – areas that have received extra health care funding because they were considered to be in special need. Under the provisions of these schemes, EHC has been available to clients free of charge, as part of a government initiative to reduce the rates of teenage pregnancy. In 2001, Levonelle was reclassified as a P medicine, permitting OTC sale by the pharmacist. A detailed information book was produced and circulated to members of the RPSGB,[53] and should be used as a training resource by every pharmacist working in the community. A service specification for the supply of EHC as a P medicine is included in part 3 of the MEP.[43] It seems likely that the HAZ schemes will continue, since the high cost of EHC may put it out of the reach of teenagers in disadvantaged areas.

The supply of EHC by pharmacists generated debate within the profession, not only because at least one pilot scheme was started before the law changes had taken effect, but also because some pharmacists had doubts about expanding the role of the profession into diagnosis and prescribing. The RPSGB Council has now issued a statement about contraception and sexual health in which it supports the involvement of pharmacists: 'a significant improvement in public health could be made by developing the role of pharmacists working with other health care professionals'.[54] The policy statement identifies four areas where pharmacists can make a bigger contribution to contraceptive health care:

- emergency contraception;
- contraceptive medicines management;
- contraception and sexual health services;
- sexual health strategy development at locality, area and other levels.

The Council acknowledges that some pharmacists may personally object to supplying contraceptive products on religious or moral grounds. Advice for such pharmacists is included within the Code of Ethics and Standards.[43]

Ear piercing

Another area in which some pharmacists have become involved is in the provision of an ear-piercing service. For this, a dedicated area is needed, in which the procedure can be carried out in privacy, and with regard to the prevention of cross-infection. The procedure must be carried out with all precautions to prevent infection from the operator or contaminated equipment. Local authorities have the option to enforce the registration of all premises in which ear piercing and other 'special treatments', such as acupuncture, aromatherapy or chiropody, are carried out; pharmacists planning such services should contact the local authority to check whether they should register.[55]

Supply of 'alternative' medicines and complementary therapies

Many pharmacists will choose to sell at least some 'alternative' medicines, usually in the form of herbal medicines. Others may choose to specialise in this field, and may include other forms such as homeopathic medicines. The sale of such preparations is governed by regulations under the Medicines Act which are detailed in *Dale and Appelbe's Pharmacy Law and Ethics*,[56] and with which all involved pharmacists should be aware. Pharmacists may also come across such preparations on prescriptions on form FP10 written by GPs, as some choose to integrate these more traditional preparations with allopathic medicines.

Apart from the legal considerations on the supply of 'alternative' medicines, it is important for all pharmacists, and especially those who choose to specialise in this area, to have a thorough understanding of the forms and actions of the preparations they supply. The service specifications section of the MEP[43] gives standards for the provision of advice in this field, and requires pharmacists to give advice only if they have undertaken suitable training or have specialist knowledge. From time to time, the *Pharmaceutical Journal* includes articles on complementary therapies, e.g. articles describing homeopathy[57] and aromatherapy[58] by Barnes. There is also a journal, edited by Ernst,[59] giving a new evidence-based approach to this field, which until recently has mainly been supported by anecdotal evidence of efficacy. A database of information accessible only to health care professionals on complementary health topics has been established with a website (HealingOnline.co.uk). The upsurge in public interest in complementary therapies has led to a corresponding professional response, with sessions at national and international conferences. Speakers often counter with scientific facts about the products the enthusiastic claims made by practitioners, which may be adulterated or of dubious identity. One recent example was a session devoted to volatile oils at the 2000 World Congress of Pharmacy, reported in the *Pharmaceutical Journal*.[60]

Supply of veterinary medicines

Most pharmacies stock a few remedies for animals, and some specialise in this field. Pharmacists recommending treatments for animals should be aware that human medicines are not licensed for animal use, although the use of some human products in animals has been authorised. Information about prescribing and preparations suitable for animals will be found in *The Veterinary Formulary*.[61] There is a membership group within the RPSGB – the Veterinary Pharmacists Group – and also a higher qualification, a diploma that can be obtained by examination.

In 2000, the government ordered an independent review of the dispensing of prescription-only veterinary medicines, in the wake of complaints about a lack of transparency about charging by veterinary practitioners for their supply. The background to the review was discussed at a Veterinary Pharmacists Group meeting[62] and at a British Veterinary Association meeting.[63] In 2001, the review was completed, and it recommended that veterinary surgeons should normally provide animal owners with prescriptions which could be dispensed by the veterinary practice, by a pharmacist or, in some cases, by an agricultural merchant. The report also proposed some changes to the legal classification of veterinary POMs.[64] If the recommendations of the report are adopted, more opportunities for pharmacists to become involved in animal treatment should arise. A review of veterinary ailments and prescribing was published by Kayne *et al.* in the *Pharmaceutical Journal*.[65] The same issue included in a *Veterinary Pharmacy Bulletin* a warning that breaking bulk from a licensed product into smaller repackaged items for sale may be considered as the illegal production of an unlicensed product, unless an Assembly Licence is held.[66]

Organisation of a community pharmacy

Opening a pharmacy

A retail pharmacy business is defined by the Medicines Act 1968. The Act stipulates that the business must be under the personal control of a pharmacist who must exhibit conspicuously his or her certificate of registration. In addition, for retail activities, the premises must be registered with the RPSGB, to whom an annual retention fee is payable. Details of these regulations can be found in the book *Dale and Appelbe's Pharmacy Law and Ethics*,[56] or summarised in the *Chemist and Druggist Directory*.[67] Pharmacists who are planning to open a new pharmacy, including a dispensary within existing premises such as a surgery or health centre, must familiarise themselves with the many regulations which control this situation, which extend beyond the Medicines Act. Merrills and Fisher cover some of the business aspects,[68] and there may be aspects to consider under the Town and Country Planning Act, outlined in an article by Appelbe.[69]

In addition to registration with the RPSGB, a pharmacist who wishes to dispense NHS prescriptions must apply to the local HA to have the premises included in the List of Chemist Contractors for the area. Such an application may be refused under regulations made in 1987[70] and subsequently modified.[71] If the application is successful, the business must be conducted in accordance with the terms of the NHS contract, e.g. specified hours of opening (see Chapter 12).

Design of premises

Detailed design of a pharmacy is probably best carried out in conjunction with a specialist firm of shopfitters, several of whom advertise regularly in the *Pharmaceutical Journal*. Advice on planning a pharmacy can also be arranged through the NPA Planning Department; the NPA also offers other services to aid proprietor pharmacists in setting up and managing their businesses. There are certain points of which all pharmacists practising in the community should be aware, and a special feature in the *Pharmaceutical Journal* under the title 'Refitting your pharmacy'[72] discusses many of these, including the important aspect of obtaining planning permission.

Since 1999, the Disability Discrimination Act requires service providers, including community pharmacies, to make 'reasonable adjustments' to enable disabled people to have access to services. The associated Code of Practice requires the 'provision of a reasonable alternative method of making the service available where the physical features of the premises make it impossible or difficult for disabled individuals to make use of the services'. Where it is not possible to build a wheelchair ramp, e.g. where planning consent cannot be obtained or for other reasons, this requirement might be met by, for example, providing a bell at wheelchair height with a sign telling disabled people that they can be served at the door.[73]

Patient areas

Many of the customers in a pharmacy wish either to have supplies of medicines from prescription or from retail sale, or to receive advice on health matters. The pharmacy must therefore be of a standard expected by the public for a place associated with health care. This must influence not only the standard of cleanliness of the premises, but also their design. Guidance on basic standards for pharmacy premises and their upkeep is given in the MEP.[43] The area for sale of medicines or for the dispensing of prescriptions should be designed for easy communication between pharmacist and customer. Space should be made available for patient advice and counselling in relative privacy.

Whilst designing the pharmacy to give good access for the customer, it is obviously important to consider security. This will include general aspects such as design against shoplifting, the need to be able to supervise the sales of P medicines, and statutory requirements for the storage of Controlled Drugs. A comprehensive burglar alarm system, regularly maintained, is usually a requirement, and the advice of the local police crime prevention officer or Drugs Squad officer should be sought.

Administration of a community pharmacy

Computer technology

Much of the labour involved in the routine administration of a pharmacy can be reduced by the use of computers and related technology. The *Pharmaceutical Journal* regularly carries advertisements for computer systems for pharmacies, and developments in their use appear in the news pages almost as routinely. There is detailed guidance on the selection of computer software and its use, including aspects concerned with the maintenance of patient medication records, in the MEP[43]. If information is held relating to individuals, then registration under the Data Protection Act 1998 is mandatory. Details of the effect of this new Act, which replaces the original 1984 Act, will be found in an article by Wingfield.[74] Unlike the previous Act, it covers every type of data storage system, including paper records. Data controllers, i.e. persons who manage the filing system, have to register with the Data Protection

Commissioner, and have to comply with a set of principles; these are listed in the article mentioned above.

Supply and control of medicines

Stock control

Perhaps the most important function of a community pharmacy is to be able to supply a customer promptly – whether it is a sale or a dispensed medicine. For the majority of items, this requires the item to be in stock in the pharmacy. This has cost implications, as the stock value of a pharmacy will usually form the largest single item amongst its assets, and represents capital tied up. All good pharmacy managers will therefore try to reduce the amount of stock held whilst endeavouring not to run out of stock of items. This may be achieved by monitoring the stock levels and the range of items carried. The turnover should be calculated, and a minimum target set, and stock holdings reviewed on a regular basis, with consideration being given to eliminating slow-moving items. This requires an analysis of stock item by item, and can be helped by the use of computerised systems. These will mechanise the use of stock cards for individual items – a system perhaps rarely used in community pharmacies because of the large number of items held. If cards are used, they usually record for each item:

- name;
- description;
- pack size;
- sources of supply;
- quantity ordered;
- date and quantity received.

In addition, for ideal stock control, the cards will include:

- details of issues;
- cumulative stock balance.

More details of using stock records, and how this method may be used to evaluate the profitability of stock lines, will be found in articles by Vanns[75, 76] in the 'Business Focus' series (which includes papers on related topics in the same issues). However, stock calculations can only give a guide, as the appropriate stock level and turnover will vary with each item, and may also be subject to variation, e.g. seasonal. It can, however, be useful in an accounting analysis of a business. In assessing the stock level for each item, it is important to consider not only its normal frequency of issue, but also its shelf-life and related factors. It is obviously inappropriate to keep large stocks of slow-moving short-dated items, but it may also be prudent not to keep excessively large stocks of drugs subject to misuse (including Controlled Drugs). Bulky items, e.g. sterile fluids and stoma care items, may impose their own limitations on stock holding.

As mentioned, in a community pharmacy the measure of effectiveness is often the ability to supply a customer. For many items, this can be achieved without holding large quantities of stock by the use of pharmaceutical wholesalers. As most will deliver at least once daily, it is possible to reduce stock levels of some items to a minimum and thus improve cash flow.

Thought must also be given to minimising the loss of stock by theft. So-called professional thieves may take some items, but ordinary customers may pilfer given the opportunity. It may be cost-effective to install closed-circuit television and security mirrors, which permit surveillance of otherwise invisible areas. These should be kept to a minimum so far as possible, and core product ranges, such as hair products, baby products and budget toiletries, should be located in the direct view of staff. There should also be robust procedures dealing with staff purchases, cash handling, refunds and discounts to deter and minimise thefts of stock and money by staff. These topics are considered in more detail in an article by Gott.[77] There should also be a written policy for dealing with staff suspected of theft.

Purchasing

The identification of the need to purchase an item may arise as a result of a routine check of stock levels, or from a specific request for an item not in stock, e.g. an unusual prescription item. The reason for an order will influence the ordering process. If the item is required urgently, then the choice of supplier will depend on ability to meet the necessary deadline. The order will probably be placed over the telephone; it may be advisable to ask the supplier to confirm ability to deliver before finalising the order, otherwise all one may receive later in the day is a delivery note with the item marked 'to follow' or 'cancelled'. Most wholesalers cancel orders automatically if they cannot be delivered at the first attempt, and expect the item to be reordered. If it is a routine order, then speed and delivery date may not be as relevant.

Most supplies to a community pharmacy come from one of two sources – the manufacturer or a wholesaler. Some multiples run their own licensed wholesaling operation, having a centralised buying point, and redistributing stocks to the branches. Manufacturers will usually be used for supplies in quantity, but they will be able to supply urgently only in exceptional cases. Wholesalers, however, are organised to give a once- or twice-daily delivery service of a wide range of items. Many community pharmacies rarely order directly from manufacturers as they keep their stock levels low by frequent small orders from wholesalers. The advantages of direct ordering to manufacturers normally arise from competitive prices for larger quantities, or from bonus offers. Bonus offers are normally restricted to items for OTC sale, and are an incentive for the pharmacist to promote that product. An example might be a 'bonus parcel' of 12 packs of a travel sickness remedy just prior to the holiday season. The cost to the pharmacist might be the normal trade price for 10 packs, whilst the retail price of individual packs remains the same. Another type of 'bonus parcel' gives favourable rates for a mixed order of a company's products – it is to simplify ordering to qualify for such offers that some dispensaries are set out with all the products of one company grouped together.

In any area there may be up to five wholesalers available to the community pharmacist. Most however will not routinely use more than two. The choice will depend on factors including time of delivery and time in advance that orders need to be placed, reliability for having items in stock and financial aspects such as price information delivered with goods, settlement date for invoices and any discounts offered. While the stock and delivery aspects are self-explanatory, the financial aspects may need further explanation. A significant proportion of pharmaceuticals ordered will be for resale – either on private prescription or OTC. The pharmacist therefore needs to know at the point of sale the trade and retail price of each item in order to make the appropriate charge. This information can be found in catalogues, but a priced delivery note from a wholesaler can be advantageous. Such information also gives the pharmacist up-to-date information on the cost of purchases made, i.e. his/her own outstanding bills. Invoices may be presented for payment by the wholesaler at weekly or monthly intervals. The latter gives greater credit advantages, and if timed for payment to be in line with the monthly credit payment from the HA for previous prescriptions dispensed, will have significant cash flow advantages.

Another reason for the selection of a wholesaler might be the provision of an automated method of ordering. Several now have computer systems which can take direct orders from pharmacies by computer links. These may include facilities to warn the pharmacist if an item is out of stock, and also which can work remotely so that the pharmacist does not need to waste time in making the telephone connection.

Receipt of goods

When goods are delivered, the receiver should make several checks. The first, and most elementary, is to check that the parcel is the correct one. In a busy pharmacy it is easy to sign for goods only to find later that they are for another destination, with resultant delays which are annoying to pharmacist and customer or patient. At this stage, if Controlled Drugs are included in the delivery, a full check of them should be made, the appropriate register entries should be made and they should be locked away without delay. For all items, the following checks should be made:

* correct item (against both order and delivery note);
* correct pack;
* correct quantity;
* pack undamaged;
* expiry date acceptable;
* special storage conditions, e.g. refrigerator.

In addition, if stock records are kept, these should be completed. The delivery note should be signed and dated, together with a note of any problems with the delivery; this should be kept at least until the invoice for these goods has been received and paid. Goods for counter sale should be priced immediately upon receipt.

Goods returned for credit

Any goods for return should be processed immediately. Some wholesalers give their customers a special book for recording the details of returned stock; note that a credit will not be forthcoming if the packaging has been damaged or disfigured with stamps or labels. Normally, goods will not be accepted for return by wholesalers, but there are certain exceptions to this rule under the terms of a formal policy agreed between the National Association of Pharmaceutical Distributors and the Medicines Control Agency. Goods will be acceptable only for the following reasons:

* Where there has been an error in delivery or ordering. Such goods must be returned within 3 working days of receipt; for items

needing temperature-controlled storage, return will be permitted only in the case of wrong delivery, and they must be returned not later than the next working day. The goods must be in perfect original condition, not marked in any way and with no evidence of tampering. The goods must be accompanied by a returns note (usually furnished by the supplier).

- Product or batch recall by the manufacturer. The arrangements are made by the product licence holder and vary according to circumstances.

- Alleged faulty product or pack. Such goods must be packed separately and accompanied by a returns note, which should include the batch number. The van driver should be asked to pass them to the depot manager immediately upon return. Where the product itself is believed to be faulty, the depot manager should be alerted by telephone, in addition to any steps the pharmacist may take to discuss the problem with the manufacturer to ensure patient safety.

Financial controls

As with any business, good financial control is essential to the running of a pharmacy. Much of the expertise required will be provided by an accountant or, in the case of a purchase or sale, by an agent specialising in the purchase and running of pharmacies. The multiple retail organisations run management courses for their prospective managers which include a substantial element of finance, and the NPA can advise the independent pharmacy. A review of the financial services which a pharmacy may need, and how they may be applied to the business, will be found in an article by Blyth in the 'Business Focus' series in the *Pharmaceutical Journal*.[78] This section will highlight some of the more important aspects of financial control in a pharmacy.

Invoices

Many suppliers send the invoice for the goods either with the goods or at the same time; the invoice must be distinguished from the delivery or contents note, which lists the items in the delivery but often does not give cost information. Others may forward monthly statements. The timing of payment of invoices will depend on any settlement terms stated – there may be a discount offered for prompt payment, e.g. within 1 week of invoice date – in conjunction with the business's cash flow. Although it is good practice to pay invoices promptly, if there is no discount available, too early payment may have an adverse effect on the pharmacy's cash flow.

Cash flow

In simple terms cash flow can be compared to the position with cash in one's pocket. If cash is available, then purchases can be made. If not, then no matter how much capital is available – in the bank or in the form of credits – then no cash purchases can be made. Similarly, if an invoice is due for settlement before credits, e.g. from the HA, are received, then the business will go into debt and incur bank interest charges. If goods can be purchased and invoiced so that payment is not required until after the normal date when credits are received, then this is to maximum cash flow advantage. The successful handling of cash flow is a major element in any profitable business, and is a topic for detailed discussion with experienced managers and accountants rather than for this book. Similarly attention should be given to bookkeeping and Value Added Tax (VAT) – especially as the regulations relating to VAT are subject to frequent change.

Accounting

It is essential for all businesses, no matter how small, to keep a detailed account of their activities. Such information will be required either to satisfy statutory requirements, e.g. income tax, VAT, shareholders (financial accounting), or to provide information to help run the business (management accounting). In any case, as mentioned above, the requirements for any particular business will best be determined in discussion with an experienced manager or accountant.

References

1. Nuffield Foundation. *Pharmacy: The Report of the Committee of Inquiry Appointed by the Nuffield Foundation.* London: Nuffield Foundation, 1986.
2. Joint Working Party Report. *Pharmaceutical Care: The Future for Community Pharmacy.* London: Royal Pharmaceutical Society of Great Britain on behalf of the Department of Health and the pharmaceutical profession, 1992.
3. *Pharmacy in a New Age: The New Horizon.* London: Royal Pharmaceutical Society of Great Britain, 1996.
4. Department of Health. *Choice and Opportunity: Primary Care: The Future.* White Paper. London: Department of Health, 1996.
5. Department of Health. *Pharmacy in the Future – Implementing the NHS Plan.* London: Department of Health, 2000.

6. Department of Health. *The NHS Plan.* London: Department of Health, 2000.

7. Forum report. Building the future through PDGs. *Pharm J* 1999; 263: 960–961.

8. Mason P. Pharmacy development groups – what next? *Pharm J* 2000; 264: 414–415.

9. Report. Society makes awards totalling £72 000 to support PDGs. *Pharm J* 2000; 265: 87.

10. News item. Call it medicines management, not pharmaceutical care, President says. *Pharm J* 2000; 265: 808.

11. Heppler D, Strand L. Opportunities and responsibilities in pharmaceutical care. *Am J Hosp Pharm* 1990; 47: 533–543.

12. Simpson D. Pharmaceutical care: the Minnesota model. *Pharm J* 1997; 258: 899–904.

13. Mason P. Pharmaceutical care in Minnesota – a profoundly different experience. *Pharm J* 1999; 262: 705–708.

14. Cipolle R J, Strand L M, Morley P C. *Pharmaceutical Care Practice.* Maidenhead: McGraw-Hill, 1998.

15. Report. Pharmaceutical Care Awards 1996. *Pharm J* 1997; 259: 18–27.

16. Report. Pharmaceutical Care Awards 1997. *Pharm J* 1998; 261: 20–30.

17. Report. Pharmaceutical Care Awards 1998. *Pharm J* 1999; 263: 17–25.

18. Cairns C. Practice research in the community. *Pharm J* 1998; 261: 318–319.

19. Alexander A M. Pharmacy practice research: designs and methods becoming "more robust". *Pharm J* 2000; 265: 406–410.

20. Department of Health. *The Health of the Nation: A Consultative Document for Health in England.* London: Her Majesty's Stationery Office, 1991.

21. Hudson S, McAnaw S J, McGlynn S *et al.* Pharmaceutical care: (2) sinusitis and otitis media. *Pharm J* 1998; 260: 868–871.

22. McGlynn S, Reid F, McAnaw J *et al.* Pharmaceutical care: (9) coronary heart disease. *Pharm J* 2000; 265: 194–205.

23. Bond C, ed. *Evidence-based Pharmacy.* London: Pharmaceutical Press, 2000.

24. News item. Pharmaceutical care opportunity for community pharmacists. *Pharm J* 2000; 264: 868.

25. News item. GP – pharmacy referral trial in Bootle. *Pharm J* 2000, 264: 168.

26. Sharpe S E, Norris G W, Ibbitt M L *et al.* Protocols: getting started. *Pharm J* 1994; 253: 804–805.

27. Hawksworth G. Pharmacy protocols. *Pharm J* 1994; 253: 759–761.

28. Mitchell D. The scope for OTC medicine sales in pharmacy: a question of balance. *Pharm J* 1997; 259: 68–70.

29. News item. Pharmacists give good advice, assistants do not – latest *Which?* survey. *Pharm J* 1999; 262: 454.

30. Edwards C, Stillman P. *Minor Illness or Major Disease?* 3rd edn. London: Pharmaceutical Press, 2000.

31. Li Wan Po A, Li Wan Po G. *OTC Medications.* London: Blackwell Science, 1997.

32. Nathan A. *Non-prescription Medicines*, 2nd edn. London: Pharmaceutical Press, 2002.

33. Mason P N. *Nutrition and Dietary Advice in the Pharmacy,* 2nd edn. London: Blackwell Science, 2000.

34. Department of Health and National Assembly for Wales *Drug Tariff*, published monthly. London: Stationery Office.

35. Harman R J. *Patient Care in Community Practice*, 2nd edn. London: Pharmaceutical Press, 1998.

36. Report. Guidance for the development of health promotion by community pharmacists. *Pharm J* 1998; 261: 771–775.

37. Anderson C, Greene R. The Barnet High Street health scheme: health promotion by community pharmacists. *Pharm J* 1997; 259: 223–225.

38. Ghalamkari H H, Rees J E, Saltrese-Taylor A, Ramsden M. Evaluation of a pilot health promotion project in pharmacies: (1) quantifying the pharmacist's health promotion role. *Pharm J* 1997; 258: 138–143.

39. Harman R, ed. *Handbook of Pharmacy Health Education*, 2nd edn. London: Pharmaceutical Press, 2001.

40. Department of Health. *National Priorities Guidance 2000/01–2002/03*. HSC 1999/242.

41. Department of Health. *New NHS Smoking Cessation Services*. HSC 1999/087.

42. Raw M, McNeill A, West R. Smoking cessation guidelines and their cost effectiveness. *Thorax* 1998: 53 (suppl. 5).

43. Royal Pharmaceutical Society of Great Britain. *Medicines, Ethics and Practice: A Guide for Pharmacists*, published yearly. London: Royal Pharmaceutical Society of Great Britain.

44. Special feature. Getting prepared for No Smoking Day. *Pharm J* 2001; 266: 151–154.

45. Special feature. Kiss smoking goodbye – how pharmacists can help. *Pharm J* 2001; 266: 319–321.

46. Moffat T. Point-of-care testing in the community pharmacy. *Pharm J* 2001; 267: 267–268.

47. Anderson S. "The most important place in the history of British birth control" – community pharmacy and sexual health in 20th century Britain. *Pharm J* 2001; 266: 23–29.

48. Department of Health, London. *Report on the Supply and Administration of Medicines under Group Protocols*. HSC 1998/051.

49. News item. New legislation paves the way for patient group directions. *Pharm J* 2000; 265: 219.

50. Department of Health. *Patient Group Directions [England only]*. HSC 2000/026.

51. News item. Emergency contraception trial in Manchester pharmacies. *Pharm J* 2000; 264: 44.

52. O'Brien K, Gray N. Supplying emergency hormonal contraception in Manchester under a group prescribing protocol. *Pharm J* 2000; 264: 518–519.

53. Centre for Pharmacy Postgraduate Education. *Emergency Hormonal Contraception Information Booklet*. London: Stationery Office, 2000.

54. Council Policy Statement. Contraception and sexual health. *Pharm J* 1999; 262: 873.

55. Law and ethics bulletin. Registration of premises for 'special treatments'. *Pharm J* 1999; 263: 669.

56. Applebe G E, Wingfield J. *Dale and Appelbe's Pharmacy Law and Ethics*, 7th edn. London: Pharmaceutical Press, 2001.

57. Barnes J. Homoeopathy. *Pharm J* 1998; 260: 492–497.
58. Barnes J. Aromatherapy. *Pharm J* 1998; 260: 862–867.
59. Ernst E, ed. *Focus on Alternative and Complementary Therapies*. London: Pharmaceutical Press, issued four times a year.
60. Conference report. What pharmacists should know about volatile oils. *Pharm J* 2000; 265: 628 –629.
61. Bishop Y, ed. *The Veterinary Formulary*, 5th edn. London: Pharmaceutical Press, 2001.
62. Conference report. Access to veterinary medicines. *Pharm J* 2000; 265: 697–700.
63. Congress report. Dispensing under scrutiny. *Pharm J* 2000; 265: 700.
64. News item. Vets should write prescriptions, says review. *Pharm J* 2001; 266: 700.
65. Kayne S, Shakespeare M, Jepson M, Cockbill S. New opportunities in veterinary pharmacy. *Pharm J* 2001; 267: 159–166.
66. Veterinary Pharmacy Bulletin. Breaking bulk in veterinary pharmacy. *Pharm J* 2001; 267; 178.
67. *Chemist and Druggist Directory*, published annually. Tonbridge, Kent: United Business Media Information Services.
68. Merrills J, Fisher J. *Pharmacy Law and Practice*, 2nd edn. Oxford: Blackwell Science, 1997.
69. Appelbe G E. Pharmacies and the Town and Country Planning Act. *Pharm J* 1987; 238: 143.
70. Statutory Instrument 1987 no. 401. National Health Service (General Medical and Pharmaceutical Services) Amendment (No. 2) Regulations.
71. Department of Health. *Pharmaceutical Service Revised Arrangements for Considering Applications to Dispense*. HSG(92)13 Annex.
72. Special Feature. Refitting your pharmacy. *Pharm J* 1997; 259: 843–852.
73. Elson, V. Pharmacy and the Disability Discrimination Act. *Pharm J* 1999; 263: 716–717.
74. Wingfield J. The Data Protection Act 1998. *Pharm J* 2000; 265: 131.
75. Vanns D. Stock control. *Pharm J* 1998; 260: 909–913.
76. Vanns D. Principles of merchandising. *Pharm J* 1998; 261: 274–277.
77. Gott J. 'Good afternoon, can I help you?' *Pharm J* 2000; 264: 372–373.
78. Blyth J. Financial services for pharmacists. *Pharm J* 2000; 264: 778–781.

5

Dispensing prescriptions

It is impossible to learn dispensing from a book: one can learn how to make individual preparations in this way, and how to pack and label products, but the whole process, which transforms a brief written request into an effective treatment, can be learned only by practice and working with an experienced practitioner to act as a role model. However, the authors have taught many students themselves, and have included in this chapter many of the aspects of dispensary management and dispensing that they find that students need to know to bridge the gap between the largely theoretical knowledge acquired during their degree course and its practical application on a day-to-day basis in the dispensary. Prescribing and dispensing each form part of a process which can easily lead to errors and young doctors and pharmacists are often made anxious by their responsibilities; some common causes of problems are identified so that safe systems of work can be employed, and the potential hazards of inexperience reduced. This chapter is intended to be read in conjunction with the many relevant entries in the Royal Pharmaceutical Society of Great Britain's (RPSGB) *Medicines, Ethics and Practice* (MEP) guide.[1]

From January 2005, the RPSGB is to introduce a requirement for pharmacists in both hospital and community to develop and put into practice standard operating procedures (SOPs) covering the whole of the dispensing process and the transfer of prescribed items to patients. Each SOP will have to be developed with the knowledge of the competence of the staff working in that pharmacy. At the time of writing, consultation is in progress on a draft guidance document,[2] which was reproduced in an article in the *Pharmaceutical Journal*. Although details may be altered during the consultation process, the underlying principles are unlikely to change, and pharmacists would be wise to address the task of preparing SOPs for dispensing and other key processes. Advice on approaching this task was given in an article by Bellingham.[3]

Receiving the prescription

The person who receives the prescription must ensure that the patient's name, including forename, and address is complete and legible. This is the moment to check whether it has been handed in by the patient in person, and should the patient be a child, to verify the age. These checks must be completed while the person who hands in the prescription is still there. Charges and exemptions should be sorted out now, too, since otherwise this will dominate the scene when the prescription is given out and distract the attention from any needs the patient may have for counselling about the use of the medicine. One must also remember that it is surprisingly easy to give out finished prescriptions to the wrong person – often patients do not hear very well and may answer to the wrong name. There may even be two patients waiting with the same name. It is safest to use a numbered receipt system; in busy dispensaries that form part of large establishments, or for hospital outpatient waiting areas this may be combined with a prescription-ready indicator that displays at remote locations. An alternative or additional safeguard is to ask patients to give their addresses when they present themselves to collect finished prescriptions. It is helpful to give customers an idea of the time needed to fulfil the prescription so that they can go for a cup of coffee or do some shopping while they are waiting.

In 1997, a NHS Executive efficiency scrutiny report[4] made 100 recommendations to reduce the incidence of prescription fraud. A summary of the report was published.[5] Since then a number of the proposals have been adopted. These have included improving the design of prescription forms to make it difficult to photocopy them, serially numbering them to make it possible to follow an audit trail and emphasising the need for security for pads of prescription forms to prevent theft. The Prescription Pricing Authority (PPA) set up a Fraud Investigation Unit, and one of the first issues to be addressed was prescription charge evasion, which was believed to be losing between £70m and £100m annually. In April 1999, both community and hospital pharmacies were directed to institute checking procedures for patients claiming exemption.[6,7] Pharmacies must check that the declaration of exemption is fully completed and signed, and are expected to check that the patient holds a valid prepayment certificate, or to see evidence that the patient or his/her partner is receiving income support, family credit, job-seeker's allowance (income-based), disability working allowance or a National Health Service (NHS) charges certificate for full help. A book, *The Pharmacists' Guide to Prescription Exemption*,[8] has been distributed to pharmacies. In the case of FP10 forms, if the exemption claim is incomplete or unsigned, normally the contractor will be penalised by having the items prescribed treated as chargeable, although there may be some latitude in the case of age exemptions where the patient's age has been entered by the prescriber's computer.[9] In cases where patients cannot produce proof of exemption, prescriptions may be dispensed, but marked 'no evidence' and submitted separately to the PPA for additional checks. In hospitals, patients may be asked to pay and given a receipt on form FP57, which enables a patient who can prove exemption to reclaim the charge.

Further measures to combat fraud include a reward scheme for pharmacists who save money by detecting fraudulent prescriptions[10, 11] and computer software at the PPA which allows comparison between prescribing patterns at neighbouring practices, and also the proportions of exempt prescriptions returned by pharmacies in the same locality.

Sometimes, as a result of checking the prescription, it becomes necessary for it to be altered or endorsed. The RPSGB Professional Standards Directorate has warned pharmacists that the PPA may suspect any alteration that has not been endorsed by the prescriber of being fraudulent. Likewise, the prescribing doctor should sign alterations in the surgery before the form is sent to the PPA.[12]

Private, or non-NHS prescriptions

The Professional Standards Directorate of the RPSGB has issued guidance on private prescriptions. The points included are:

- Prescriptions for prescription-only medicines (POMs) are valid for 6 months from the date of issue. The pharmacist must retain the prescription for 2 years.
- A repeatable prescription is a prescription that contains a direction that it may be dispensed on more than one occasion. The first time must be within 6 months of the date of issue. When the supply is complete, the pharmacy dispensing the final supply must retain the prescription for 2 years; if a prescription bears more than one item, it must be retained by the last supplier once any POM request has been completed, even if more repeats are available for other items.
- There is no limit to the number of repeats that may be requested by the prescriber, but a prescription that has the direction to repeat but does not specify the number of times should not be dispensed on more than two occasions, i.e. the first dispensing and one repeat,

unless it is for an oral contraceptive, in which case it may be dispensed six times before the end of the period of 6 months from the date of issue.

- Prescriptions for Controlled Drugs may not be repeated, but a direction for dispensing in instalments on specified dates may be included by the prescriber.

Reading and checking prescriptions

The next stage is to read and assess the prescription. Most general practice FP10 forms are now computer-generated, but forms written in hospital outpatient clinics are not, and these often present more difficulty to the pharmacist, particularly as items may be prescribed which are unfamiliar. There are two stages to the checking process. The first stage is intended to clarify the prescriber's intentions for this patient; the second may be termed a pharmaceutical assessment. This has been defined as the application of pharmacists' knowledge to establish safety, quality, efficacy and possibly economy of drug treatment specified by a prescriber.[13] The protocol for checking prescriptions is shown in Table 5.1. (See also sections on infants and children and services for drug addicts, below.)

Potential prescription problems

Many problem prescriptions are intercepted by pharmacists every day. In a survey of community pharmacies undertaken in 1995, Greene[14] found an overall detection rate of problems of 0.062%. Of these, about two-thirds were judged to represent a serious or very serious risk to the patient. Greene extrapolated his findings to show that, nationally, 280 000 potentially serious errors are detected annually. In another survey, of 23 general practice prescribers, Shah et al.[15] found an error rate of 7.46 per 100 items prescribed. The paper included an analysis of the types of error: the commonest, with an incidence of 25%, was the omission of directions, with a further 11% being incomplete, illegible or written 'as directed'. The prescribed item had not been requested in 18% of prescriptions. Pharmaceutical assessment draws on clinical pharmacy skills and knowledge. In the community pharmacy and outpatient dispensary, its scope may be somewhat limited by the pharmacist not being aware of the diagnosis, but possible areas for pharmaceutical intervention are identified in the following sections.

Table 5.1 Protocol for checking prescriptions.
Work systematically through every section listed:

Is it valid, including date?	Forename or at least initials required Surname Address: a legal requirement for POMs; in-house hospital prescriptions often have unit/registration number instead Age if under 12 years; essential for checking dose One patient only on NHS prescription, unless bulk prescription (*Drug Tariff* Part VIII para 6[63])
Check prescription	Name of drug must be legible without doubt Dose form must be stated if there is more than one (this is important if dosage varies between forms, e.g. dihydrocodeine tablets and DHC Continus) Exact local preparation: creams and ointments are not necessarily interchangeable If strength not stated, check that there is only one available For CDs, prescriber must insert every legally required detail in his/her own handwriting. Prescriptions may not be computer-generated For short-shelf-life products, ensure that quantity ordered will not last longer than 'life'. Either contact prescriber, or arrange collection in instalments Check PMR for allergies, contraindications or interactions Never supply an item or formulation which seems wrong or unusual without checking because it is said to have been supplied before. Each pharmacist on each occasion must verify that all is well to the best of his/her ability

POMs, prescription-only medicines; NHS, National Health Service; CDs, Controlled Drugs; PMR, patient medication record.

Drugs with similar names

Certain drugs have names that may appear similar when carelessly written; others are liable to confusion for other reasons. Problems are particularly likely if the strengths and doses of the two preparations are similar. Doubts should always be resolved by checking with the prescriber. Sadly, in most cases where mistakes have occurred, it has been because the item was dispensed without a second thought. Some recently noted examples that illustrate the pitfalls are:

- chlorpropamide/chlorpromazine;
- disopyramide/dipyridamole;
- Inderal/Indocid;
- Lasix/Losec;
- Metatone/methadone;
- methyldopa/levodopa;
- Priadel/Parlodel/Parnate.

Prescriptions for local-use preparations and wound care products present particular difficulties. Unfortunately, many doctors do not appreciate that every word in the title may be significant, and a slight change may in fact signify a different product. The only way to be sure is to find out exactly how the item is to be used, and then to ascertain that it has been correctly prescribed – in fact this is the golden rule for all dispensing, and the pharmacist who does this will rarely make a mistake or allow the prescriber to do so.

Abbreviations

Although widely used in prescription writing, abbreviations can kill. This is because in health care there are no recognised standards for abbreviations and prescribers invent their own. The problems are outlined in a paper by Cousins.[16] He gives some examples:

- HCT 250 mg was intended to mean hydrocortisone 250 mg, but hydrochlorothiazide was supplied.
- AZT can mean zidovudine or azathioprine (additionally, MTX can mean methotrexate or mitoxantrone/mitozantrone).
- CPM can mean chlorpromazine or chlorphenamine.
- The abbreviation 'U' for unit is dangerous; it has been read as zero and has caused 10-fold errors with insulin doses.
- A slash mark (/) has been read as 1 (one). A patient received 120 units of isophane insulin which was prescribed as '6 units soluble insulin/20 units isophane insulin'.

Chemotherapy drugs

This section must be read in conjunction with the section on cytotoxics or chemotherapy dispensing in Chapter 7.

There are particular dangers in prescribing and administering chemotherapy, i.e. cytotoxic drugs. Most prescriptions are seen in hospitals; Cousins[17] has illustrated the problems and suggests some solutions.

Table 5.2 Key recommendations of the Woods Report[19]

An immediate action plan should be introduced, implemented by national
  guidance on safety procedures and reinforced by clinical governance
There should be formal designation within each trust of medical staff competent
  to give intrathecal chemotherapy; the named individuals must have received
  training on the protocol to be followed
Steps should be taken to ensure that intrathecal and intravenous chemotherapy are
  given at different times by different people and in different clinical locations.
  Drugs should be checked by two members of staff with chemotherapy training

It is good practice to draw up protocols for all chemotherapy regimens
that are held both on the ward and in the pharmacy, and to permit no
deviation from the protocol without stringent checking with senior
medical staff familiar with the chemotherapy in use. In the community,
problems can arise with unfamiliar products, and it is particularly important to check whether drugs are to be given daily, once a week or once every
2 weeks. In a serious incident which was the subject of an enquiry, failure
to check the patient medication record or confirm an unusually high dose
for a patient with a prescription for methotrexate led to her receiving a
daily dose instead of a once-weekly dose; she died 3 weeks later. Although
this was only one in a series of errors in the management of this patient,
the fact is that the tragedy could have been prevented at this stage.[18]

Following a later incident resulting in a patient death subsequent
to an erroneous intrathecal injection, the Department of Health (DoH)
commissioned a report on chemotherapy safety. This report (the Woods
Report) made several recommendations to prevent a recurrence.[19] The
most important of these are reproduced in Table 5.2.

One of the recommendations relates to staff competent to give
chemotherapy. In August 2001 a training package was launched for
medical staff undertaking such procedures.[20] This package includes an
independent assessment leading to accreditation of staff – including
medical staff – who undertake these procedures.

In 2001 national guidance on the intrathecal administration of
chemotherapy[21] was issued under the cover of a circular[22] which directed
NHS trusts to assess their performance against a checklist of good practice, and to implement the guidance immediately. The guidance, which
like all official circulars can be downloaded from the RPSGB website
(www.rpsgb.org.uk) via a link to Health Circulars, is too detailed to
summarise here. All pharmacists managing or involved in the running
of chemotherapy services *must* familiarise themselves with it.

Incorrect or ambiguous dose

Drugs that have a very wide dose range are potentially dangerous. It may be difficult to detect inappropriate doses, and extra vigilance is needed. An example might be MST Continus morphine tablets, with a range of tablet strengths from 5 to 200 mg. Doses at the high end of the range would only be suitable for a patient who had been on opiates for some time and had developed tolerance.

Some dose forms of the same drug have different bioavailability and hence dose. Thus, drugs with liposomal delivery systems have different doses from their non-liposomal counterparts. Amphotericin products illustrate the point, with different dosage schedules for lipid complex and liposomal preparations. Another example is doxorubicin, where the dose of the liposomal product is one-third of the conventional product.

The use of the word 'normal' to denote strength has caused fatal mix-ups in the past when applied to sodium chloride solutions. Unfortunately still in common use in hospitals, the title 'normal saline' means sodium chloride solution 0.9%, and not 'normal' in the chemical laboratory sense. The use of the expression 'twice normal' and 'one-fifth normal' for 1.8% and 0.18% sodium chloride solutions is also hazardous. In a survey conducted by the author (PS), a high proportion of student nurses asked to multiply 0.9% by two to interpret a request for twice-normal saline produced the answer 0.18%.

Repeat prescriptions

Attention is drawn to the guidance given in the Code of Ethics and Standards;[1] there is also a relevant Law and Ethics Fact Sheet.[23] Repeat prescriptions require monitoring carefully. Table 5.3 illustrates some of the potential pitfalls.

Since repeats form a large proportion of general practice prescribing, there have been many initiatives in which pharmacists undertook audits of repeats. In one such study, reported by Burtonwood et al.,[24] 845 interventions were considered necessary on 2515 items surveyed. The most common intervention was the removal of items no longer being taken by the patient. In all, 20% of the interventions represented fine-tuning of the medication, but for 30% it was important that action be taken.

The government intends[25] to implement repeat dispensing of prescriptions for chronic conditions by 2004. General practitioners (GPs)

Table 5.3 Possible repeat prescription problems

Repeats may be ordered too early or too late

The wrong item may be selected, and the prescription signed unnoticed by the
    doctor

Patient with worsening symptoms may use the repeat system as way of avoiding
    contact with doctor

Patient may not be using all the items repeated

Repeat may not reflect changes initiated at hospital visits

One-off item may be repeated

Therapeutic duplication

Patients may reinstate medicines previously discontinued

Dose adjustments may be needed as patient ages and, e.g., renal function declines

---

will issue prescriptions that may be dispensed in instalments; at present
this is not allowed for NHS prescriptions. It is believed that this will
reduce wastage of medicines, since pharmacists will have the opportunity to confirm that patients understand their medicines and still
require them. The pitfalls listed in Table 5.3 will be equally applicable
in most cases.

Unlicensed or 'off-label' prescribing

At times doctors may prescribe licensed products to be used in a way
outside the terms of the marketing authorisation – so-called 'off-label'
use. An example might be a request to take orally the contents of an
ampoule of an injection, or at a dose not recommended within the
marketing authorisation. Such prescriptions should be discussed with
the doctor to confirm that he/she is aware of the implications, since the
professional liability of the prescriber could be greater in the event of an
adverse reaction. Readers are strongly advised to consult the appropriate RPSGB Fact Sheet[26] for more information. The sheet advises 'that
the pharmacist should bring to the attention of the patient that the
product does not have a marketing authorisation or is being used outside
the terms of its marketing authorisation, as the case may be. As far as
possible this should be done without undermining the patient's confidence in either the prescriber or the prescribed medicine'. When possible,
'off-label' use should be avoided. It is most often encountered in prescriptions for children, where appropriate licensed products may not
exist. (See also the section on Infants and children, below.)

Contraindications and interactions

While these should be considered when dispensing all prescriptions, some groups of patients are particularly vulnerable, and extra vigilance is required. This would include, for example, asthmatics, who should not receive beta-blockers or non-steroidal antiinflammatory drugs (NSAIDs) and diabetics, who should avoid medicines containing sugar. Known allergies should be checked, particularly for antibiotic prescriptions, where prescribers may fail to consider cross-sensitivities within groups of drugs, e.g. semisynthetic penicillins.

Prescriptions for extemporaneously dispensed items ('specials')

'Specials' may be supplied only when there is no suitable product with a marketing authorisation. Modern doctors rarely write prescriptions for extemporaneously prepared items, and as a result they are on unfamiliar ground and are liable to make many errors. There is no systematic tuition in prescription writing in most medical schools. Unfortunately, many pharmacists have little experience in dispensing such prescriptions. Table 5.4 illustrates some common problems.

Table 5.4 Common extemporaneous preparation prescribing errors

Formula not specified	May happen when an obsolete/imprecise title such as 'Brompton mixture' is used. Synonyms are an adequate description only when they appear in a monograph in an official formulary
Dose in wrong units	e.g. 100 mg not 100 mcg: a particularly dangerous error, since it is all-too-easy to dispense such a prescription
Wrong dose volume specified	e.g. formula calls for 5 mg in 5 ml, but label directions give a 15 ml dose. This may be intentional, but more often is not
No preservative	Vehicle given as water only
Excessive quantity prescribed	Duration of prescription exceeds shelf-life
Chemical incompatibility; lack of stability data	Consider if an ingredient is to be added to a proprietary product. Also important for TPN, IV additives
Overdilution of preservatives	Liable to occur if proprietary products are mixed or diluted – a practice which should be discouraged as stability data are rarely available

TPN, total parenteral nutrition; IV, intravenous.

Table 5.5 Pharmacists' role in medication risk management

Detecting, recording and reporting medication risks and events
Educating staff to avoid repetition of risk and improve quality of prescribing
Focusing on details and analysing risks in prescribing
Advocating best practice which is evidence-based and safe
Neutralising, eliminating or reducing risks in the medication process
Designing out the risk of bad practice through guidelines and the auditing of
    compliance with them

The author (PS) as a student was taught that 'all prescriptions were guilty until proved innocent'. This principle is a sound one on which to base checking prescriptions for extemporaneous products. (See also the section on dispensing extemporaneous preparations, below.)

Operating a safe system of work

No one would travel by air if they thought safety had been left to chance. Passengers enter a commercial airliner secure in the knowledge that systematic procedures have been followed to ensure that the crew have been adequately trained, the aircraft has been correctly maintained and traffic controls are in place to prevent mix-ups on the runway and in flight. This is a useful model to consider when developing safe systems of work in a pharmacy – safe practices do not come about by chance, but procedures have to be developed, and safe methods of work have to be designed into them. There is an element of risk to the patient in taking medicines, and the pharmacist has an important role to play in managing that risk and keeping it within professionally acceptable limits. Tomlin[27] identifies the key features of this role. She points out that disasters occur most commonly when a poorly trained and uncoordinated team makes a series of mistakes. Table 5.5 summarises points from her paper.

The Council of the RPSGB has decided that from 1 January 2005, all dispensing staff should be appropriately trained and all dispensaries should have SOPs in place. The background to this decision and details of the recommendations will be found in a paper in the *Pharmaceutical Journal*.[28] By that date, anyone involved in dispensing, i.e. the assembly of a prescription, including the generation of labels, in both community and hospital pharmacies, will have to be trained or be training for at least a (to be developed at the time of writing) Level 2 National Vocational Qualification (NVQ) or the Scottish Vocational Qualification (SVQ) in Pharmacy Services. Although at the time of writing there is an

NVQ/SVQ Level 3 in Pharmacy Services, the Council recognises that qualification to this level may not be achievable or necessary for all dispensing assistants. Additionally, pharmacists must ensure that all dispensing staff are kept up-to-date.

Council has also stated that there will be a professional standard requiring that pharmacists ensure that there are written guidelines or SOPs for all dispensaries, including those where there are normally no support staff, since they will be of value to locums. To quote from the paper: [28]

> Standard operating procedures should specify the range of activities which may be undertaken by support staff and thus provide a framework enabling pharmacists to delegate tasks to support staff up to and including those which their level of training permits. They must comply with legal and ethical requirements and should address the pharmacist's underlying responsibilities and accountability in relation to dispensing. They should therefore specify the point at which the pharmacist normally undertakes the pharmaceutical assessment. This is the point at which the pharmacist uses his or her knowledge to establish the safety, quality, efficacy and, perhaps, cost-effective use of the drug treatment(s) specified by the prescriber.

For several years it has been the practice in hospital pharmacies to train and accredit pharmacy technicians reaching a required standard to carry out accuracy checks on dispensed items. These technicians are known as 'checking technicians', and a number of accreditation schemes have been developed. One such scheme is described in a paper by Perrett.[29]

In addition to the measures discussed above, good dispensary management requires attention to a number of further aspects of practice, outlined in the following paragraphs.

Interruptions and distractions

It is preferable to organise the dispensary so that the patients cannot speak directly to the staff while they are working. In large dispensaries with several staff, idle chatter during working should be discouraged. Likewise, radios and televisions are unacceptable. Busy dispensaries are rarely peaceful places to work, and it is important to adopt a systematic method of working so that when the dispensing process is interrupted, it can be resumed without confusing the orderly sequence of: read prescription/check prescription/print label/locate stock/dispense item/affix label/read stock container label again/check by second person/replace stock/consider reordering stock/final check/hand out or set aside to await collection.

Labels and patient information leaflets

Labels should always be produced as soon as the prescription has been read; the act of concentrating on the directions may reveal some hitherto unperceived problem. Additionally, the label can be applied to the pack as soon as it is prepared, which eliminates the potential hazards of transposition of unlabelled containers left lying around. Spoiled or surplus labels must be destroyed immediately, and particularly not left on the label printer where they may be used inadvertently. It is a potentially dangerous practice for one person to read the prescription and generate the labels, and for a second person to prepare the drug containers; although said to be fast, this method of working has been responsible for many errors over the years, and should never be employed.

Some new labelling hazards have been introduced with the advent of computer-generated labels. Some systems write the number of tablets in the container on the same line as the name of the drug. This is readily confused with the strength of the product, and has recently emerged as a cause of inaccurate repeat prescriptions. The use of 'pop codes', i.e. single-key entries for popular label directions, can mean that a mis-hit key may put a totally inappropriate direction on the label, which may be overlooked at the final check – a patient returned to us clomethiazole capsules labelled 'one to be inserted vaginally'! When setting up the labelling system, it is important to check whether the computer is to enter the pharmacy name and address; if not, preprinted labels must be used.

Under the provisions of the Marketing Authorisation Regulations, pharmacists have a legal obligation to provide a manufacturer's Product Information Leaflet (PIL) each time a medicine is sold or supplied. More detailed information is given in the RPSGB Professional Standards Directorate Fact Sheet 3.[30] In hospitals PILs do not have to be supplied to hospital inpatients, but they must be available to patients on request. The Professional Standards Directorate has advised[31] that when insufficient leaflets are supplied, pharmacists must do their best to obtain extra supplies from the manufacturer. When producing their own leaflets, pharmacists should ensure that they do not contravene the Medicines Advertising Regulations.

Giving the patient a leaflet does not mean that the pharmacist can opt out of counselling to ensure that the patient understands how to take or use the medicines supplied. According to a survey carried out by the Consumers' Association,[32] patients would prefer to receive advice about their treatment from doctors and pharmacists, or to go through the leaflets with them. (For more about compliance, see the section on concordance, below.)

Dispensary layout and housekeeping

There are various methods of arranging the stock – alphabetical, grouping of a manufacturer's products, frequently used items close to hand, pharmacological or functional. Most pharmacies use a combination of methods. It does not matter what system is employed, so long as the dispensary is tidy and clean. Used containers must be returned to their place as soon as possible, and not be left cluttering the work area. This must be done with care, since a container put away in the wrong place may be selected in error for a later prescription if it resembles the item usually kept in that location – this is particularly a hazard for some product ranges, where the manufacturers use identical containers and minuscule print on the labels of a whole range of similar-looking generics.

Stock rotation is important, and new items must always be placed behind older ones. On occasions, one may find two or more stock containers of the same drug in use at a time. The temptation is to tidy up by combining them into one; this is permissible only if the operation is done carefully and only if products of the same batch number are mixed. Regular checks of stock to identify out-of-date items should be undertaken.

Refrigerators should be defrosted regularly and records should be kept of regular maximum and minimum thermometer readings. Ideally, no foodstuffs should be stored in drug refrigerators. Where this is impossible, food, e.g. milk and dairy products, should be kept separately and not allowed to contaminate pharmaceuticals or their packaging. Stock requiring refrigeration should be unpacked and put away promptly. Dispensed items requiring cold storage should be kept in the refrigerator until collected.

Dealing with a dispensing error

The shroud of secrecy that has formerly surrounded failures of health care is now being stripped away. Recommendations in a report[33] published by an expert group on learning from adverse events in the NHS include:

- unified mechanisms for reporting and analysis when things go wrong;

Table 5.6 Role of the National Patient Safety Agency

To collect and analyse information on adverse events from a range of NHS
  sources, and patients and carers
To assimilate safety-related information from a variety of existing reporting
  systems and other sources in the UK and abroad
To learn lessons and ensure that they are fed back into practice, service organisation and delivery
Where risks are identified, to produce solutions to prevent harm, specify national
  goals and to establish mechanisms to monitor progress

NHS, National Health Service.

- a more open culture, in which errors or service failures can be
  reported and discussed;
- mechanisms for ensuring that, where lessons are identified, the
  necessary changes are put into practice.

In 2001, a further report[34] was published which set out the details of the
new national mandatory reporting system for adverse health care events
and near misses. The report identifies some of the deficiencies of former
methods of investigating and reporting major adverse events by a wide
range of bodies, such as local investigations, internal and external
enquiries and reviews, which leads in some cases to duplication. It states
that, in future, there will be only two ways of responding: an independent investigation commissioned by either the DoH or by the Commission for Health Improvement. The government's plan[25] for pharmacy
states that incidents involving pharmacists or the use of medicines will
be included. The new system will introduce an integrated approach to
learning from adverse events, and will capture adverse event information
from a variety of sources. It will depend on the establishment of local
reporting systems which, by feeding selected reports to a national
system, will enable clusters and trends to be identified. A new body, the
National Patient Safety Agency, has been established. Its functions[35] are
set out in Table 5.6.

Many hospital pharmacies and some multiples already have dispensing incident reporting schemes, but how a national scheme will be
operated is not yet known. The subject of dispensing errors and their
reporting is discussed in an article by Cox and Marriott.[36]

In the previous section, we have discussed methods for making the
dispensing process as safe as possible. Nolan[37] stated that designers of
systems of care can make them safer by attending to three key tasks:

- Design the system to prevent errors.
- Design procedures to make errors visible, so that when they do occur, they may be intercepted.
- Design procedures for mitigating the adverse effect of errors when they are not detected or intercepted.

The examples he gives for making errors visible include pharmacists checking doctors' prescriptions, and also educating patients so that they may spot errors; they should be encouraged to ask questions and to speak up when unusual circumstances occur. Few studies of the incidence of dispensing errors have been published, but in a survey of five hospitals reported by Bower[38] 119 errors were detected in 6 months; 19.3% of these were detected after the item had been issued from the pharmacy ('external errors'). The external error rate was calculated at 16.3 per 100 000 dispensed items. It is apparent that mistakes will occur, and this fact must be acknowledged, and pharmacists must be prepared to deal with them in an effective way.

Wu[39] discusses the effects on doctors of discovering that a serious mistake has been made. His comments apply equally to pharmacists who realise that they have made a dispensing error. There is a sickening feeling when the realisation dawns; there may be a lack of true support from colleagues and confession is thus discouraged. It would be better to deal with the incident with a problem-solving focus, and to explore what might have been done differently.

It follows that every pharmacy should have a procedure in place for dealing with both the immediate effects of an error and with any possible reporting requirements. This should be based on the RPSGB Fact Sheet on the subject.[40]

Dispensing extemporaneous preparations

A pharmaceutical product with a marketing authorisation must always be prescribed and dispensed when available rather than formulating a 'special'. Guidance issued by the Professional Standards Directorate[41] states that as a request for a special can be made only by a doctor or a dentist, pharmacists are under no legal obligation to establish that there is a need for the special, or that licensed products available are not suitable. However, the pharmacist should alert the prescriber to the unlicensed status, preferably before the product is ordered, and in any event before the product is administered. If there is no appropriate licensed product, the doctor and pharmacist may decide that the patient's condition justifies the prescribing of an extemporaneously prepared preparation. Rather than attempting to make the preparation in-house, it is usually preferable to purchase such items from a licensed 'special-order' manufacturer, since there will then be guarantees of the quality of the ingredients and of the dispensing process. Special-order manufacturers in each region are listed in the *British National Formulary* (BNF).[42] The pharmacist will have to make a professional judgement about whether the possible resulting delay would be against the patient's best interests in each case.

'Specials' may be ordered only from a licensed 'specials' manufacturer. The conditions governing their supply are set out in guidance published by the Medicines Control Agency (MCA) in Guidance Note 14,[43] which can be downloaded from the MCA website (www.open.gov.uk/mca/mcahome.htm). This guidance states that items dispensed extemporaneously according to prescriptions or to pharmacopoeial formulae are not considered as 'specials' by the MCA. In spite of this, they may, however, be obtained from a special-order manufacturer. It is common practice for parenteral nutrition solutions and intravenous antibiotics to be supplied to patients at home in this way by specialist contractors. The guidance requires pharmacists to keep records of supplies of 'specials' to patients for 5 years; these records should be available on request for inspection. The details to be recorded are the source; the person to whom the product was supplied and the date; the batch number; and details of any adverse reactions to the product of which the pharmacist is aware. Any suspected adverse reactions to specials should be reported to the MCA via the Yellow Card scheme. (See also section on unlicensed or 'off-label' prescribing, above.)

At this point, we should consider why dispensing extemporaneously, traditionally an activity undertaken by pharmacists, is now considered as a high-risk activity. The reason is that just as few doctors regularly prescribe formulae for extemporaneous dispensing, the majority of pharmacists have little experience of preparing them. This may lead to unsafe practices that in turn can lead to defective or dangerous products. In pharmacies that rarely undertake this type of work, safe procedures, equipment and ingredients of the required quality may be lacking. Table 5.7 lists problems that may be expected to occur when inadequate procedures are followed.

The RPSGB Council has set standards for good professional practice in extemporaneous dispensing in the 'Service Specification' section of the MEP,[1] and these must be followed at all times. Additionally, if records of master formulae are kept in the pharmacy, e.g. a book

Table 5.7 Potential extemporaneous dispensing hazards

Formula	Out-of-date; not updated to reflect changes in ingredients
	Wrong ingredient selected, e.g. wrong phosphate salt
	Unvalidated formula; stability data not available
	Expiry date miscalculated
Calculation	Errors in calculation
	Dose units misinterpreted
Ingredients	No identity or strength checks; no certificate of analysis supplied
	May have deteriorated or become contaminated during storage
Dispensing process	Wrong ingredients selected
	Ingredients transposed/wrongly measured
	Ingredients omitted or duplicated
	Made up to wrong volume
Labelling	Wrong patient's name (and/or ward for hospital inpatients)
	Labels transposed between products
	Wrong dosage instructions

containing a record of the ingredients and perhaps quantities of regularly prepared items, these must be validated by a pharmacist who should sign and date each record, thereby accepting professional responsibility for its accuracy. Records must be updated properly if any changes to any of the ingredients take place. An example might be the decision to use concentrated chloroform water rather than double-strength chloroform water as an ingredient, with a consequent change in volume to be measured. Such a change must be made by cancelling the old formula and rewriting it, rather than by making informal alterations, which may be subsequently misread. A pharmacist must take professional responsibility for checking that the correct master formula has been selected, and that calculations are correct on each occasion. When dispensing repeats or instalments, the formula must always be checked with the original source and not derived from the label of a returned container.

Dispensing pharmaceuticals: packaging

There are British Standards (BS), which give the design characteristics of containers suitable for pharmaceuticals and measures to be used both in dispensing and by patients. These are listed in Tables 5.8 and 5.9.

Table 5.8 British Standards (BS) for pharmaceutical containers

Paperboard containers for strip and blister packs	BS 1679: Part 1: 1976 (1994)
Plastic containers for tablets and ointments	BS 1679: Part 8 (1992)
Eye-dropper bottles	BS 1679: Part 5: 1973 (1994)
Glass medicine bottles	BS 1679: Part 6 (1994)
Ribbed oval glass bottles	BS 1679: Part 7: 1968 (1977)
Glass and plastic containers for solid dosage forms, semi-solids and powders	BS 1679: Part 8 (1992)
Metal collapsable tubes for eye ointments	BS 4230: 1967 (1992)
Packaging: child-resistant packaging – requirements and testing procedures for non-reclosable packages for pharmaceutical products	BS 8404: 2001
Packaging: child-resistant closures – requirements for non-reclosable child-resistant packaging for pharmaceutical products	BS EN 28317: 1993
Code of Practice for non-reclosable packaging for solid-dose units of medicinal products	BS 7236 (1989)

Information supplied by British Standards Institute.
The dates in brackets are the years in which Standards have been updated.

Table 5.9 British Standards (BS) for medicine measures

Glass dispensing measures for pharmaceutical purposes	BS 1922: 1987 (1999)
Medicine measures of 50 mL total graduated capacity	BS 3221: Part 1: 1985 (1990)
Free-standing plastic medicines measuring spoons of 5 mL capacity	BS 3221: Part 6: 1987 (1992)
Oral syringes delivering doses of less than 5 mL	BS 3221: Part 7: 1995

Information supplied by British Standards Institute.

Items complying with the relevant standard should be specified when orders or contracts are placed. Dispensing measures are required by the Weights and Measures Act 1985 to be tested, passed for use in trade and stamped by an inspector of Weights and Measures before they can be used; cylindrical measures as used in laboratories are not available thus stamped and, according to Lund,[44] introducing this would be very expensive as the cost of testing is related to the number of graduations. In 1997, the RPSGB Law Department[45] drew pharmacists' attention to the fact that plastic cylindrical measures, although stamped with the code ISO 6706, are not suitable for dispensing. The British Standards Institute stated that these measures do not conform to the appropriate BS.

Caps for liquid products should be flanged, i.e. wadless, to mini-mise microbial contamination hazards, and to prevent interaction between contents and liner material. For adequate leak-proof closure, it is important to use caps compatible with the threads of the container body, and of a depth that ensures that the flange is in contact with the rim of the bottle. Certain imported non-BS bottles have a different neck configuration, and it is impossible to get a satisfactory seal with British-designed child-resistant closures when fitted to such bottles. More detail about this problem, which presumably could recur, was reported in a news item.[46]

Concordance: a more liberal approach to taking medicines

Background to concordance

For many years pharmacists have been aware that patients often do not take their medicines as prescribed. The term coined for this was 'non-compliance'. Originally, the solution to this problem was seen in fairly simplistic terms, and research was undertaken to find ways of improving patient compliance or adherence to their doctors' treatment regimens by methods such as counselling and improved instruction leaflets. There is now a growing awareness that the problem is far-reaching and requires more fundamental solutions. At a meeting of the Parliamentary All-Party Pharmacy Group held in June 2000,[47] it was reported that half of all patients with chronic diseases do not take their medicines as prescribed. In addition to the cost of wasted medicines, there were further costs to the nation: extra treatment required, lost production and earnings and other knock-on costs that could exceed £1bn. In 1995, the RPSGB in partnership with Merck Sharp & Dohme began an enquiry into the prob-lems surrounding patient compliance. When the working party formed had undertaken a wide-ranging consultation exercise and reviewed research findings, a report was published in 1997.[48] It is essential reading for all health care workers wishing to take their studies of this problem further. An article in the *Pharmaceutical Journal* summarised many of the report's main recommendations.[49] Included in the findings is the fact that, apart from the practical difficulties that patients face, 'the most salient and prevalent influences on medicine taking are the beliefs that people hold about their medication and about medicines in general. These beliefs are often at variance with the best evidence from medical science and consequently receive scant, if any, attention from the prescriber. For the

Table 5.10 Why patients fail to get their prescription dispensed

Disagree with diagnosis
Reject doctor's plan of treatment
Have different perception of risk of illness from doctor
Psychological resistance to taking medicines
Cannot afford prescription charge
Forgetfulness
Incompetent because of illness or social factors

prescriber simply to reaffirm the views of medical science, and to dismiss or ignore these beliefs, is to fail to prescribe effectively'. In the past, the aim had been to influence the patient to follow his/her doctor's orders. It is now believed that there should be a negotiation between doctor and patient as equals to achieve a therapeutic alliance; the outcome of the negotiation may even be an agreement to differ. This approach may be termed concordance. The working party proposed that in future the use of the terms 'compliance' or 'adherence' should be reserved to signify the theoretical intention of the prescription, while 'concordance' should imply the practical and ethical goal of treatment.

The *Pharmacy in the Future*[25] plan alludes to the importance of the concordance approach to medicines management and makes plans for a national strategy for implementing partnership in medicines taking.

Having defined the terms, the report presents more facts. For example, up to one in five patients fail to get their prescriptions dispensed. Possible explanations are set out in Table 5.10.

An extensive survey of published work identifies reasons why patients, having got their medicines, may not take them according to the directions. In many cases, non-compliance is not total – patients may sometimes forget doses, while others may at times have 'drug holidays' when they suddenly stop taking their medication, only to start again at a later date, which may have serious consequences. Table 5.11 gives some possible reasons for this type of behaviour.

The pharmacist's role in concordance

For a satisfactory outcome to the patient's treatment, a team approach is essential. The team will include doctor, practice nurse, pharmacist and, ideally, a fully informed patient. The pharmacist is ideally placed to be the team member who informs patients about the place of their medicines in managing the disease process. This is not a new idea. As far back as

Table 5.11 Factors affecting compliance/adherence

Physical or social vulnerability	Being elderly, infirm or partially sighted
	Belonging to an ethnic minority
	Psychotic illness
Antidrug attitude	Fear of addiction or of developing drug resistance
	Belief that drugs are 'unnatural'
	May stop to check if symptoms still persist
Adverse drug reactions	Experienced by patient
	Feared because of PIL emphasising side-effects
Unable to follow regimen	Especially with increasing numbers of medications
	If frequency more than twice a day
	Unable to open containers or read directions

PIL, patient information leaflet.

1984, Smith and Stephenson[50] surveyed the information needs of patients, and in their paper list factors associated with non-compliance. Headed by misunderstanding of the prescription – poor labelling/packaging/instructions – their list also includes complex drug regimens, and frequency and severity of side-effects. As the RPSGB working party found, there are further factors somewhat outside the field of influence of the pharmacist, such as failure to appreciate the seriousness of the illness or the benefits of treatment, social isolation and dissatisfaction with the doctor–patient relationship. The authors point out that it is important to get the intellectual level of information right and, in particular, to cater for patients in the lower socioeconomic groups, since better-educated patients already have at their disposal a wider range of information sources. They also warn that, handled insensitively, patient information could conflict with what the doctor wants the patient to know. Pharmacists should, of course, ensure that they know how to use all the various products themselves, so that they can give advice as needed. In the case of inhalers where many treatment failures are caused by poor technique, a practical demonstration including supervised practice may be needed; it is possible to obtain placebo inhalers for this purpose from the suppliers.

Compliance aids

A number of compliance aids are commercially available, e.g. Dosette, Medidos and other monitored dosage systems (MDSs); these are not

Table 5.12 Patients eligible for monitored dosage system (MDS)/medication review

---

Anyone with mental or physical disability
Anyone confused by regimen
Patients living alone and needing help with medication
Those with conditions that make taking medicines difficult, e.g. Parkinson's
    disease, dementia
Patients on complicated regimens
Those discharged from hospital and needing help
Tuberculosis patients

---

available on FP10 prescription. The RPSGB Report[49] found no convincing evidence that patients were in fact helped by such compliance
aids, but it seems possible that certain patients, where forgetfulness is a
problem, are in fact likely to find them useful. Nunney and Raynor surveyed pharmacists and compliance aid users, but concluded that in many
cases the use of MDSs was not focused on the patients' real needs.[51]

Typically, these aids contain compartments corresponding with the
days of the week and meal times, and are prefilled by the patient or by
a relative; others are intended to be prefilled at a pharmacy. Standards
for the filling of MDSs are given in the MEP; [1] although they are given
in the context of providing a service to residential homes, they would
equally apply to any service offered to individual patients living in their
own homes. There is a Law and Ethics Fact Sheet on labelling MDSs
and compliance aids.[52]

Until recently, there was no way of remunerating pharmacists for
filling these aids, but now some health authorities have initiated schemes
where payments may be made for pharmacists to undertake medication
review services and to provide MDSs for patients for whom failure to
adhere to therapy could have serious consequences. One such scheme
was outlined in a news item.[53] The scheme identified seven main groups
of patients who might be helped by a MDS. These have been reproduced
in Table 5.12 and may serve as a guide to potential MDS users.

In many cases, pharmacists' only contact with patients is via a carer
– a home help or warden of residential accommodation. Many tasks
which were formerly undertaken by the district nursing service are now
considered to fall into the category of social care and be carried out by
carers (either family members or paid employees) with no formal qualifications. Paid carers are likely to be employees of social services providers, volunteers and private agencies. Although employers may have
policies that their carers should not administer medicines, in practice

- All hospitals should implement a one stop 'dispensing for discharge' scheme and self-medication schemes for older people where appropriate.

By 2004:

- Every primary care trust will implement schemes to ensure that older people get more help from pharmacists in taking their medicines.

It is clear that pharmacists can contribute a great deal to these objectives; an overview of the ways in which this may be achieved was given in an article by Ewing[60] (see also Chapter 3).

Smith and Stephenson's paper[50] showed that many patients do not get the best from their medicines because they do not understand how to use them. An earlier study of the information and counselling needs of hospital outpatients by Knowles[61] showed a 70% non-compliance rate overall, and in particular a decrease in the knowledge of treatment and the correct use of medication in elderly patients. In fact, in her study group, no patient over 71 years was able to answer four simple questions about their drugs, and only 14% were taking their drugs correctly. The problems of elderly patients received further study by Horner,[62] who listed reduced visual acuity, poor hearing and impaired memory and mental capacity which, coupled with diminished manipulative skills, may combine to interfere with taking medicines correctly. Horner found that improvements could be achieved with counselling, and by supervised self-medication before discharge from hospital. Keeping compliance charts and carrying a medication record card also helped. She also considered the type of containers used for dispensing; larger containers than usual may be advantageous and certainly it is better to avoid the use of child-resistant closures where patients find them a problem to remove. Patients may overcome this difficulty by asking someone to remove the cap, and then leave it off, or alternatively empty the drugs into another bottle, often inappropriately labelled. Simplified dosage instructions, with large print on a separate card if necessary, using symbols or references to mealtimes, have been found helpful in some centres.

Patients with poor sight may be helped by the provision of large-type labels and/or PILs. Braille labels are available giving dosage instructions, but very few elderly patients whose sight has failed can read Braille, unless they have been blind from childhood and attended a school for the blind. Partially sighted or blind diabetics may be helped by a preset insulin syringe. These are available on the *Drug Tariff*,[63] but not as disposable items.

Infants and children

A number of problems may arise when the young need medicines. For most drugs, the only evidence about their clinical pharmacology in children has been obtained by extrapolation from their use in adults, since regulatory authorities will not license drugs for indications, nor for groups of patients, for which no clinical trial data exist. For either ethical or commercial reasons, clinical trials of drugs in children have been rare, and thus few dosage or paediatric indications are given in product literature, other than for drugs routinely used for children. Furthermore, many drugs are not routinely made in a paediatric dose form and this may create difficulties for prescribers and pharmacists. This has led to widespread 'off-label' prescribing in paediatric practice. To protect themselves, drug companies may include a statement in the PIL that the drug is not recommended for use in children, and this means that parents will need reassurance when such leaflets are supplied. The legal and ethical problems caused by this situation are beginning to be addressed only recently. In the USA the Food and Drug Administration (FDA) now requires drug companies to include paediatric usage and dosage information where relevant for both new and existing drugs.[64] No such regulations currently exist in the UK, but it is to be hoped that pressure from concerned professionals will encourage the MCA to follow suit. (For a discussion of 'orphan drugs', i.e. drugs available only on a named-patient basis, see Chapter 2.)

A recent development has been the production of a national paediatric formulary, a joint venture between the Royal College of Paediatrics and Child Health and the Neonatal and Paediatric Pharmacists Group.[65] At the time of writing, an updated edition is in preparation. The book includes a therapeutic section, a section giving information on licensed and unlicensed indications and a table of dietary products that are borderline substances. An abbreviated paediatric formulary has recently been published by the same group.[66] Community pharmacists can obtain information about paediatric medicines from their local hospital drug information centre – a useful contact point if the child in question has recently been a patient there. There is a national specialist paediatric and neonatal drug information Drug Information Advisory Line (DIAL) provided by the Alder Hey Children's Hospital.[67] Contact details are given in Table 5.14.

Table 5.14 Contacting Drug Information Advisory Line (DIAL) (hours 08.45–1700, Monday–Friday)

Telephone 0151 252 5837	E-mail: info@dial.org.uk
Facsimile 0151 220 3885	Web site: http: //www.dial.org.uk

Reproduced from Nunn *et al.*[67] by permission.

For pharmacists working in the field of paediatrics, there is a Neonatal and Paediatric Pharmacists Group, with an official journal, *Paediatric and Perinatal Drug Therapy.*

Calculating dosage for infants and children

The only accurate methods of calculating dosage for children are by calculating mg/kg body weight, or by surface area, which may be derived from a nomogram or calculated from the formula given in the BNF. If a recent weight is not available, average or ideal values may be found in the section on prescribing for children in the BNF. For potent medicines with a low therapeutic index, it is preferable to use recent actual measurements, particularly as a child with a chronic serious illness may be small for its age. The problems of determining doses for children were surveyed by Nunn.[68] He emphasises an important fact about how doses are expressed in reference texts such as the BNF and manufacturers' summaries of product characteristics, namely that some give the total daily dose, to be divided by the dose interval given, and others show the individual dose, to be repeated at the intervals shown. Errors have been known to occur because readers have confused the two systems.

Presentation of drugs for children

Many drugs are not available in a dose form intended for children. It is usually considered preferable to give a liquid preparation to children under 5, although tablets may be swallowed by some younger children. Tablets are preferable for long-term conditions if at all possible, to avoid the necessity for the parents to keep returning to the pharmacy for repeat supplies. Indeed, this may result in the less well-motivated parent abandoning treatment. Those tablets which are not sustained-release or enteric-coated may be crushed. The taste may be masked with jam or honey, or possibly yeast extract or cheese. Some medicines that are formulated for children contain sucrose. This is a disadvantage for diabetics, and also may lead to dental caries if use is prolonged. If needed, the manufacturer's medical information department will give the sucrose content of any preparation. The child should brush the teeth or rinse the mouth after each dose if possible.

Where a suitable dose form for a child does not seem to exist, the drug manufacturer will be able on occasion to provide a formula to make a suspension using either the powdered drug or by crushing tablets. Formulae should not be improvised locally without reference to the manufacturer, who will have stability and compatibility data on file – and who may, on occasion, be able to supply a ready-made preparation on a 'named-patient' basis. On occasions, there may be no alternative but to make individually weighed and wrapped powders from crushed tablets with a diluent such as lactose, provided this is tolerated by the child. When a child's treatment has been started in hospital, the hospital pharmacy will be able to give details of the preparation for continuing treatment. Medicines should not be added to bottles of feed, since if the child does not finish the bottle (which is likely if it tastes strange), part of the dose will be lost, and anyway some medicines are incompatible with milk. In young children, compliance depends on the parents, who should be given every encouragement to maintain compliance. At the same time, parents should be warned not to leave medicines lying about the home and, in particular, not to leave them in the child's room. Similarly, medicines should not be left within the reach of unsupervised babies and toddlers in prams.

Medicines in schools

Pharmacists should always consider the difficulties that may face school-age children on medication. The Scottish Executive has published a booklet containing guidance about the administration of medicines in schools.[69] While acknowledging that community services pharmacists may give advice about the management of medicines in schools, this also states that when schools draw up policies about the storage and handling of medicines, they should be able to get help from primary care trust chief pharmacists.[70] In 1997, the Pharmacy Community Care Liaison Group developed guidelines[71] for dealing with medicines for schoolchildren. The document sets out the responsibilities of the parties involved. Key points directly affecting the pharmacist are summarised here. Parents are responsible for medicine administration to younger children, and should make arrangements for either themselves or a representative to administer medicines during the school day. If the school agrees to provide the representative, the parents should make a written request including all necessary information; any changes must be communicated in writing. Medicines should be provided in an original dispensed container with the following information on the label:

- name and strength of the medicine and dose;
- time of administration, e.g. lunch, between 12 noon and 1 p.m.;
- length of treatment or stop date as appropriate;
- expiry date whenever possible.

The medicine should have been dispensed within the last 3 months. It follows that parents should be advised to ask their doctor to prescribe a supply to be dispensed separately for school use.

Pharmacists can provide support in a number of ways, including contacting local schools to offer help and advice. Pharmacists who plan to do this are advised to consult the original document,[71] which has much more information about developing policies and procedures. They may advise on safe and appropriate storage of medicines, and assist by labelling inner containers of medicines so that the directions are still available to school staff even though the outer packaging may have been disposed of by the parents. Pharmacists may also consider whether alternative medication could avoid the need to administer doses during the school day, and should liaise with the doctor to suggest this if possible.

Services for drug addicts

As drug addiction becomes an escalating problem in the UK, increasing numbers of addicts are receiving treatment and more community pharmacists are offering services – instalment dispensing, supervised self-administration of prescribed medication and syringe and needle exchange. According to an RPSGB working party report, the number of NHS prescriptions for methadone as a drug of dependence more than doubled in England between 1991 and 1996, and in Scotland between 1992 and 1996.[72] It also stated that, by 1995, 50% of pharmacies in England and Wales were dispensing Controlled Drugs to misusers, with a higher proportion in Scotland. The working party was set up to identify problem areas for pharmacists in the existing framework for treatment. The report, which was extensively summarised in the *Pharmaceutical Journal*,[73] makes 59 recommendations ranging from improvements in practice to changes in the law. One identified problem, of concern to English community pharmacists, was the fact that, unlike

Scotland, in England NHS instalment prescriptions could be written only for methadone and some other Schedule 2 drugs. It was recommended that this should be extended to cover other drugs liable to misuse or licensed for prescription for the management of opiate withdrawal. From April 2001, an amendment of the NHS (General Medical Services) Regulations 1992 has allowed the prescription of Subutex Sublingual Tablets brand of buprenorphine in instalments on forms FP10HP(Ad) and FP10(MDA).[74]

Any pharmacist contemplating providing services for drug misusers is advised to read the report or its summary. Also important are the guidelines on clinical management, which replace the 1991 guidelines.[75] On supervised consumption, the guidelines state:

> In order to ensure compliance and reduce diversion, it is good practice for all new prescriptions to be taken initially under daily supervision for a minimum of three months, and supervision should be undertaken at any stage during a prescription if there are any doubts about compliance.

In the section on approaches to maintenance, there is a warning:

> There are a number of drugs listed in the clinical guidelines which are used outside the licensed indication. It is important to note that prescription of licensed medications outside the recommendations of the product's licence alters (and probably increases) the doctor's professional responsibility.

Roberts,[76] in reviewing the guidelines, identified a key role for pharmacists as part of the multidisciplinary team needed to manage the drug misuse problem. In particular, she welcomed the recommended arrangements for effective dispensing:

- Wherever possible, prescribers should liaise with the dispensing pharmacist about specific patients and the prescribing regimen.
- If a prescriber has a special prescribing licence or handwriting exemption the pharmacist should be informed.
- As a general principle, substitute drugs should be dispensed on a daily basis.

The prescribing of substitute and other drugs for drug addicts is subject to a number of regulations over and above those made under the general run of the Misuse of Drugs Act 1971. Only doctors holding a licence from the Secretary of State may prescribe diamorphine (heroin), cocaine and dipipanone (in Diconal) to addicts other than in the short term, for the relief of pain. Such doctors usually work in specialist treatment centres, usually in hospital outpatient departments. GPs and non-specialist hospital doctors may prescribe other drugs in this class for addicts, but are strongly advised to treat addicts only in conjunction with specialist advice, either from a treatment centre or from a hospital-based consultant psychiatrist. The rules for prescribing for addicts are complicated, and a number of special FP10 prescription forms exist which distinguish prescriptions for addicts, and also permit dispensing in instalments. In England and Wales the pink forms FP10(AD) are mainly issued by drug addiction centres; GPs use light-blue forms FP10(MDA). In Scotland, pink HBP(A) forms are used. Forms issued in Scotland may be dispensed in England. There are additional NHS rules about what other items may be prescribed on these forms, and pharmacists planning to supply addicts should familiarise themselves with the relevant RPSGB Professional Standards Directorate Fact Sheet.[77] Some pharmacists may be reluctant to participate in such schemes because they themselves feel threatened by the clients, or because they think that other patients or customers will be intimidated. To address both these problem areas, Boots the Chemists has drawn up a form of agreement for clients of drug misuser services, which sets out standards of conduct and also explains some of the features of the service provided.[78]

Some drug addicts are treated privately and are thus not eligible for NHS prescriptions. Problems can arise which are peculiar to these patients, who may have difficulty in paying for their prescriptions, and may demand credit. If granted, this can lead to them selling part of their supply to raise funds to pay off the debt. The problems have been addressed by agreeing guidelines to be followed by two London health authorities.[79]

Matheson[80] sought the views of drug users about the services they received from pharmacies. She found that they felt stigmatised by their condition, and this was closely related to the level of privacy in the pharmacy. In particular, they would have appreciated a private area for supervised methadone consumption. Several of her study subjects valued the fact that the pharmacist acted in a discreet manner. She suggests that when it is impossible to have a private area, discussing with the client whether it is possible to visit the pharmacy at a quiet time might lessen the problem.

Needle and syringe exchange schemes

The spread of the acquired immunodeficiency syndrome virus (AIDS or human immunodeficiency virus (HIV)) through needle sharing by addicts has led to the introduction of needle and syringe exchange schemes. There are detailed guidelines for running such schemes in the MEP,[1] and all pharmacists should be familiar with them whether they work in a participating pharmacy or not, since they may receive requests to supply injecting equipment in any pharmacy.

Drug users may develop a number of health problems as a result of their habit, and the needle exchange pharmacist may be the most accessible member of the primary care team. Scott and Bruce[81] have undertaken a literature review on the subject and, reinforced by their own experience, have compiled a paper with practical advice which should be read by pharmacists dealing regularly with injecting drug users, to enable them to offer appropriate advice as necessary.

Wound management products

Forms FP10NC/C (GP10 in Scotland) and FP10(HP) may be used to prescribe only those wound management products that are listed in the *Drug Tariff*;[63] in Scotland, the hospital prescription form HBP may be used only for drugs. Additionally, wound management products are listed in the *Nurse Prescribers' Formulary* (NPF),[42] and may be prescribed on forms FP10CN, FP10PN (Scotland) and HS21(N) in Northern Ireland. No payment to the contractor would be made for the supply of items not included in the *Drug Tariff* or NPF. Within hospitals, many non-*Drug Tariff* wound management products are in use. These are not therefore available to patients within the community, and this may cause considerable problems when patients leave hospital if treatment is to be continued by community nurses. Sometimes, arrangements are made to continue to supply from the hospital, although this may not be via the pharmacy, since most hospital pharmacies handle only antibiotic-impregnated or other medicated dressings, the rest being issued by the stores organisation or the central sterile supply department.

Surgical equipment, appliances and reagents

Those items of surgical equipment, appliances, stoma care requisites, trusses and elastic hosiery which are included in the *Drug Tariff*,[63] may be prescribed on form FP10 by GPs. These prescriptions may be dispensed by a surgical appliance contractor who is not necessarily a pharmacist. Many pharmacists do however supply such items, and those who do so should familiarise themselves with the excellent handbook of non-medicinal health care by Harman.[82] Most hospitals refer in- and outpatients to a surgical fitter (a contractor who attends the hospital regularly) for these items, and would not therefore use form FP10(HP), although there is nothing in the regulations to preclude it. A further range of items can be supplied on the NHS only by referral to a hospital consultant, who will in turn refer the patient to a hospital fitter, a specialist department such as audiology, a limb-fitting centre or specialist nurse. The list includes orthopaedic appliances like surgical corsets and surgical shoes, mastectomy and other prostheses, artificial limbs, wheelchairs and hearing aids.

Reagents

Those most commonly prescribed are blood sugar and urine sugar monitoring reagent strips for patients to monitor treatment in diabetes. Some test strips rely on a visual colour comparison, but others are used in conjunction with a meter; the various strips are not interchangeable and can only be used with the corresponding meter supplied by the same company. In fact, in some cases, the meters require prior calibration with the batch of test strips to be used. Although the reagent strips may be prescribed on form FP10/FP10(HP), the meters may not. Hospitals may loan meters to diabetics requiring particularly intensive monitoring for a period, perhaps immediately after diagnosis or during pregnancy, and some patients are prepared to buy their own.

Medical gases

Medical gases are considered to be pharmaceuticals, and pharmacists are involved in their supply and use in both hospitals and in the community. Only oxygen is listed in the *Drug Tariff*[63] for supply on form FP10/FP10(HP). In hospitals, a wide variety of gases is used, including nitrous oxide for anaesthesia, Entonox (a proprietary mixture of nitrous oxide and oxygen) for analgesia, various gas mixtures and helium for respiratory function tests, compressed air for nebuliser therapy, and finally, of course, oxygen. Besides being inhaled via a mask by patients with poor respiratory function due to chest infection or airways disease, oxygen is used in conjunction with anaesthetic gases via anaesthetic machines, during mechanical ventilation in recovery rooms and intensive therapy units, in hyperbaric oxygen chambers and incubators for babies. Medical gas cylinders are colour-coded according to BS 1319: 1955. Additionally, liquid nitrogen and carbon dioxide snow are both used for cryotherapy (see below).

Some hospitals have a piped oxygen system to all patient areas or to certain high-use areas; this may be fed from a tank of liquid oxygen outside the building. In addition, operating theatres often have a piped supply of nitrous oxide, which is fed from one central large bank of cylinders via a manifold. Strict procedures have to be followed in running manifold rooms to prevent the supply running out; warning lights are provided within the theatre suite, where they can be seen constantly by a responsible person during normal working. Manifolds are arranged so that there is always a reserve set of cylinders attached, which may be brought into use either manually or automatically when the first set is empty.

The main supplier of gas in cylinders is BOC Gases, which delivers regularly medical gases in cylinders which are rented. Normally an equivalent number of empty cylinders has to be returned when a delivery is made. It is advisable to minimise stock holdings of cylinders and to try to stop them being hidden away in odd corners of hospitals, otherwise excessive rental charges will be incurred. Gas cylinders come in a range of sizes designated by letters, e.g. oxygen cylinders range from size C (170 litres) to J (6800 litres). Full cylinders are sealed with viscose seals. There are various hazards associated with gas cylinders. They are heavy, e.g. size J weighs 69 kg, and easily toppled. To prevent accidents, retaining chains should be provided *and used* in cylinder stores, and transport should be on proper trolleys or cylinder stands. Safety precautions for the safe handling and storage of oxygen cylinders are given in the MEP.[1] Oxygen cylinders must be stored away from flammable substances, and no smoking allowed in the vicinity during storage, transport or use. Cylinder stores should be away from other buildings and specially constructed and maintained in a clean condition. Full details of the requirements for these, and many other important aspects of medical gas storage and safety in use will be found in the then Department of Health and Social Security Code of Practice.[83] Further important information about medical gas pipeline installations will be found in a series of Health Technical Memoranda no. 2022.[84–86] Medical gas cylinders must not be used for non-medical purposes, e.g. oxyacetylene welding. (See also section on quality control of medical gases, Chapter 7.)

In use, the cylinder is connected to a reducing valve and flow meter, which incorporates a cylinder contents gauge. In hospitals, valves giving variable flow rates up to 15 litres per minute are usually used; those prescribable on form FP10 for home use give two rates only: 2 and 4 litres per minute.

When pharmacy staff visit wards and departments – particularly those which may not use oxygen regularly – it is good practice to check the storage facilities for cylinders and the expiry date, which is usually found on a label on the valve.

Domiciliary oxygen

Certain community pharmacists are contracted to provide oxygen according to the terms specified in the *Drug Tariff*.[63] They undertake to stock cylinders and accessories, and to arrange to deliver them to the patient's home, set them up and give instructions for their use. The MEP[1] sets out professional standards for this activity. Only size F (1360 litres or 48 cu. ft) cylinders are included in the *Drug Tariff*.[63] The cylinders and reducing valves remain the property of the pharmacist, who pays for or rents them. The plastic mask belongs to the patient, and has to be represcribed on form FP10 should a replacement be needed. On cessation of treatment, the pharmacist takes back the equipment from the patient's home. Expenses incurred in delivering oxygen are claimed from the health authority. If the equipment cannot be recovered and reused, e.g. if it has been lost or broken, the pharmacist can submit a claim for reimbursement of its value.

The prescription of an oxygen concentrator is a better way of supplying oxygen to patients who require long-term treatment for more than 15 hours per day. Oxygen concentrators separate nitrogen from air and deliver a gas enriched in oxygen. The DoH has awarded contracts to deliver and set up concentrators to a number of firms on a regional basis; pharmacists are not involved. A list of contractors and details of the arrangements are listed in the *Drug Tariff*.[63] Hamid Husain[87] outlined the prescribing for, and selection of, suitable patients for this approach to therapy.

Nebuliser therapy

In diseases characterised by airways obstruction, it is usual to prescribe inhaled bronchodilators, corticosteroids or sodium cromoglicate. Most patients are satisfactorily treated using aerosol inhalers, possibly moving on to a patent dry-powder inhaler if their disease or concomitant problems like arthritic hands make use of an aerosol difficult. For most patients, every attempt should be made, by counselling and trying the various devices and aids available, before concluding that a jet or ultrasonic nebuliser is needed. One exception would be when patients who normally manage an inhaler are admitted to hospital for an operation, when their dosage requirements may be higher, and they will be unable to use an aerosol around the time of their anaesthetic. Jet nebulisers form an aerosol when oxygen or air is fed into the chamber into which a dose of inhalation solution has been measured. The gas may come from a cylinder or from an air compressor. *Drug Tariff*[63] reducing valves do not give an adequate flow rate to work these satisfactorily; the dose will be incomplete, and the time taken excessively long. Patients' respiratory function will decline if they are thus forced to inhale high concentrations of oxygen for long periods. The *Drug Tariff* specifically warns pharmacists against the potentially dangerous practice of attempting to modify oxygen sets to increase the rate of flow.

Considerable dose variations have been recorded in studies that measured the output of nebulisers driven in different ways, and it is important to match the equipment carefully. Advice is available from the manufacturers of the inhalation solutions. An alternative is the ultrasonic nebuliser, which is self-contained and requires no compressed-gas source. Nebulisers are not prescribable on the *Drug Tariff*, but hospitals often arrange to loan them to selected patients for home use. Some patients may buy their own, but not necessarily acting upon medical advice. There are hazards – patients may not fully understand their use, and may try to treat acute exacerbations by increasing use of their nebulisers, when hospital admission may be more appropriate. Several studies, including that by Hilditch *et al.*,[88] have shown potentially dangerous practices in the use of nebulisers at home.

Liquid gases

Pharmacists may have to order and supply liquid gases, particularly nitrogen, to hospital clinics where its main use is for freezing off small lesions in dermatology. The supplier is BOC Cryospeed, which delivers from a tank into a large Dewar flask. Liquid gases are hazardous to handle and use; contact with tissues causes lesions similar to burns; extremities will rapidly suffer from frostbite and tissue destruction. All staff who handle liquid gases must be aware of the hazards and safety precautions. This includes staff such as porters and drivers. The containers used must be designed to vent to the atmosphere; domestic vacuum flasks with tightly fitting screw caps are not suitable. Hospital pharmacists should try to ensure that no unauthorised unsafe decanting operations are taking place: in one hospital it was found that local GPs were being encouraged to collect liquid nitrogen from the outpatients department in domestic vacuum flasks for use in their surgeries. Dewar flasks must be kept, protected from accidental spillage, in a well-ventilated store in which there is a proper emergency exit, since it is possible for nitrogen to layer from the floor upwards. For the same reason, personnel should not travel in lifts with large volumes of liquid gases. Users are strongly advised to read the safety precautions published by BOC.[89,90]

References

1. Royal Pharmaceutical Society of Great Britain. *Medicines, Ethics and Practice: A Guide for Pharmacists*, published yearly. London: Royal Pharmaceutical Society of Great Britain.
2. Guidance document: consultation on SOPs for dispensing. *Pharm J* 2001; 266: 616–619.
3. Bellingham C. How to write a SOP without tears. *Pharm J* 2001; 266: 615.
4. NHS Executive. *Prescription Fraud: An Efficiency Scrutiny*. London: Stationery Office, 1997.
5. News item. Scrutiny team wants pharmacists to check prescription charge exemptions. *Pharm J* 1997; 258: 890–891.
6. NHS Executive. *Countering Fraud in the NHS: Prescription Charge Evasion*. HSC 1999/209.
7. NHS Executive. *Security of Prescription Forms*. HSC 1998/062.
8. Department of Health. *The Pharmacists' Guide to Prescription Exemption*. London: Department of Health, 1999.
9. News item. Temporary fix agreed for prescription switching problem. *Pharm J* 2000; 265: 116.
10. Department of Health and National Assembly of Wales *Drug Tariff*. Reward scheme – fraudulent prescription forms, part XIVC, published monthly. London: Stationery Office.
11. NHS Executive. *Pharmacy Reward Scheme*. HSC 1999/133.
12. Law and ethics bulletin. Prescription alterations. *Pharm J* 1999; 262: 839.
13. Council of the Royal Pharmaceutical Society of Great Britain. Consultation document. Making the best use of pharmacists and their support staff. *Pharm J* 1998; 260: 743–745.
14. Greene R. Survey of prescription anomalies in community pharmacies: (1) prescription monitoring. *Pharm J* 1995; 254: 476–481.
15. Shah S N H, Aslam M, Avery A J. A survey of prescription errors in general practice. *Pharm J* 2001; 267: 860–862.
16. Cousins D H. Abbreviations in health care. *Hosp Pharm* 1997; 4: 108.
17. Cousins D H. Reducing the risks of chemotherapy errors. *Hosp Pharm* 1995; 2: 117–120.
18. Cambridgeshire Health Authority. *An Inquiry into the Death of a Cambridgeshire Patient in April 2000*. Cambridge: Cambridgeshire Health Authority, 2000.
19. Woods K. *The Prevention of Intrathecal Medication Errors: A Report to the Chief Medical Officer*. London: Department of Health, 2001.
20. *Safety in the Clinical Use of Cytotoxics*. Bath: S & J Health Consulting/CoAcS, 2001.
21. Department of Health. *National Guidance on the Safe Administration of Intrathecal Chemotherapy*. London: Department of Health, 2001.
22. NHS Executive. *National Guidance on the Safe Administration of Intrathecal Chemotherapy*. HSC 2001/022.

23. Royal Pharmaceutical Society of Great Britain Professional Standards Directorate Fact Sheet 7. *Prescription Collection, Home Delivery and Repeat Medication Services*. London: Royal Pharmaceutical Society of Great Britain.

24. Burtonwood A M, Hinchcliffe A L, Tinkler G G. A prescription for quality: a role for the clinical pharmacist in general practice. *Pharm J* 1998; 261: 678–680.

25. Department of Health. *Pharmacy in the Future – Implementing the NHS Plan*. London: Stationery Office, 2000.

26. Royal Pharmaceutical Society of Great Britain Professional Standards Directorate Fact Sheet 5. *The Use of Unlicensed Medicines in Pharmacy*. London: Royal Pharmaceutical Society of Great Britain.

27. Tomlin M. Medication risk management – the pharmacist's role. *Hosp Pharm* 1999, 6: 314.

28. Royal Pharmaceutical Society of Great Britain Council. Professional standards and training for dispensary staff from January 2005. *Pharm J* 1999; 262: 351–352.

29. Perrett A T. The West Midlands accredited checking technician course. *Pharm J* 1999; 263: 952.

30. Royal Pharmaceutical Society of Great Britain Professional Standards Directorate. Fact Sheet 3. *The Medicines for Human Use (Marketing Authorisation etc.) Regulations 1994, and the Effect Thereof*. London: Royal Pharmaceutical Society of Great Britain.

31. Royal Pharmaceutical Society of Great Britain Professional Standards Directorate. Requirement for patient leaflets (law and ethics bulletin). *Pharm J* 2000; 264: 401.

32. News item. Patients want information from people, not paper, says Consumers' Association. *Pharm J* 2000; 265: 117.

33. Department of Health. *An Organisation with a Memory*. London: Stationery Office, 2000.

34. Department of Health. *Building a Safer NHS for Patients*. London: Stationery Office, 2001.

35. Department of Health website (2001). www.doh.gov.uk/buildingsafenhs (accessed 10 June 2001).

36. Cox A, Marriott J. Dealing with dispensing errors. *Pharm J* 2000; 264: 724.

37. Nolan T W. System changes to improve patient safety. *BMJ* 2000; 320: 771–773.

38. Bower A C. Dispensing error rates in hospital pharmacy. *Pharm J* 1990; 244: R22–R23.

39. Wu A W. Medical error: the second victim. *BMJ* 2000; 320: 726–727.

40. Royal Pharmaceutical Society Professional Standards Directorate. Fact Sheet 11. *Dealing with a Dispensing Error*. London: Royal Pharmaceutical Society of Great Britain.

41. Law and ethics bulletin. Supply of unlicensed medicinal products ("specials") for individual patients. *Pharm J* 2000; 265: 513.

42. Mehta D K, ed. *British National Formulary*, published twice-yearly. London: British Medical Association/Royal Pharmaceutical Society of Great Britain.

43. Medicines Control Agency Guidance note no. 14: *The Supply of Unlicensed Relevant Medicinal Products for Individual Patients*. (Previously MAL 14.) London: MCA, February 2000.

44. Lund W. Measuring liquids. *Pharm J* 1987; 238: 576.
45. Law and ethics bulletin. Use of plastic measures in dispensing. *Pharm J* 1997; 258: 335.
46. News item. Pharmacists urged to check that they only use compatible caps on liquid medicine bottles. *Pharm J* 1993; 250: 76.
47. News item. NICE effort wasted if patients will not take the medicine. *Pharm J* 2000; 264: 938.
48. Working Party Report. *Achieving Shared Goals in Medicine Taking: From Compliance to Concordance.* London: Royal Pharmaceutical Society of Great Britain, 1997.
49. News item. "Concordance" should replace compliance, says Society working party. *Pharm J* 1997; 258: 333–334.
50. Smith J M, Stephenson J. Information for patients: general principles and a survey on hospital outpatients and the general public. *Proc Guild* 1984; 18: 21.
51. Nunney J M, Raynor D K T. How are multi-compartment compliance aids used in primary care? *Pharm J* 2001; 267: 784–789.
52. Royal Pharmaceutical Society Professional Standards Directorate Fact Sheet 9. *Labelling of MDS and Compliance Aids.* London: Royal Pharmaceutical Society of Great Britain.
53. News item. HA pays £120 000 for MDS services. *Pharm J* 1999; 262: 827.
54. Pharmacy Community Care Liaison Group. Pharmacist support for home carers. *Pharm J* 1998; 260: 879–882.
55. McGraw C, Drennan V. District nurses and compliance devices. *Pharm J* 2000; 264: 368.
56. Stewart D, Ogilvie E, Kennedy E *et al.* Medication devices in primary care: activities of community-based nurses. *Int J Pharm Pract* 2001; 9: 91–96.
57. NHS Executive. *National Service Framework for Older People.* HSC 2001/007; LAC (2001)12. Available at www.doh.gov.uk/nsf/olderpeople.htm (accessed 17 March 2002).
58. News item. Blueprint for care of older patients highlights roles for pharmacists. *Pharm J* 2001; 266: 415–416.
59. NHS Executive. *Medicines for Older People: Implementing Medicines-related Aspects of the NSF.* Available at www.doh.gov.uk/nsf/olderpeople.htm (accessed 17 March 2002).
60. Ewing A B. NSF for older people – a starting point to improve care. *Hosp Pharm* 2001; 8: 150.
61. Knowles J. The evaluation of the need for pharmacist counselling in outpatient clinics at the Birmingham General Hospital. *Proc Guild* 1981; 10: 56.
62. Horner R. Medication and the elderly. *Proc Guild* 1986; 21: 18.
63. Department of Health and National Assembly for Wales *Drug Tariff*, published monthly. London: Stationery Office.
64. Timmins J G, Barr L M A. Paediatric hospital pharmacy practice – current issues. *Hosp Pharm* 1999; 6: 134–138.
65. *Medicines for Children.* London: Royal College of Paediatrics and Child Health Publications, 1999.
66. *Pocket Medicines for Children.* London: Royal College of Paediatrics and Child Health Publications, 2001.
67. Nunn A J, Barker C E, Caitens G R. Paediatric pharmacy – the Alder Hey national paediatric drug information advisory line (DIAL). *Hosp Pharm* 1999; 6: 139–142.

68. Nunn A J. Drug dosage in childhood. *Pharm J* 1982; 229: 419.

69. Scottish Executive. *The Administration of Medicines in Schools.* Edinburgh: Stationery Office Bookshop, 2001.

70. News item. New school medicines role for pharmacists. *Pharm J* 2001; 267: 315.

71. Pharmacy Community Care Liaison Group. Medicines in schools: implementing good practice in mainstream schools – a guide for pharmacists. *Pharm J* 1997; 258: 69–72.

72. *Report of the Working Party on Pharmaceutical Services for Drug Misusers.* London: Royal Pharmaceutical Society of Great Britain, 1999.

73. Article. Working Party Report: services for drug misusers. *Pharm J* 1998; 260: 418–423.

74. Department of Health. *Instalment Prescribing of Buprenorphine for the Treatment of Drug Addiction.* PL/CMO/2001/2, PL/CPHO/2001/2.

75. Department of Health. *Drug Misuse and Dependence: Guidelines on Clinical Management.* London: Stationery Office, 1999.

76. Roberts K. Revised drug misuse guidelines: pharmacists must get more involved. *Pharm J* 1999; 263: 203–205.

77. Royal Pharmaceutical Society of Great Britain Professional Standards Directorate Fact Sheet 1. *Controlled Drugs and Community Pharmacy.* London: Royal Pharmaceutical Society of Great Britain.

78. Wingfield J, Evans V. Reaching agreement with drug misusers. *Pharm J* 1999; 262: 131.

79. Carson T, Stimson K. Guidelines on good practice for the dispensing of controlled drugs to drug misusers on private prescriptions. *Pharm J* 1997; 259: 184–185.

80. Matheson C. Privacy and stigma in the pharmacy: illicit drug users' perspectives and implications for pharmacy practice. *Pharm J* 1998; 260: 639–641.

81. Scott J, Bruce L. Practical advice on medical complications of intravenous drug misuse. *Pharm J* 1998; 260: 957–960.

82. Harman R. *Patient Care in Community Practice*, 2nd edn. London: Pharmaceutical Press, 2002.

83. Health Equipment Information no. 163, *Code of Practice: Safety and Care in the Storage, Handling and Use of Medical Gas Cylinders on Health Authority Premises.* London: Department of Health and Social Security, NHS Procurement Directorate, 1987.

84. NHS Estates Health Technical Memorandum no. 2022. *Medical Gas Pipeline Systems: Operational Management.* London: Stationery Office, 1997.

85. NHS Estates Health Technical Memorandum no. 2022. *Medical Gas Pipeline Systems: Design, Installation, Validation and Verification.* London, Stationery Office, 1997.

86. NHS Estates Health Technical Memorandum no. 2022. *Medical Gas Pipeline Systems: Management Policy.* London, Her Majesty's Stationery Office, 1994.

87. Hamid Husain M. General practitioners to prescribe oxygen concentrators. *BMJ* 1985; 291: 1543.

88. Hilditch P I, Horsley M G, Rees J A, Barnes P C. The use of domiciliary nebulisers. *Pharm J Pract Res Suppl* 1987; 239: R7.

89. BOC Gases. *Safety Data Sheet: Liquid Nitrogen.*

90. BOC Cryospeed. *Guidance Notes: Transport by Vehicle of Liquid Nitrogen in Containers of less than 450 litres Capacity.*

6

Hospital pharmaceutical services

The hospital pharmaceutical service provides medicines, pharmaceutical advice on every aspect of medicines management and drug information for hospital in- and outpatients, and also for hospital-based personnel who are treating patients in their own homes, e.g. midwives and some community nurses. There are also many types of health clinic that need pharmaceuticals, either to treat patients on the spot such as dental clinics, or to provide items for later use at home, such as head lice shampoos and family planning requirements. This chapter surveys the varying needs and methods of supplying the differing units. It is important to remember that a flexible approach is needed, and a genuine interest in and concern for the users' needs is essential for a successful service. It is a good philosophy to adopt the principles of the Medicines Act 1968, i.e. to control the safety, quality and efficacy of medicines, and to extend this to the point of use as far as possible. To achieve this, advice must be given on storage, stock management and methods of drug use and prescribing, as well as administration methods. Pharmacists can hope to achieve this only by making the most of opportunities to visit users and by building up a good working relationship. It is not necessary or desirable to have a pharmacy in every unit. Typically, large National Health Service (NHS) trusts will have one central pharmacy in the district general hospital (DGH) providing pharmaceutical services not only to its own wards and departments, but also often on a contract basis to neighbouring trusts.

For some years, it has been health care policy to discharge patients from inpatient care into the community. This has led to greater integration between community and hospital pharmaceutical services. In parallel with this, the introduction of new treatment models such as home care teams and early discharge schemes has generated a need for the provision of aftercare, and also, in some cases, ongoing care for acutely ill patients in their own homes. Treatments that would have necessitated hospital admission in the past, such as cytotoxic chemotherapy, dialysis, intravenous (IV) therapy for human immunodeficiency virus (HIV) patients, parenteral and enteral nutrition, are all now regularly undertaken in the home. Considerable pharmacy support may be needed to deliver such treatment modes successfully. In this and in other ways, the hospital pharmaceutical service has evolved and diversified, with the development of new specialities and services.

Pharmacy managers have to compete for scarce funding to maintain and develop their services. They have to convince non-pharmacists of the value of professional services, since traditionally pharmacy has been regarded simply as a supply function. Other workers are not always aware of their own needs for pharmaceutical advice and may not value other services that can be offered relating to the use of medicines. A powerful tool is now available to support the role of the pharmacy within the organisation. This is an NHS Executive Controls Assurance Standard:[1] an audit document listing standards for handling medicines at every stage within the organisation, clearly defining the key responsibilities of the chief pharmacist. This document refers to an earlier document giving guidelines for medicines management within hospitals – the Duthie Report.[2]

Ward and department stock drugs

Hospital pharmacies usually supply commonly used items to wards as ward stocks and less frequently used items on an individual-patient basis. Other systems of supplying wards are in use, either using exclusively ward stock packs, or alternatively entirely individualised dispensed packs on a daily basis for each patient. The latter is known as 'unit dose dispensing', and was originally developed in the USA to meet the needs of a service where treatment costs must be invoiced to the patient with accuracy. In this system, the ward medicine trolley has a separate drawer for each patient, and the pharmacy places the doses needed for each day's treatment into it. Few NHS hospitals in the UK have adopted this labour-intensive system, although it is used in the private sector where, as in the USA, the additional staff costs can be passed on to the patient. This may change with the need to assign accurately the costs of patients' treatment to clinical directorates, and to enable accurate cost data to be captured for contracting. The main difficulty with the traditional method is the problem of accurately apportioning the costs of ward and departmental stocks to individual consultants in mixed-speciality wards, and in facilities such as operating theatres and diagnostic imaging departments.

As well as to wards, stock supplies are made to virtually every department and clinic within a trust, and thus the processing of stock orders may form a major part of the work of the pharmacy. Ward stock items are issued as original packs. Child-resistant closures should be avoided, since nurses find them inconvenient. The pack's contents are administered to every patient on the ward at the time for whom that item has been prescribed, unlike an individually dispensed item, which may be administered only to the patient whose name appears on the label. Other ward stocks will be items used by nurses without a pre-scription – for example, disinfectants and staff antiseptic hand scrub – so-called 'nursing items'. In departments dealing with outpatients or casualties, as well as items to be administered by nurses, there may be items to be issued by nurses, either as a result of nurse prescribing or under the authority of a patient group direction. In all cases, the quan-tity in the pack will be chosen with regard to the shelf-life, turnover and availability of commercial packs. Where no suitable commercial pack exists, repacks produced in large batches in the hospital's own produc-tion unit or purchased from a licensed repacking unit are used. By con-trast, individually dispensed items bear the patient's name, should be administered only to that person and should accompany him/her if transferred to another ward. Here the quantity supplied relates to the expected length of the course of treatment or to the anticipated stay in the ward. Such items should not be allowed to become ward stocks by default.

Control of ward stock lists

The stock list must be drawn up in consultation with the ward staff, but in so doing some control over the items included must be exercised. Nurses like to have as many items as possible as stocks since they see them as being more convenient than individually dispensed items. Stock lists should be reviewed on a frequent regular basis, using retrospective data about turnover and usage, which will permit the removal of slow-moving or obsolete items and the adjustment of stock levels up or down. It is important to be clear about the intended use of items since this may affect their presentation and labelling. Some potential pitfalls are listed in Table 6.1.

A typical ward stock item would be a medicine that at least five or six patients would be receiving at a time, not too expensive, with a good shelf-life and no major contraindications. It is important to remember that, even with regular ward pharmacy visits, many doses will be admin-istered before a pharmacist has checked the prescription. Thus it is not wise to give ward stocks of drugs which are often the subject of

Table 6.1 Control of stock lists – factors to consider

All departments	Consider **policies**, e.g. antibiotic, control of infection, agreed nursing and medical procedures
	Are items to be **supplied** or **administered** under patient group directions? Have these been legally drafted?
	Risk management: avoid known hazards, e.g. undiluted potassium chloride ampoules
Diagnostic imaging departments	Bowel preparations may be issued with appointment letters – are they suitably packaged and labelled for individual patients?
Chiropodists	May **supply** patients – caution required with POMs, labelling
Opticians	May **supply** patients – caution required with POMs, labelling
Occupational health departments	Are there current signed authorisations for qualified occupational health nurses for items to be administered or supplied?

POMs, Prescription Only Medicines.

prescribing errors. An example might be nystatin tablets – many inexperienced doctors do not realise that they are not suitable for systemic infections.

Creating stock orders

It is common for nurses to reorder ward supplies, but other methods are being explored, with the aim of saving nurse time and achieving better stock management. One tried-and-tested method is a top-up service, run by pharmacy technicians or assistants, who visit the ward regularly to monitor and reorder stock. This system uses more pharmacy staff time, but according to a 1985 study by Collins et al.,[3] this is more than offset by the savings on drugs wasted on the wards. Then it was an experimental system, but now its worth is acknowledged by the medicines management standards document.[1] The value of wards' drug stocks is high – between £2000 and £3000 for an average surgical or medical ward respectively – and even a modest reduction across all the stock-holding departments of a large hospital may result in substantial savings on money tied up in stock. Langham and Boggs[4] recently described the work of ward-based technicians within a medical directorate. Their role was wider than simply running a top-up service, since they also

Table 6.2 Ward-based technicians' stock management role

Orders stock drugs; unpacks and puts away deliveries
Organises and rationalises drug items in drug trolleys, ensuring current items only
Keeps stock cupboards tidy and returns unwanted items to pharmacy
Updates stock lists in liaison with clinical pharmacists and ward managers

undertook some monitoring of patients' charts and supply of individually dispensed items. Their duties in connection with ward stocks are summarised in Table 6.2.

These authors did not attempt to quantify the saving of nursing time in processing drugs, but were able to demonstrate a number of other benefits. Elsewhere, methods of reordering using electronic data capture have been piloted (see below).

How often ward stock orders are delivered depends on local circumstances, such as the rate of use and the capacity of storage facilities. Infrequent deliveries may encourage nurses to hoard because they feel insecure and in the long run they may prove uneconomical because of stock wastage. If stock levels are set too low, wards will run out at busy times and will have to order on a one-off basis. These items must be provided, since by definition stocks are frequently used items and failure to make them available will mean that wards will borrow and improvise. However, such practices are unsafe and inefficient for both the ward and the pharmacy.

Processing ward stock orders

Traditionally, in-house ward stock order assembly has been the norm, with a technician-led team operating in a centralised bulk distribution area arranged like a supermarket. Alternatively, instead of having a separate area devoted to assembling ward orders, order processing may take place within the local DGH pharmacy store to avoid double-handling of stocks. In either case, this may not be the most cost-efficient method. Various new models of stock distribution are being developed, some utilising direct supply from an outside supplier, and it is not yet clear which, if any, of these will become established universally. Karr[5] makes a case for stock distribution from a centralised NHS pharmaceutical store (CNPS). This method utilises the existing facility of a large centralised store under pharmacy management, which supplies several hospitals clustered around it, although not all within the same trust.

Medicines cost reductions are achieved by bulk buying many items direct from manufacturers. One of the less obvious operational benefits Karr cites is that neighbouring units are likely to use the same computer system, with compatible data files. Such systems, where supplies for at least the clients within the same trust may be requisitioned rather than ordered, may reduce the administrative workload by reducing the need for official orders and invoice-matching procedures. (See Chapter 11 for ordering procedures.) This model has the advantage of maintaining pharmaceutical control of the supply chain, a principle upheld by both the Controls Assurance Standard – Medicines Management[1] and the Duthie Report.[2]

Another option being piloted is similar to the CNPS, with the exception that the centralised store is under the management of the NHS supplies organisation rather than under pharmacy management. Although superficially similar to the previous system, this method may create problems for users as the staff operating it have not had a background in pharmacy and ward procedures.

There are other pilots in progress of ward distribution direct to the users from wholesalers, now known as ward order assembly. One such pilot at Perth Royal Infirmary is described by Low *et al*.[6] Data were captured during top-up visits using hand-held terminals; these were downloaded and subsequently edited using the AAH Hospital Service Mediate System. More details of the method and costing are to be found in the paper.[6] Results showed that there were some excess medicines costs compared with the previous conventional method of distribution; to offset this, there were savings in pharmacy staff costs, stock holdings and space requirements. The various ways of undertaking ward distribution are summarised in a paper by Radley.[7]

Whatever method of assembly is used, safe and prompt distribution to the users must be assured. Stocks must be protected from pilferage in transit: the usual way is to use a lockable ward pharmacy box. Training should be provided for portering staff. The trust transport policy should contain specific references to transporting medicines and medical gases. Written procedures for transport drivers should cover aspects such as security, handling temperature-sensitive supplies and safety procedures for spillage.

Controlled Drugs

The Professional Standards Directorate of the Royal Pharmaceutical Society of Great Britain (RPSGB) Fact Sheet *Controlled Drugs and*

Hospital Pharmacy[8] covers the legal aspects, but may not prepare one for the scale of the operation in a busy DGH pharmacy, where around 100–150 Controlled Drug (CD) requisitions may be processed each week. Carefully drafted procedures are required for every stage in the supply and delivery process, and these should be audited regularly and with a high profile to act as a deterrent to staff contemplating theft. Sadly, this is all too common, and thus a high level of awareness is necessary. (See the section on monitoring Controlled Drugs, below.)

Supplying Controlled Drugs

Most CDs are issued as ward stocks. Although in law there is no requirement for nurses to keep a stock record book showing details of use, in fact it is recommended good practice for them to do so.[2, 9] Supplies made to individual patients are often entered into the ward CD stock record book in order to record their administration. There is no objection to this, provided that the drug is not given to anyone else. Order/requisition and stock record books for both wards and pharmacy have been standardised nationally and are available from the Stationery Office. Unused books should be kept in a secure place, preferably serially numbered and issued against a signature to an authorised person. This prevents audacious thieves from providing themselves with an order book and ordering their supplies openly from the pharmacy – as has been known to happen! CDs must be delivered to wards in a locked box; the standard order gives a space for the messenger to sign a receipt, and to obtain a signature upon handing over the drugs to the ward. Individual prescriptions may also be dispensed; these are ordered by the ward nursing staff in the same order book as ward stocks. No such order is needed when the drugs are handed directly to the patient or his/her representative, e.g. when the supply is to an outpatient.

Storing Controlled Drugs

CD storage in hospital pharmacies must comply with the Safe Custody Regulations 1973; steel cupboards connected to a burglar alarm system are usually used, but alternatives giving equal protection would be permissible. Advice should be sought from the crime prevention officer of the local police.

In wards, a wall-mounted cupboard with a warning light that is activated when the door is open must be used. Dead locks which will not permit the key to be removed unless it is turned are required to prevent the cupboard from being closed but not locked. In some departments such as operating theatres, there may be a repeater warning light in, for example, the theatre manager's office. Irrelevant items such as patients' wedding rings and spare laryngoscope bulbs may *not* be stored in the CD cupboard.

Unwanted Controlled Drugs

In law, ward managers are allowed to destroy CDs held as ward stocks without a witness, but it is good practice for such transactions to be witnessed by a second person; many hospitals require this to be a pharmacist. Entries should be made in the CD stock book, and signed by both parties. It is good practice for pharmacists to write (pharmacist/ MRPharmS) after their name, since they cannot later be identified from the nursing rota. The Misuse of Drugs Act 1971 permits nurses to return unwanted CD stocks to the pharmacy, where they may be returned to stock and reissued (always supposing that their quality is assured). It is important to impress on nurses that unwanted stocks are still subject to control, since in the author's experience (PS), they are likely to return them thoughtlessly to the pharmacy in the ward box. Drugs not suitable for reissue, including drugs brought in by patients, may be surrendered to a pharmacist but will ultimately have to be destroyed under supervision. Both their return and destruction must be documented in the pharmacy CD register.

The destruction of unwanted pharmacy stocks of drugs must be witnessed by an authorised person (Table 6.3). Those marked with an asterisk (*) were authorised for England only by a 1997 circular.[10]

Storage of pharmaceuticals on wards

Storage areas have to be adapted to local circumstances, but usually medicine cupboards are placed in the clean utility (or treatment) room. The cupboards listed in Table 6.4 are usually in use.

There is a detailed account of the requirements for the security and storage of medicines in hospital wards and departments in the Duthie guidelines.[2] Most wards also have a drugs trolley, which is used to transport the medicines around the ward during medicine administration rounds. This should be securely locked to the wall when not in use, well away from radiators.

Table 6.3 Controlled Drugs in hospitals: persons who may witness destruction

RPSGB inspectors
Police chemist liaison officers
Home Office Drugs Branch inspectors
Chief executives of NHS trusts[*]
Senior officers in an NHS trust who report directly to the chief executive and who
    have responsibility for health and safety, security or risk management[*]
Pharmaceutical advisers to health authorities[*]
Supervisors of midwives (midwives' Controlled Drugs only)

RPSGB, Royal Pharmaceutical Society of Great Britain; NHS, National Health Service.
[*]Authorised for England only by a 1997 circular.[10]

Table 6.4 Ward drug storage

Internal medicines cupboard	
Controlled Drugs cupboard	Often within internal medicines cupboard
External medicines cupboard	
Disinfectants cupboard	Sometimes called 'lotions' cupboard by older nurses
Drugs refrigerator	Large enough for TPN if appropriate
Urine-testing reagent cupboard	Often in sluice
Clean area for IV and irrigation fluids	Only this need not be lockable

TPN, total parenteral nutrition; IV, intravenous.

Monitoring ward stocks

The pharmacist's responsibility for the quality of the pharmaceuticals used in a hospital extends to the point of use, and thus it is his/her lot to arrange for the regular inspection of ward and departmental stocks by pharmacy staff and to advise on storage conditions. There should be a written procedure to follow and a record of findings and dates of visits. A written report of inspections with comments should be produced; this should be discussed with and signed by the ward sister/charge nurse or a responsible staff nurse. On subsequent visits, it is then possible to undertake follow-up.

The following points should be considered when training staff to undertake this task:

* Uncritical demeanour: the approach should be a friendly offer of help, without a lofty air of criticism. Nurses are more likely to ask for help and cooperate with reducing stocks if they do not feel

threatened by the visit, which should always be at a time arranged with the ward manager and convenient for the ward. Problems should be discussed in private with the ward manager who will not want the juniors to hear your views on any shortcomings, however tactfully expressed.

- Cleanliness and hygiene: overcrowded storage areas are difficult to clean, and heavy boxes of fluids may obstruct cleaners. Spilt sugary liquids attract cockroaches in old, cold buildings and pharaoh's ants in new, warm buildings.
- Stock rotation: it is often difficult to convince busy nurses that new stock must be put away behind old. It pays to check that they have.
- Correct stock levels: it should be possible to assess stock levels by checking issue dates and reviewing stock orders. Unused stock should be taken back in time to reissue it where appropriate. Both ward and finance managers will be interested to receive details of the money with which they have been credited in this way – an easy way to justify expenditure on a quality pharmacy service.
- Appropriate storage: check that items are stored in the correct cupboard. Check flammables – are they well away from oxidising agents; properly closed; dangerously close to or inside electrical apparatus, e.g. refrigerators; well-labelled; stored near oxygen cylinders or combustible materials such as stocks of dressings? Advise against taking cardboard or other potentially contaminated outer containers into clean areas such as dialysis rooms. Remember that stocks must not be stored directly on floors with under-floor heating.
- Refrigerators: a separate, lockable refrigerator with temperature monitoring must be provided for medicines, and it should never be used for foods, pathological specimens, including blood and urine samples, or anything else. A suitable design is available on NHS Supplies contract, but this model may not be large enough for some users. Adequate dedicated refrigeration should be provided for total parenteral nutrition (TPN) solutions and cytotoxics. Many nurses refrigerate items that could be stored at room temperature such as heparin, and this explains some of the complaints that ward refrigerators are too small. It is advisable to check that items such as antibiotic syrups are being returned to the refrigerator after the medicine round, as they are often overlooked and left at room temperature for hours on end in the medicine trolley.

Monitoring Controlled Drugs

The CD cupboard must be inspected only by a pharmacist, in the presence of a nurse, to protect the pharmacist from suspicion should a stock discrepancy come to light. It is the ward manager's responsibility to account for the stock on a day-to-day basis; only with the Duthie guidelines[2] has it been considered that the pharmacist should audit that every item is correct. The stock record book should be examined to see that it is being correctly maintained. The possibility of theft should be borne in mind; unfortunately, many people are so unsuspecting that this may go undetected for long periods.

Pharmacists should be aware of some of the ways in which misappropriation of ward stocks may occur. The author has observed all of the following:

- false entries in ward stock book (extra doses recorded for genuine patients; doses recorded but not administered; doses of two drugs apparently given to same patient at the same time; fictitious patients; doses continued after the patient has died or has been discharged);
- wrong totals carried forward when new stock book started;
- stock book lost under mysterious circumstances;
- pages torn out of stock book or obliterated by spillage;
- ampoules broken or substituted and even powder replaced with another substance;
- forgery of pharmacist's entry recording drugs returned or destroyed;
- theft of individually dispensed items, patients' own drugs and take-home items.

A roll call of all the items listed in the stock book should be completed in case anything has disappeared altogether. Any problems must be investigated immediately, and if unresolved must be reported to senior nurse management. If preliminary investigation points to theft, the hospital management must be informed, and advised to call in the police.

Midwifery services

Hospital obstetrics units in general are run like ordinary hospital wards, ordering their pharmaceuticals in the usual way. Although registered midwives attending a home delivery may prescribe certain drugs, after the 1958 Aitken Report,[9] midwives working in hospitals ordered and administered only medically prescribed drugs in the same way as other registered nurses. Since 1984[11] midwives have been able to administer drugs during labour under the authority of standing orders signed by medical staff, thus being ahead of their colleagues in other branches of nursing. Patient group directions[12] are applicable to midwifery as to other branches of the profession, and should be drafted as set out in the circular. (See Chapter 1 for details of patient group directions and nurse prescribing.)

Community midwives

Although home deliveries are now unusual, the hospital maternity unit will probably be the practice base of a team of community midwives. Their work mainly consists of providing aftercare to mothers recently discharged home with their babies. They obtain stock drugs from the hospital pharmacy using an ordinary ward stock list and a ward box. Small pack sizes of drugs are needed, since they use very small quantities of most items, and slow turnover is likely to be a problem.

Midwives may order those CDs which they are allowed to possess and administer (currently pethidine and pentazocine) using a Midwife's Supply Order, usually countersigned by the local supervisor of midwives, who will be the senior midwifery nurse manager in the trust. Drugs ordered may be supplied by a community pharmacy, but more often are supplied by the hospital pharmacy that provides their other drug requirements. Unwanted drugs may be returned to the pharmacy that supplied them for reissue or destruction as above. Alternatively their destruction may be supervised by the supervisor of midwives.

Midwifery 'flying squad'

In the event of an obstetric emergency arising suddenly in the home, midwives are able to summon a 'flying squad' – a doctor with extra equipment and drugs to resuscitate the mother or infant before transfer to hospital by ambulance. Pharmacists should be aware of the local arrangements for this, and should ensure that the drugs are properly presented and regularly checked for expiry dates, like other emergency kits.

Hospital inpatients

Prescribing for inpatients

In hospital wards medicines are prescribed sequentially on prescription sheets which, in addition to recording all current medication, also allow

Table 6.5 Specialised prescription sheets

Anticoagulant therapy	
Intravenous therapy	Fluids and electrolytes plus drug additions
	Total parenteral nutrition
	Cytotoxic regimens
Irrigation solutions, e.g. bladder irrigations	May include input and output data
Diabetic	For sliding scales of insulin
Subcutaneous analgesia	Must comply with the Misuse of Drugs Act 1971
Patient-controlled analgesia	Must comply with the Misuse of Drugs Act 1971
Continuous epidural analgesia	

nurses to record the doses as they are administered. There is no standard design for such sheets, which may vary even between wards within the same trust, since lay-outs appropriate for acute services may not be suitable for long-stay patients. In addition to the standard medicines prescription sheet, there are likely to be others designed to meet special requirements. Some possible examples are listed in Table 6.5, although not all will be in use on every ward.

Hospitals have been slow to introduce electronic prescribing, because there are many difficulties to overcome. There have been a number of pilots, most using modified software originally designed for the USA, where the requirement to charge treatment to individual inpatients has given impetus to the development of hospital information systems. These have required substantial modification to function satisfactorily in the UK. Doctors in the USA rarely enter their own prescriptions into computers; they write 'doctors' orders' on slips of paper, and these are transcribed by ward clerks, or in some cases by nurses or ward pharmacists. Systems relying on transcription by non-medical staff were banned by the Gillies Report[13] in the UK following work analysing and quantifying medication errors undertaken in the 1960s.[14–17] Since hospital computer systems in the UK are not standardised, junior medical staff will have to be taught to use differing systems as they work in various hospitals during their training. A further complication is that within the hospital service there is no nationally recognised database for drugs, so nomenclature is liable to vary as locally developed drug files are used. The database used by the Prescription Pricing Authority (PPA) for FP10s omits many drugs used in hospitals and, as it records every presentation of the drugs it does include, does not readily support formulary management.

Prescribing systems should be compatible with the main hospital information system, which handles patient registration data and records admissions and discharges. They also have to be compatible with the pharmacy systems handling stock control, labelling and drug cost data. In the NHS plan for pharmacy,[18] the government states that electronic prescribing will become routine in hospitals by 2004, which leads one to hope that resources may become available to address the problems discussed. In 1998, a conference on the subject of electronic prescribing was held at the Royal Pharmaceutical Society. Its proceedings were later reported in a series of papers.[19] Speakers covered many aspects, including the ethical and legal issues, such as the handwriting requirements for CD prescriptions and the need to have strictly controlled access to prescribing and confidential patient data.

In many hospitals, medical students may gain experience by being attached to medical and surgical teams ('student assistantships'). Their terms of employment are set out in a circular.[20] They are not allowed by law to initiate treatment or write prescriptions, and any nurse who administered a 'prescription' for a Prescription Only Medicine (POM) written by a medical student would be committing an offence under the Medicines Act 1968. Although the circular does not specifically say so, medical students should not write treatment on prescription sheets for later signature by a qualified doctor, since the signing may never happen, or there may be a substantial delay during which the drug may be administered. Hospital authorities should issue students with a guidance statement when they commence duties.

An important difference between hospital and community pharmacy practice is that, by prior agreement with the medical staff, usually through the Drug and Therapeutics Committee, brand or generic substitution takes place in most hospitals. This is acknowledged in the RPSGB Code of Ethics. Usually only one brand of a drug is stocked, and this may have been bought at a favourable price through a regional or local contract. Only if a consultant insists on a certain brand or if there is a bioavailability difference would a particular brand be supplied. In some cases the contract may be for the national brand leader – it is a common fallacy among lay persons that all drugs could be made available in cheap non-branded forms made by obscure drug companies!

Administration of medicines to hospital inpatients

The standard scenario is for ward nurses to give out medicines from a lockable medicines trolley during a medicine round of the ward which takes place at set times during the day. Reference is made to the doctor's prescription for every administration, and no drugs are given unless prescribed by a doctor. This includes even simple remedies, which outside the hospital would be available over-the-counter. In some situations, patient group directions may be in force, but they are not intended to replace prescriptions for individual patients, and would be difficult to justify in acute units with medical staff giving 24-hour cover. In 1986 the UK Central Council for Nursing, Midwifery and Health Visiting in an Advisory Paper (*Administration of Medicines*) recommended that qualified nurses should administer medicines on their own without a second person checking. This conflicted with the view expressed previously by the Aitken Report that medicine administration should be checked by a second nurse. Each administration is recorded at the time, to prevent inadvertent omissions or duplications. Only one prescription sheet of each type is used for a patient at a time, and it should be a chronological record of all current treatments. A way is needed for non-stock items to be dispensed without sending the prescription sheet away from the ward; ideally a clinical pharmacist visits the ward on a regular basis and notes what is required. At the same time, it is convenient to discuss problems and offer advice. From such simple origins 30 years ago, the modern concept of clinical pharmacy developed.

Under certain circumstances, patients may self-administer their medicines. There is no reason why competent patients should not look after and administer long-term medication, although at times they may require assistance, e.g. postoperatively. Sometimes supervised self-medication is introduced prior to discharge, e.g. for patients with learning difficulties who may be preparing for life in the community. Self-medication schemes require some planning. Written procedures should be agreed to include as a minimum the following points:

- Criteria must be set for patient admission to the scheme (or exclusion from the scheme).
- There must be lockable storage available at each bed space (the patient in the next bed may be wandering and confused).
- Staff should not abdicate their professional responsibility, and should check that medicines are being administered correctly.
- Medicines must be individually dispensed and labelled with directions, rather than administered from ward stocks.
- If patients are to use their own medicines brought into hospital, checks of identity and quality should be carried out by a competent member of staff; this applies equally when the nursing staff are to administer the drugs.

In 1991, the Standing Pharmaceutical Advisory Committee produced a policy document[21] about the extended use of patients' own drugs in hospitals; this remains in force. Recently, Dua[22] described a scheme introduced in Southampton where treatment was continued using patients' own drugs, although not self-administered. This paper includes an excellent algorithm to be followed when determining whether medicines are suitable for continued use.

It should be noted that, in law, patients' own drugs remain their property unless voluntarily surrendered; they should not be destroyed until it is reasonably certain that their return will not be demanded; without safeguards, the hospital may have to compensate irate patients who are aggrieved by their loss. Under no circumstances may patients' drugs be added to ward stocks and used for other patients.

Dispensing for individual inpatients

Most pharmacy departments have either one dispensary handling both in- and outpatient prescriptions or a separate dispensary for outpatient prescriptions. Some hospitals have, however, adopted an American idea, having satellite pharmacies situated within units – 'near-patient dispensing' or, when part of a broader picture, 'patient-focused care'. This appears to have advantages, in that the staff become integrated with the ward team, and can supply their requirements in a timely fashion. In 1994, Bunn et al.[23] and Blain et al.[24] described the setting-up of patient-focused pharmacy services at St Helier NHS Trust and Kingston Hospital respectively. In each case, the concept was adopted not only for pharmacy, but also for other services normally provided from a central base, e.g. at St Helier, X-ray and hotel services. On the face of it, this seems an excellent idea, but there are major resource implications, since satellites require adequate staffing and also duplication of stocks and, in some cases, equipment. Bunn,[25] commenting 3 years later on the operation of satellites in the UK, considers that the staffing levels required to operate efficiently are neither prevalent nor attainable, except perhaps in some teaching hospitals.

Wherever items are dispensed, the principles remain the same. Except in hospitals where prescriptions are transmitted to the dispensary electronically, individual inpatient items are dispensed by reference either to the doctor's prescription or to a ward pharmacy slip. These prescriptions are written mainly by the house officers since they are responsible for the day-to-day medical care of ward patients. The house officers in general medical and surgical wards are often in their preregistration year, i.e. provisionally registered. As they are inexperienced, many errors and ambiguities creep in – in a survey conducted by the author (PS), about 20% of prescriptions needed some intervention by the pharmacist. Considerable tact is needed when dealing with these problems, since at this stage doctors will form an impression of the pharmaceutical profession that may colour their attitude for the rest of their career.

The work of the dispensary must be organised so that prescriptions and ward pharmacy orders are dispensed in rotation, without undue delay. This will not happen if it is left to chance. A pharmacist should check all prescription sheets as they are received, and deal with queries as soon as possible. If an item is not available, it is worth considering any possible alternatives in stock and offering them to the prescriber, who would often prefer treatment to start immediately. Items that take a long time can then be started promptly, and if there are several queries for one doctor, one telephone call will suffice. Juniors must be supervised to see that they do their fair share of the unpopular items.

The following list gives a procedure for checking prescriptions, whether on the ward or in the dispensary. (See also Chapter 5.)

- Check patient's name for legibility; one forename plus surname must go on the label in case there are two patients with the same name on the ward.
- Check age, weight and drug allergies.
- Check ward name – this will be needed for delivery.
- Check consultant's name – this gives clues about diagnosis and may be needed for costing.

By now a mental picture of the patient should have been formed, and, with practice, a good idea of the range of likely diagnoses.

- Read the prescription; make sure it is still current.
- Check the dose, bearing in mind the age, weight, possibility of poor renal or liver function and other relevant factors.
- Read the other prescriptions and think of interactions/additive side-effects/two agents with similar activities or two compounds with the same ingredients. Check the 'when required' section of the chart as well.
- Check the availability and presentation of the drug. Consider which preparation is most suitable for the patient: for example, tablets are no use if the patient has a nasogastric tube or is 2 weeks old.

- Work out the quantity needed. Prepare the label so that the container can be labelled immediately it is filled. Prepare work sheets and calculations.
- Dispense the item; complete one item before starting the next. Leave items and original containers together for checking.
- Take an interest in the checking: there may be useful lessons to be learned.

'Take-home' and 'weekend-leave' prescriptions

Many hospitals use a form which combines the 'take-home' (TTA/O or 'to take away/out') prescriptions with a brief discharge summary for the general practitioner (GP). The pharmacy should annotate this legibly with any details that will be needed for a repeat prescription, such as the tablet strength or preparation used. TTA prescriptions *must* be checked against the inpatient prescriptions and any variations queried, since transcription errors at this stage are some of the commonest prescribing errors encountered.

These items should be dispensed as though they were for outpatients, although they will probably be sent to the ward and not handed to the patient directly. This means that instructions for use must be really clear and detailed, since there is rarely a chance to counsel the patient first-hand. The ward pharmacist may have had a chance to do this, and should assess the need for dose aids (such as the Dosette – useful in the forgetful elderly), foreign-language instructions and lessons in the use of inhalers.

Intravenous fluids and additives

In 1976 the Breckenridge Report[26] was published, which made important recommendations about IV practice: where possible, admixtures should be prepared in the pharmacy, or bought ready-made, e.g. potassium chloride; the then health authorities (now trusts) were to establish policies about which medical and nursing staff were allowed to add drugs to IV infusions on the wards, and training was to be provided for them.

Most pharmacies have TPN compounding and cytotoxics reconstitution services, or obtain these services commercially, possibly from a licensed production unit in another trust. Many have set up a central intravenous additive service (CIVAS) for a wider range of drugs. After fatalities arising in 1994 from contaminated IV solutions,[27, 28] a study of unlicensed facilities was undertaken by Farwell.[29] This, and further studies of unlicensed aseptic dispensing facilities by the Medicines Control Agency, led to recommendations about quality control and standards in unlicensed units. (See Chapter 7.)

Some drugs, including antibiotics, electrolytes, vitamins, heparin and aminophylline, may be added to infusions on the ward. The regimen should be prescribed on a specially designed prescription sheet giving the sequence and volume of the IV solutions, the drip rate, and dose and method of administration of any added drugs. A separate prescription sheet should be used for each site if the patient has more than one infusion running at a time. This often happens during TPN when the hyperosmolar nutrition solutions are administered via a central venous catheter that delivers the fluid into the right atrium, and a peripheral line is used for the administration of other drugs. No substance intended for any other method of administration, e.g. bladder irrigations or enteral feeds, should be prescribed on the same sheet, since this could lead to inadvertent administration of an unsuitable drug by the IV route. For the same reason, IV containers must never be used for other types of preparation. Failure to observe these precautions has caused fatalities.

Clinical pharmacists working on wards should familiarise themselves with the various methods of giving IV drugs, particularly those which should be administered as a continuous drip, and which should be given as a bolus. Information is given in the *British National Formulary* (BNF),[30] and in manufacturers' summaries of product characteristics. Stability data will also be found in the *CIVAS Handbook*;[31] a further information source is the American *Handbook on Injectable Drugs*.[32] IV prescriptions should be checked for compatibility, taking into consideration the shelf-life of the admixture, particularly in slow-running infusions. Drug additions on the ward are often undertaken in far from ideal conditions, so contamination may be expected. Langford[33] has highlighted causes of IV contamination in Table 6.6.

Although nurses are supposed to be trained to make IV additions, in practice this training may be sketchy or omitted. Many drug administration errors by nurses have been recorded, some with serious consequences. The journal *Pharmacy in Practice* has a regular feature on drug-related errors. Cousins and Upton[34] illustrate an article about preventing IV drug administration errors with a table giving examples of errors reported at ward level.

Although it is possible to regulate the flow rate of infusions using a standard giving set, this is quite inaccurate, and it is increasingly common to use infusion pumps and syringe pumps to deliver an accurate

Table 6.6 Causes of microbial contamination in intravenous systems

Hairline cracks in bottles
Cumbersome and unwieldy bottle and closure systems, and difficulty in attaching
  administration sets, causing leaks
Flexible plastic containers, which are difficult to manipulate, and risk of touch
  contamination when attaching administration sets
Wrong administration set used
Dirty preparation area
Omission of hand washing
Touching of needle hubs and other critical points
Failure to swab vial top
Failure to close container or replace air filters on administration sets
Omission of cleaning procedures
Filling multiple syringes from one vial or infusion bag
Preparing syringes hours in advance of use, or on the night before use
Reusing syringes and pump lines on multiple patients
Misuse of vacuum pumps
Inadequate aseptic filtration
Inappropriate storage conditions
Inadequate transfer procedures into clean air devices
Long-term use of administration sets and filling lines
Leaking isolator covers and general failure to maintain equipment
Combination of several of the above practices on any one occasion

Adapted with permission from Langford S A. Mortality and morbidity from the in-use microbial contamination of intravenous products. *Hosp Pharm* 1999; 6: 104–109.

flow rate when drugs are being administered intravenously. Clinical pharmacists should ensure that they understand the devices in use in their hospital, and are able to check that prescriptions are appropriately written. Some drugs are commercially available in prefilled syringes suitable for use in common makes of syringe pump. If the pharmacy is planning to fill syringes, or purchase them ready-made, compatibility with ward equipment must be confirmed. There was a special feature on infusion devices in the *Hospital Pharmacist* in 1998, in which the various types available, including those used for patient-controlled analgesia, were described.[35, 36]

Hospital outpatients

Many patients who consult hospital doctors in outpatient clinics require supplies of medicines, either for long periods if they are hospital-only products, or until they can return to the care of their GP. Patients attending accident and emergency (A&E) departments may also require medicines. Prescriptions may be dispensed by the hospital pharmacy, or the hospital doctor may prescribe on an FP10(HP) prescription form to be dispensed at a community pharmacy. Most hospitals use both methods of supply at times; the decision whether to use one or the other is based on the presence of an adequately staffed pharmacy on site, numbers of pharmacy staff and timing of clinics. Either way, the cost of the service is borne by the hospital, since the cost of the FP10(HP) prescriptions is calculated by the PPA as for GP prescriptions, then charged to the health authority, which reclaims the money from the trust.

The relative economics of the two methods have been hotly debated for many years. Most people now consider that in-house dispensing is cheaper. To offset the staff salaries, cost of stock and overheads, savings arise from various factors. For example, generally hospitals practise brand/generic substitution even when branded drugs have been named on the prescription. (N.B.: community pharmacists must not.) The medical staff must have agreed to this policy, but nowadays it is almost universally accepted, unless a consultant has a reason for excluding a certain item. It is thus possible to minimise the range of brands stocked and to negotiate, either regionally or locally, better prices for bulk purchases. It is also easier to monitor that prescribing conforms with locally agreed policies when dispensing is done in the hospital pharmacy – for example, in many places the length of time for which drugs may be prescribed is limited. When attempting to make comparative costings, it is important to be aware that Value Added Tax (VAT) is paid on drugs purchased for hospital dispensing, but not on drugs purchased for use in community pharmacies. This means that prescriptions with a high ingredient cost will be significantly cheaper on FP10(HP); it is necessary therefore to calculate the relative numbers of cheap and expensive drugs in the study sample to get a true figure. (See Chapter 3 for a discussion of prescribing issues at the hospital–general practice interface.)

Although there have been attempts to standardise hospital documents nationally, no design has achieved national acceptance, and prescription sheets for in-house prescribing are designed locally. Many hospitals favour a card sheet cut to insert into the standard A4 case-note folder, since this provides a chronological record of items supplied at previous attendances. An alternative method is to use a one-off sheet for each occasion. Either way the sheet must be filed in a way which retains it for reference – within the pharmacy department, or preferably in the patient's case notes. While the Medicines Act 1968 requires the retention of prescriptions for POMs for 2 years from the date of supply, it is important to remember that hospitals are required by the Public Records Act 1958 and the Department of Health (DoH),[37] to retain patients' medical records, including prescriptions, for a minimum 8 years from the date of the last entry, and for some cases, e.g. maternity records, for 25 years.[38]

The heading of the prescription sheet must provide the following details:

- patient's surname;
- patient's forenames;
- sex;
- date of birth;
- hospital registration number (sometimes called unit number);
- consultant in charge of patient.

There should also be space to enter drug allergies and, particularly for children, weight at a given date.

Use and abuse of FP10(HP) prescription forms

It is important for hospitals to have good audit and security procedures for FP10(HP) prescription forms.[39] Quite apart from the obvious hazards of prescription forgery and drug abuse should the forms be stolen, their misappropriation can lead to major financial losses to the trust – both in paying for drugs for unauthorised persons and staff time spent in investigating fraud. Unused forms must be kept in a secure place and issued only to authorised users, keeping accurate records of serial numbers. Doctors must be aware of the need to guard against theft and should also be warned about the restrictions in use of the forms. The regulations for their use, originally stated in two early Department of Health and Social Security circulars[40,41] but not changed since, are:

- where a hospital or clinic has no dispensary of its own and it has not been possible to make regular and convenient arrangements for dispensing outpatient prescriptions at another hospital;
- where hospital pharmacies have had to restrict the services provided due to shortages of staff;
- clinics such as family planning clinics.

An earlier circular,[42] still relevant although not current, listed various irregularities in use that were to be avoided. These include:

- prescriptions for inpatients (this would include drugs to be taken home at discharge);
- prescriptions for persons who were not registered patients of the hospital, e.g. by doctors for themselves or their families, for other hospital staff other than in an emergency, for patients at other hospitals and for persons presumed to be private patients;
- prescriptions by doctors who were not members of the hospital staff.

The PPA returns the FP10(HP) forms to the Director of Finance of the trust when pricing procedures have been completed. The forms are accompanied by a summary statement of the charges and a computer print-out which lists all the items dispensed by each chemist contractor and the individual charges incurred. Unfortunately, there is a delay of several months. Taking a sample, auditors should check that the doctors' signatures are genuine, and that the doctor was employed by the trust at the time of writing. Hospital medical records are then checked to make sure that the patients were genuine and were seen on the day stated. A senior pharmacist should check either all or a sample of forms for evidence of forgery or misappropriation. When suspicions are aroused, the matter is reported to the hospital management and auditor for further investigation and action. Experience shows that misuse to a greater or lesser extent is quite common; wrongdoers are traced and disciplined as appropriate. In serious cases, prosecution ensues.

Dispensing for outpatients

Patients must always be welcomed with a friendly smile and a greeting; their view into the pharmacy should reveal tidily dressed busy staff behaving in a professional manner. Their opinion not only of this pharmacy but also of the profession at large may be formed at this moment. The pharmacy is often the last place to visit after a series of terrifying and embarrassing experiences – don't be surprised if patients begin to be irritable and aggressive, and do your utmost to send them away in a calmer state of mind.

Hospital prescriptions are charged in exactly the same way as those dispensed in a community pharmacy,[43] and hospital pharmacies are expected to carry out point-of-dispensing checks for exemption in the same way as community pharmacists.[44] In addition to these circulars, there is an NHS Executive publication, *The Pharmacist's Guide to Prescription Exemption*. There is an information leaflet for patients about exemptions, coded HC11. No charge is made for items administered on the premises. Exempt patients sign declarations on special hospital exemption forms, similar to the reverse of FP10 forms. These forms are returned to the trust's finance department where a sample should later be checked for veracity. Hospitals are supposed to provide a person – not a pharmacist – to give patients advice on claiming exemptions; in large departments it is cost-effective to employ a prescription reception-ist. Advising patients about their rights to exemption may require tact or even caution, since the pharmacist does not know what the doctor has told patients about their diagnosis and moreover there may be other people within earshot. Cash receipts should be recorded in a way that avoids the necessity for the pharmacy to keep accounts and be subject to detailed audit. This is usually achieved by having a ticket machine or a cash register. The latter method is simpler now that statutory charges change so frequently. Items prescribed and supplied by nurses under the authority of patient group directions are also subject to prescription charges, and arrangements must be made to levy them and deal with exemptions where this is taking place.

On occasions, patients may refuse to pay for their medicines or claim that they are unable to do so. In cases of genuine need, it may be possible for financial aid to be provided by the Department of Social Security. Some patients will promise to return with the money or send a cheque – as with other debtors, a record should be kept and reminders sent by the management. At times, considerable ethical dilemmas arise. Before refusing to supply a medicine to a patient who appears to be 'trying it on', the pharmacist should check with the doctor. At all times when the patient refuses the medicine, from any cause, the prescription sheet should be endorsed, to protect the pharmacist from an accusation of refusal to supply by the patient at a subsequent visit, and also so that the doctor is aware of the problem.

A numbered receipt system should be used to avoid handing out medicines to the wrong patient. It is surprisingly common for patients to answer to the wrong name or for two patients with the same name to be waiting at the same time. Many departments use a 'prescription-ready' indicator that displays the numbers in the waiting room.

The person receiving the prescription should also try to anticipate potential problems that may arise: for example, the arthritic patient will not be able to cope with a child-resistant closure, the partially sighted or those who may have language difficulties.

Because traditionally drugs were supplied to last from one appointment to the next, quantities are indicated by days or weeks.

Hospital doctors rarely indicate amounts to be dispensed for external preparations; a discreet enquiry to find out the site of application and reference to the section on guidance on prescribing of the BNF is needed.

Hospitals can supply non-*Drug Tariff*[45] items if prescribed for in-house dispensing (but not on FP10(HP)), but it must be remembered that the patient will then have to return to the clinic for all future supplies, unless he/she is willing to buy them outside the hospital, since repeat prescriptions cannot be made by his/her GP on form FP10. Because of the potentially serious results for the hospital's drugs budget, it is usual to supply non-*Drug Tariff* items only to exceptional cases.

Items are labelled with full directions; child-resistant closures or strip packaging are used. Patient information leaflets are supplied. The pharmacist must always check that the patient has any necessary ancillary equipment such as inhalers or syringes/needles, and is fully conversant with their use and upkeep. It is as well to confirm that arrangements have been made for injections to be given by the GP or community nurse. Water for Injections must always be supplied where needed – although few doctors think to prescribe it, and are surprised at its POM status. On an FP10/FP10(HP), the community pharmacist cannot supply this unless specifically prescribed.

At times, items will be owed to a patient. This may arise because patients choose to return later to avoid waiting or because they have no money, because the item has a short shelf-life, or because it had to be ordered. Owing slips should be issued for patients to produce when collecting their medicines. These should be cross-referenced with a carefully kept record of outstanding items, checked by a pharmacist, since this record will act as a surrogate prescription later. The record should include an indication of the urgency and the eventual method of supply – at times it may be necessary to post or deliver the item by hand. This record must be inspected regularly to ensure that items are not overlooked. If a patient fails to collect an essential item as arranged, the prescriber should be alerted.

Handing out the prescription should be done by the person who has dispensed the prescription if possible, and never by lay receptionists. After checking the patient's identity, the directions should be carefully explained. Well-designed pharmacies have a patient advisory cubicle where more detailed counselling and personal details can be discussed in privacy. However far from the truth it might be, the pharmacist or technician should always appear as if time were no object at this stage, as only then will the patient have the confidence to ask questions and fully benefit from the interview.

Hospital staff as patients

According to HSC 1999/082,[39] it is up to each trust to decide whether they will dispense prescriptions for their own staff. The usual practice is for hospital staff, including doctors, to be supplied only if they are registered patients of the hospital, or on prescriptions written by occupational health department doctors. If the pharmacy is registered with the RPSGB, private prescriptions for staff could of course be dispensed, but unless the pharmacy has an NHS contract, FP10s written by staff members' GPs should not be dispensed. All staff prescriptions must be properly documented and the appropriate prescription charge levied. Failure to do so may have serious consequences for the pharmacists involved, as reference to this report of the Statutory Committee proceedings will show.[46] Doctors should be discouraged from self-prescribing (although it is not illegal provided that FP10(HP)s are not used – even for CDs!). There should be a policy agreed with senior medical staff to regulate self-prescribing by medical staff. Preregistration house officers should not prescribe for themselves or colleagues (except on the wards if the latter are inpatients). The use of cumulative prescription sheets provides a simple method of surveillance to detect abuse at an early stage. All pharmacy staff must be aware of the need for absolute confidentiality when dealing with colleagues.

Private patients in NHS hospitals

Some NHS hospitals have accommodation reserved for the treatment of private patients, but private (paying) patients may also be treated in ordinary wards. In recent years, trusts have been permitted to use private practice as a form of income generation, and they are able to set charges on a commercial basis. There have been a number of private finance initiatives, in which trusts have entered into partnerships with commercial companies to provide facilities, with benefits on both sides. Some of these are diagnostic facilities, e.g. magnetic resonance imagers, but others provide a full range of services for inpatients. In some cases paying patients are from overseas and therefore not eligible for NHS treatment. There is a circular that sets out the criteria for eligibility to NHS treatment in the primary care setting; much of the information it contains would be equally applicable to hospitals.[47] It also explains the situation of European Economic Area nationals. The pharmacy must be familiar with the system for identifying and charging private patients within the trust, and must know whether charges are inclusive of medicines for inpatient therapy, or whether they are to be charged separately.

Outpatient treatment, if supplied from the hospital pharmacy, is usually charged on each occasion. Whatever system of documentation is used, pharmacists must expect it to be audited at regular intervals, and plan accordingly.

Intermediate care

For many years government policy has been directed towards supporting people in their own homes to minimise hospital admissions. This policy was reinforced in 2001 by the issue of guidance on the provision of such intermediate care,[48] and the allocation of £150m recurrent funding to health authorities to develop such services for older people. The service models falling into this category are:

- rapid response to illness in the home which might otherwise lead to hospital admission;
- hospital at home; either to avoid acute admission or to enable early discharge;
- short-term residential rehabilitation, e.g. in a community hospital or a rehabilitation centre;
- supported discharge, i.e. short-term nursing and/or therapeutic support in the patient's own home;
- rehabilitation in a day-care centre or a day hospital.

Such services have already been developed in many areas, with the establishment of home care teams of nurses whose practice base is within a hospital department, but whose job is to provide care for hospital patients nursed at home. The pharmaceuticals they administer are usually prescribed by hospital medical staff, and some may be supplied as ward stocks to the practice base of the team. However, shared-care policies will be agreed with local GPs, and in some cases, they may prescribe all or some of the drugs on form FP10. There may be specialist pharmacists and/or technicians appointed to manage the pharmaceutical aspects of home care, e.g. HIV pharmacists. Some examples of home care are shown in Table 6.7.

Table 6.7 Examples of home care

Postoperative wound care	Macmillan nurses (cancer patients)
Parenteral/enteral nutrition	Renal dialysis
IV antibiotics (cystic fibrosis and HIV)	Haematology

IV, intravenous; HIV, human immunodeficiency virus.

Supplies of sterile disposable items and sterile dressings not prescribable on FP10 will also be obtained via the hospital service, often through the central sterile supply department.

Community services

Community clinics

A considerable amount of health care is provided through community clinics managed by NHS trusts; some of these are changing their status to become primary care trusts. Community nurses, community psychiatric nurses, health visitors, various therapists and chiropodists staff and work from clinics, but some have doctors or dentists in attendance at certain times. Stock pharmaceuticals are supplied from a hospital pharmacy, typically by means of a weekly or monthly order delivered by trust transport in a locked pharmacy box. Individual prescriptions are dispensed at community pharmacies having been written on either form FP10(HP) or, in the case of school dental clinics, form FP10(D). Some items, such as welfare foods, vitamin tablets and family planning items, are handed out by the clinic nurses under the authority of patient group directions (see Chapter 1). Pharmacists supplying clinics should determine whether the staff are proposing to supply or administer Pharmacy (P) or POM items themselves or under the direction of a doctor, and ensure that the necessary authorisations are in place. Examples of community clinics are shown in Table 6.8.

If the trust managing the clinics does not have its own pharmacy, the service may be provided by a neighbouring trust. The contract should specify that there is a pharmacist and/or senior technician with special responsibility for providing advice to clinics. They should visit on a

Table 6.8 Examples of community clinics

Antenatal	Immunisation
Audiology/hearing aid	Mastectomy advice
Care of the elderly	Ophthalmic
Child health/assessment	Parentcraft
Chiropody	Psychiatric nurses
Dental	School clinics
Ear, nose and throat	Speech therapy
Enuresis	Stoma care
Family planning	Welfare foods

regular basis and assess needs, review stock lists and monitor the storage and use of pharmaceuticals. Such a service was described by Rambow.[49,50] Although written in 1985, the work is equally valid now, since she illustrates the benefits of regular visiting, by rationalising the range of stocks and promoting adherence to policies such as the local disinfectant policy.

The catalogue of items used by clinics is vast, and ranges from medical gases, anaesthetics, vaccines, 'the pill' and intrauterine devices, to medicated shampoos and chiropody supplies. The need for pharmaceutical advice is correspondingly large.

Childhood immunisation programme

Distribution of vaccines for the childhood immunisation programme has traditionally been a feature of clinic supply work. Details of the immunisation schedules may be found in the *Green Book*;[51] a new edition is expected shortly. Records of immunisations are held on computer in each health authority, both to call up patients as doses fall due, and to organise payments to GPs. The vaccines, with the exception of tetanus, are funded for by the DoH, and a central contract for the supply of vaccines has been placed, currently with Farillon Ltd, who will supply direct to both GPs and to community clinics, if required.

Close attention to maintaining the cold chain during the transport of vaccines to users is essential. Vaccines should be packed in prechilled insulated containers with cold blocks, and deliveries timed so that personnel are available to unpack and refrigerate supplies promptly. Quality assurance staff should monitor the effectiveness of the cold chain. Clinic staff must be trained in the importance of maintaining the cold chain, and should be given guidelines about returning in-use packs to the refrigerator promptly. Consideration should be given to transport between clinics and possibly to schools by nurses for vaccination sessions, and cold boxes should be used. Grassby[52] studied the storage conditions of vaccines within health authority clinics and found a number of examples of poor refrigerator performance. He proposed a number of points to address the problems of refrigerator storage he identified. These were:

- Not more than 50% of the internal space should be filled, with at least two slots of clear space allowed for on each shelf.
- One individual should be identified as responsible for monitoring and recording daily temperature readings.

- Daily temperature readings should be taken alternating between the top and bottom of the cabinet, using an external digital thermometer with internal temperature sensor.
- To prevent freezing, the coolest part should be adjusted to between 2 and 4°C, where polio vaccine should be stored.
- Each refrigerator should be independently checked every 6 months using calibrated thermocouples at three locations within the cabinet to confirm the mean temperature profile together with cyclical fluctuations, and refrigerators with excessive fluctuations or gradients should be replaced.
- Staff should be trained to understand the importance of correct storage procedures, and be aware of action to be taken after malfunctions.
- Opening and closing of refrigerators should be kept to a minimum.
- Defrosting should be carried out routinely.
- Where possible, domestic refrigerators should not be used.

Emergency procedures

Hospitals are used to dealing as a matter of routine with incidents that the general public regards as an unusual emergency; even so, some events occur so infrequently that they cannot be regarded as routine even in a hospital. Pharmacists, particularly those working in hospitals with large A&E departments, must be familiar with their role in procedures developed to cope with these, since their department may be called upon to provide extra stocks of drugs or unusual items at short notice, day or night. Some emergency plans may be required because of local circumstances, e.g. flood evacuation, but others, like the procedures for handling suspected rabies[53] and viral haemorrhagic fever[54] cases, are based on DoH publications.

Major incidents

All DGHs are required to have a major incident and service continuity plan to enable an immediate response to be coordinated with the emergency services.[55] A detailed handbook giving examples of major incidents in recent years and guidelines for planning has been published[56] and may be viewed on the NHS Executive website (www.doh.gov.uk/nhs.htm). There has to be a plan to deal with non-specific emergencies, e.g. a fire in the hospital, as well as one dedicated to major accidents. Since shortfalls in dealing with previous incidents have been identified, standards have been developed against which the effectiveness of the plan can be audited.[57, 58] Each hospital must have a plan of action, reviewed and rehearsed regularly. Departments such as the pharmacy must plan which staff will be called to the hospital, and how, should the need arise, and what they will do first when they get there.

A major incident (or accident) has been defined as one which because of the number and severity of live casualties requires special arrangements by the health service. Usually, the nearest hospital with an A&E department will be designated to receive the first wave of injured. Nearby hospitals will be informed that they are on stand-by ('support hospitals') should more casualties require treatment than the designated hospital can manage. Sometimes, hospitals more remote from the scene will be designated to receive casualties arriving by helicopter or from an airport, as happened during the Gulf War.

The emergency services set up an incident control unit at the scene, and organise the transfer of the injured to the appropriate hospital. A mobile team of medical and nursing staff may attend the incident to provide immediate medical care and also to assess the priorities for rescue and transfer. Alternatively, immediate care at the scene may be provided by specially trained GPs who specialise in dealing regularly with the badly injured in conjunction with the Ambulance Service at, for example, serious road traffic accidents. Such immediate-care doctors are organised into local teams, and may obtain certain supplies, e.g. IV fluids, from a nearby hospital pharmacy. They usually belong to the national organisation, the British Association for Immediate Care (BASICS).

Kits containing an agreed list of drugs and equipment are kept ready for mobile teams in A&E departments and should be inspected and updated regularly. CDs subject to Safe Custody Regulations 1973 and which are vulnerable to theft if kept in kits, and drugs requiring refrigeration, should be added to the kit immediately before it is taken to the incident.

Out-of-hours pharmaceutical service

Hospital pharmacy departments usually open $5^1/_2$–6 days per week during 'normal' working hours, although some have extended hours of opening during the day. There are various solutions to the problems caused by the fact that their patients are likely to need drugs on a 24-hour basis. One of these is to operate a residency scheme, in which a team of pharmacists forms a rota to provide cover round-the-clock by living in hospital accommodation on-site and being available to supply urgent items and advice. Several such schemes operate nationally, and give the participants very good experience of taking responsibility over a wide range of pharmaceutical activities.

A more usual way of providing emergency cover is to run an on-call scheme, where a number of pharmacists participate in a rota to provide advice, or to attend the hospital to supply urgently needed drugs at times when the pharmacy is closed. The usual method is for the on-call pharmacist to be contacted by the hospital switchboard via a mobile telephone or pager. Rota participants should be sufficiently experienced to be able to deal adequately with a wide range of clinical problems, and should have had specific training for their on-call duties. A portable file containing details of drug recall, major incident and other essential procedures must be provided and reviewed regularly, in addition to some basic drug information reference books.

Emergency cupboards

To avoid excessive demands on the on-call pharmacists, it is advisable to make a range of drugs available to the medical or nursing staff outside pharmacy hours. To permit access to the department is likely to be an unacceptable security risk; the best method is to provide a range of items in an emergency cupboard or small room to which access is restricted to medical staff and senior nurses. Items used must be recorded at the time, and the cupboard must be checked and replenished regularly.

Procuring drugs out-of-hours

Outside normal business hours the request for an urgently needed drug that is not in stock may cause considerable anxiety. There are a number of possibilities. The best chance is from another hospital, either via their on-call pharmacist, or by asking their switchboard to contact the medical registrar on duty. The borrower arranges transport – either hospital van or a taxi; in the latter case, if possible the driver should be furnished with a letter of identification written on headed notepaper. Clear instructions about the pick-up point and delivery point must be given. At the earliest opportunity, the borrower must contact the lending hospital's pharmacy and make arrangements for payment or replacement. Another possibility is to contact the manufacturer of the drug; many companies' switchboards are operated out-of-hours by security staff who will have home telephone numbers of senior staff for a dire emergency. Finally, some pharmaceutical wholesalers are willing for senior hospital pharmacists to have their home telephone numbers to use in a real emergency.

Cardiopulmonary resuscitation (CPR) and other emergency kits

Most wards and departments hold a special kit of drugs presented in prefilled syringes for emergencies – usually intended for the immediate treatment of cardiac arrests or anaphylactic shock. Kits can be purchased, or should be assembled in the pharmacy, and in either case, records should be kept of their locations, contents and expiry dates, so that they can be checked routinely. A standard procedure for adult advanced life support has been agreed by the European Resuscitation Council and the Resuscitation Council (UK). A flow chart based on this appears in the BNF.[30] Based on this procedure and standardised throughout the hospital, the drugs included in CPR kits must be agreed in consultation with a committee authorised to make decisions for all the medical staff, such as a resuscitation committee, which might be a subcommittee of a drug and therapeutics committee, with consultant representatives from the anaesthetic department, intensive therapy and cardiology. Opened kits should be returned to the pharmacy for reprocessing, and not topped up informally from ward stocks.

Pharmacists must ensure that paediatric CPR kits, with contents agreed in consultation with both resuscitation committee and paediatricians, are available at all locations where children may be treated or anaesthetised, e.g. operating theatres, intensive therapy units, diagnostic imaging departments and dental clinics. Anaphylactic shock kits, containing adrenaline (epinephrine) and possibly hydrocortisone are needed by community vaccination clinics, school nurses, and occupational health departments. There is official guidance[59] on the dosage schedule for adrenaline to be used in cases of anaphylaxis following immunisation. Contents of kits should be based on this advice.

Ward and clinical pharmacy

When pharmacists visited wards in the early days of ward pharmacy, they concerned themselves primarily with organising the supply of nonstock items, and with annotating the prescription sheets to prevent misinterpretation and hence administration errors. These tasks are still important, but in recent years the role of the pharmacist has expanded, and with the wide availability of clinical pharmacy training to certificate standard and beyond, many are able to participate in the clinical service as members of the ward team. Thus, the terms ward pharmacist and clinical pharmacist overlap, and it is to be hoped that in some future golden age all ward pharmacists will be competent clinical pharmacists. What exactly is a clinical pharmacist? There have been many attempts to arrive at a definition, but none is so far universally accepted. The pharmacist's unique expertise lies in supplementing a detailed knowledge of clinical pharmacology and therapeutics with the pharmaceutical aspects that are largely unfamiliar to doctors. Thus formulation science may enable the devising of a novel presentation of a drug, or a knowledge of the range of presentations available may enable the pharmacist to suggest substituting another agent where no suitable dose form exists for the original choice. Familiarity with excipients and additives will aid in the diagnosis of disease and adverse reactions. The clinical pharmacist's drug history-oriented approach may well mean that it is he/she who realises that the patient's glaucoma or urinary retention has been worsened by tranquillisers, or elucidates that his/her obstructive jaundice is a result of previous therapy for schizophrenia. Furthermore, he/she is the most likely to find that problems have been caused by non-prescription over-the-counter or 'fringe' medicines. Thus the clinical pharmacist makes a unique contribution to the therapeutic team.

Official recognition of the value of clinical pharmacy was achieved when a health circular[60] *The Way Forward for Hospital Pharmaceutical Services* set out a policy for health authorities: 'the aims are the achievement of better patient care and financial savings through the more cost effective use of medicines and improved use of pharmaceutical expertise obtained by implementing a clinical pharmacy service'. Authorities were instructed to plan for a comprehensive pharmaceutical service, including the provision of an adequate supply of trained staff.

The routine ward visit

Procedures will vary in different hospitals, but a typical ward visit is outlined below. After the initial courtesy of greeting the ward staff, the pharmacist should visit each bed and examine the prescription sheet for items prescribed since the last visit. One must *always* introduce oneself to the patient and explain the purpose of the visit. Newly admitted patients should be asked about previous drug therapy, and possible problems assessed. For example, a patient who is to have an operation may be 'nil by mouth' (see NBM sign on bed) for several days, and this will pose problems if he/she is receiving drugs for an underlying medical condition like Parkinson's disease or epilepsy. The administration record should be checked. If doses are being missed unaccountably, the pharmacist should look for a reason: a supply failure, or perhaps an inappropriate preparation of the drug; patients who vomit tablets, and those who are confused or disoriented may sometimes cope better with a liquid preparation.

Stock items are indicated – usually by writing 'S' against them – and a ward pharmacy order form completed for non-stock items. The prescription sheet should be annotated *legibly* with any details needed to ensure correct administration – Approved Names, calculations of volume and dilution instructions. Many pharmacists use red or green pens to make their notes stand out. Local practice will determine how many days' supply of inpatient treatment is ordered; it is usual to arrange matters so that all refills of continuous medicines fall due on the same day each week. On this 'top-up' day, the medicine trolley is checked and repeat supplies ordered. Doctors should be encouraged to prescribe TTA drugs in advance; these prescriptions should be checked against the inpatient regimen, and the patient given any necessary counselling.

While at the bed, other charts (Table 6.5; p.149) should be checked. This will give an overall picture of the patient. In some cases it will be helpful to refer to the patient's case notes: in an ideal situation, the pharmacist would check all notes for history of previous drugs, reason for present admission (e.g. could the symptoms have been caused by the drugs?) and other data such as renal function, blood chemistry results and microbiological sensitivities. In reality, few can spare the time, and so it is necessary to be selective. For example, renal function should be specifically checked where known problem drugs such as gentamicin have been prescribed; patients admitted for investigation of jaundice may provide clues from their drug history. On surgical wards, the operating lists are a quick way of spotting diagnoses and hence potential problems. A survey of the nursing notes also gives useful information and the reason for admission. Regular experience on a ward soon teaches how to get the most information in a brief time. Queries are dealt with where possible on the spot: these may be prescribing problems, but also the pharmacist should use every opportunity to urge compliance with local policies like the antibiotic policy. The economical use of drugs and nursing items should also be promoted. A record should be made of queries (sometimes called interventions) and their outcome in a logbook with numbered pages, cross-referenced with the prescription sheet. Logbooks should be carefully maintained, and retained for medicolegal reasons. The book should be used by any pharmacist covering that ward to avoid duplicating effort, and to provide continuity of care.

It takes training and practice to provide a fast and efficient service in the ward environment. To help inexperienced pharmacists make the best use of their time and to develop a systematic approach to prescription monitoring, Batty and Barber, then clinical pharmacy trainers in North-west Thames, devised a simple and effective scheme for clinical pharmacists which they describe in a paper[61] that could form the basis of a structured approach to the ward visit. Barber and Willson have also produced a pocket-sized handbook intended to be used as a quick reference for clinical pharmacists.[62] Pharmacists can also benefit from studying case studies such as those set out by Dodds.[63] An introduction to the theoretical principles underlying clinical pharmacy practice may be found in the book by Greene and Harris, which explains the pathology of disease states and discusses drug treatment in this context.[64]

In parallel with the development of clinical pharmacy, managers have monitored the work of clinical pharmacists on the ward. In the early days, the quantity of interventions and the time spent on the wards were studied rather than quality, since facts and figures were required to plan and justify clinical services. In the former North-East Thames region, a computer program was developed which enabled comparisons to be made between hospitals in the region.[65] Later, it was recognised that intervention data could be used for a wider range of purposes, as well as for quantifying workload. Batty and Beech[66] identified a number of possible reasons for monitoring interventions:

- providing evidence of the effectiveness of a prescription monitoring service;
- auditing drug use against agreed policies, e.g. formularies;
- providing feedback to directorates or consultants on prescribing trends;
- identifying training needs of prescribers;
- preventing litigation.

The present situation in intervention monitoring was outlined by Batty and Wind.[67] They survey the methods currently in use, including locally programmed hand-held computers and commercial software. They also speculate on the likely developments arising from the government's declared commitment to use technology to improve patient care.

Clinical pharmacokinetics service

A few pharmacy departments offer an in-house therapeutic drug monitoring (TDM) service, but many more are able to offer pharmacokinetic

Table 6.9 Therapeutic drug monitoring: drugs that are frequently monitored

Aminoglycoside antibiotics	Lithium
Carbamazepine	Phenytoin
Ciclosporin	Theophylline
Digoxin	

advice on the interpretation of drug-level assays performed by hospital biochemistry departments. This is of value in determining optimum dose regimens for certain drugs only: drugs with a fairly narrow range of effective blood levels and serious side-effects at toxic levels, with unpredictable pharmacokinetics, and where the effective dose cannot be readily assessed by clinical results. The drugs most commonly monitored are shown in Table 6.9.

For a clinical pharmacokinetics service to provide the maximum benefits to the patient, it is not enough merely to report blood levels; for these to be of any value, doctors must be given training on ideal sampling times in relation to dose times, and a purpose-designed request form should accompany the sample, giving details of diagnosis, concomitant drug therapy, reason for request and name and location of doctor for report. Once the blood level has been determined, it may be necessary to adjust the dose regimen using pharmacokinetic data, additionally taking account of factors such as the patient's renal function, to produce blood levels within the required therapeutic range. Campbell[68] gives a detailed description of all aspects of the clinical pharmacokinetics service at the Western Infirmary, Glasgow, where ward pharmacists select the patients to be screened. Protocols have been developed to facilitate interpretation of the results; in some cases, computer programs are used to calculate an optimum dosing schedule, which is then discussed with the doctor.

The clinical pharmacist's advisory role

The pharmacy student's concept of the clinical pharmacist's role is usually somewhat narrow. He/she believes that the job can be done only at the patient's bedside or the outpatient clinic, and visualises the pharmacist giving advice at ward rounds surrounded by an attentive audience of junior doctors who grasp at every fact. Real life is not like this. In fact, attendance at ward rounds will involve long periods of waiting while little of pharmaceutical significance occurs: teaching clinical signs and diagnostic skills to medical students, exploring lumps and bumps, marking out varicose veins for surgery and planning trips for the patient to other hospitals for diagnosis or treatment, for example. Many pharmacist managers feel that routine attendance on rounds is not a cost-effective way of delivering clinical pharmacy, and that a better return on staff time will be had if it is invested in areas where the results will affect a greater number of people. Opportunities for giving clinical advice and promoting effective drug usage exist in many multidisciplinary committees that work on different aspects of patient care.

One particularly fruitful area is the drug and therapeutics committee or the pharmacy users' committee. Membership is variable, and may include consultants of varying specialities, GPs, pharmacy managers, and sometimes senior nurse managers as well. A drug or medicines information pharmacist may be included. One task of the committee may be to produce a hospital or district drugs formulary. This is seen increasingly as a way of rationalising the range of drugs in use and promoting cost-effective prescribing. Linked with this may be a policy to regulate the addition of new drugs to the range in use – this is usually achieved by allowing only senior medical staff to request new drugs. This has the effect of minimising the influence of drug sales representatives on inexperienced doctors. Some committees may design prescribing documents, make rules about generic substitution and formulate other cost-containment policies – for example, in trusts where the duration of outpatient prescribing is limited, it is likely to have been the decision of this committee, made in conjunction with the local health authority prescribing committee.

Most trusts have in addition a control of infection committee whose membership includes public health, medical, surgical and occupational health consultants, nurse managers, school of nursing representatives, pharmacists and also probably the central sterile supply department (CSSD) manager. In conjunction with the control of infection nurse, it will be the pharmacist's lot to implement the policies agreed by providing the appropriate agents and monitoring and advising upon their use. Policies and procedures determined by the committee are likely to cover a variety of topics; some examples are listed in Table 6.10.

There is much scope for the clinical pharmacist with a good knowledge of ward procedures to make significant contributions to this work. Students should learn which organisms are likely to cause problems and the use and limitations of the various disinfectants available within the antiseptic and disinfectant policy.

Many hospitals have a nursing procedures committee, which draws up protocols to standardise practical nursing techniques on the wards;

Table 6.10 Typical control of infection policies

Antibiotic usage	Patient isolation/barrier nursing
Antiseptics and disinfectants	Staff vaccination
Ectoparasite infestation	Theatre cleaning/disinfection
HIV-positive patients	Wound management
Meningitis prophylaxis	

HIV, human immunodeficiency virus.

Table 6.11 Typical medicines-related nursing procedures

Bladder irrigation	Nebuliser therapy
Blood sugar monitoring	Ordering and storage of medicines
Changing giving sets	Patient-controlled analgesia
Continuous epidural analgesia	Rectal lavage
Cytotoxic drug administration	Urine testing
IV additives	Use of patients' own medicines
Medicines administration	

IV, intravenous.

many of these procedures include references to pharmaceuticals, and should be drafted with a pharmacist's advice on both clinical matters and law. Table 6.11 gives some typical examples.

Such standardisation has a number of advantages: it ensures good standards of practice, and means that nurses in training do not encounter differing methods as they rotate through different clinical areas. It also makes it easier to design a range of CSSD packs of equipment and dressings. The pharmacy should keep a complete set of procedures for reference.

References

1. NHS Executive. *Controls Assurance Standard – Medicines Management (Safe and Secure Handling)*. London: Stationery Office, 2000.
2. Department of Health. *Guidelines on the Safe and Secure Handling of Medicines: A Report to the Secretary of State for Social Services* (Duthie Guidelines). London: Her Majesty's Stationery Office, 1988.
3. Collins S R, Hyde J R G, Oakley P A, Sharott P. Are ward topping up services cost effective? *Pharm J* 1985; 235: 716–717.
4. Langham J M, Boggs K S. The effect of a ward-based pharmacy technician service. *Pharm J* 2000; 264: 961–963.
5. Karr A. Ward supplies – developing an effective NHS model. *Hosp Pharm* 1998; 5: 35–37.

6. Low J, Radley A, Dodd T, Jamieson W. Ward order assembly – "Just in time". *Hosp Pharm* 1998; 5: 109–112.
7. Radley A. Feasibility of ward order assembly. *Hosp Pharm* 1999; 6: 124.
8. Royal Pharmaceutical Society of Great Britain Professional Standards Directorate. Fact Sheet 2. *Controlled Drugs and Hospital Pharmacy*. London: Royal Pharmaceutical Society of Great Britain.
9. Report of a Joint Sub-committee. *Control of Dangerous Drugs and Poisons in Hospitals* (Aitken Report). London: Her Majesty's Stationery Office, 1958.
10. NHS Executive. *Destruction of Controlled Drugs*. EL(97) 22.
11. English National Board for Nursing, Midwifery and Health Visiting. *Administration of Drugs*. ENB(84)34.
12. Department of Health. *Patient Group Directions [England only]*. HSC 2000/026.
13. Department of Health and Social Security. *Measures for Controlling Drugs on the Wards*. HM(70)36.
14. Crooks J, Clark C G, Caie H B *et al*. Prescribing and administering drugs in hospitals. *Lancet* 1965; 1: 373.
15. Crooks J, Weir R D, Coull D C. Evaluation of a method of prescribing drugs in hospital, and a new method of recording their administration. *Lancet* 1967; 1: 668–671.
16. Crooks J, Calder G, Weir R D. Drugs in hospital. *J R Coll Phys Lond* 1967; 1: 233.
17. Hill P A, Wigmore H M. Measurement and control of drug administration incidents. *Lancet* 1967; 1: 672.
18. Department of Health. *Pharmacy in the Future – Implementing the NHS Plan*. London: Department of Health, 2000.
19. Electronic prescribing conference report. *Hosp Pharm* 1998; 5: 262–279.
20. NHS Executive. *Medical Students in Hospitals: A Guide to their Access to Patients and Clinical Work*. London: Stationery Office, 1991.
21. Standing Pharmaceutical Advisory Committee. Extended use and reuse of patients' own medicines on admission to hospital. *Pharm J (Hosp Suppl)* 1993; 251: HS49–HS50.
22. Dua S. Establishment and audit of a patients' own drugs scheme. *Hosp Pharm* 2000; 7: 196–198.
23. Bunn R J, Thomas M K, Giles L. St Helier NHS Trust's approach to patient focused health care. *Hosp Pharm* 1994; 1: 8–12.
24. Blain J, Mackay S, Rigg R, Ward V. Patient focused pharmacy services at Kingston. *Hosp Pharm* 1994; 1: 12–14.
25. Bunn R J. Satellite pharmacies. *Hosp Pharm* 1997; 4: 164.
26. Department of Health and Social Security. *Report of the Working Party on the Addition of Drugs to Intravenous Fluids* (Breckenridge Report). HC(76)9.
27. News item. Two children die after receiving infected TPN solutions. *Pharm J* 1994; 252: 596.
28. News item. Accidental death verdict on children infected by TPN at a Manchester hospital. *Pharm J* 1995; 254: 313.
29. Farwell J. *Aseptic Dispensing for NHS Patients*. London: Department of Health, 1994.
30. Mehta D K, ed. *British National Formulary*, published twice-yearly.

London: British Medical Association/Royal Pharmaceutical Society of Great Britain.

31. Needle R, Sizer T, eds. *The CIVAS Handbook*. London: Pharmaceutical Press, 1998.
32. Trissel L A, ed. *Handbook on Injectable Drugs*, 11th edn. Washington, DC: American Society of Health-system Pharmacists, 2001.
33. Langford S A. Mortality and morbidity from the in-use microbial contamination of intravenous products. *Hosp Pharm* 1999; 6: 104–109.
34. Cousins D H, Upton D R. How to prevent IV drug errors. *Pharm Pract* 1997; 7: 310–312.
35. McCarthy J P, Keay S, Gibson C. A review of pump types and applications. *Hosp Pharm* 1998; 5: 41–45.
36. Gibson C, McCarthy J P, Truran R J (1998). The safe use of intravenous infusion pumps. *Hosp Pharm* 1998; 5: 46–48.
37. NHS Executive. *For the Record: Managing Records in NHS Trusts and Health Authorities*. HSC 1999/053.
38. NHS Executive. *For the Record: Managing Records in NHS Trusts and Health Authorities*. Appendix B to HSC 1999/053.
39. NHS Executive. *Fraud: Countering Fraud in the NHS*. HSC 1999/082.
40. Department of Health and Social Security (HM(64)).
41. Department of Health and Social Security. *Use of Prescription Forms FP10 (HP) and FP10 (HP)(Ad)*. DS 306/74.
42. Ministry of Health. *Irregularities in the Use of Prescription Forms EC10 (HP)*. G/P72/2C.
43. NHS Executive. *Countering Fraud in the NHS: Prescription Charge Evasion*. HSC 1999/209.
44. NHS Executive. *Countering Fraud in the NHS*. HSC 1999/208.
45. Department of Health and National Assembly for Wales *Drug Tariff*, published monthly. London: Stationery Office.
46. Royal Pharmaceutical Society of Great Britain Statutory Committee report. Inquiry into apparent irregularities at hospital. *Pharm J* 1984; 234: 287.
47. NHS Executive. *Overseas Visitors' Eligibility to Receive Free Primary Care*. HSC 1999/018.
48. Department of Health. *Intermediate Care*. HSC 2001/001: LAC (2001)1.
49. Rambow E J. A pharmaceutical service for community clinics (part 1). *Pharm J* 1985; 235: 51–53.
50. Rambow E J. A pharmaceutical service to community clinics (part 2). *Pharm J* 1985; 235: 82–83.
51. Salisbury D M for the Joint Committee on Vaccination and Immunisation. *Immunisation against Infectious Disease*. London: Department of Health, 1996.
52. Grassby P F. Safe storage of vaccines: problems and solutions. *Pharm J* 1993; 251: 323–327.
53. Department of Health. *Rabies Prevention and Control*. London: Department of Health, 2000.
54. NHS Executive. *Management and Control of Viral Haemorrhagic Fevers: A Summary of Guidance from the Advisory Committee on Dangerous Pathogens (ACDP)*. HSC 1998/028.
55. NHS Executive. *Planning for Major Incidents – NHS Guidance*. HSC 1998/197.

56. NHS Executive. *Planning for Major Incidents: The NHS Guidance*. London: Stationery Office, 1998.
57. Department of Health. *The Standards Approach to Health Emergency Planning*. London: Department of Health, 2000.
58. NHS Executive Controls Assurance Standard. *Emergency Preparedness*. London: Stationery Office, 2000.
59. Department of Health. *Current Vaccine and Immunisation Issues*. PL/CMO/2001/1, PL/CNO/2001/2001/1, PL/CphO/2001/1.
60. Department of Health. *The Way Forward for Hospital Pharmaceutical Services*. HC (88)54/HN (FP) (88)24.
61. Batty R, Barber N. Prescription monitoring for ward pharmacists. *Pharm J* 1991; 247: 242.
62. Barber N, Willson A. *Churchill's Clinical Pharmacy Survival Guide*. London: Churchill Livingstone, 1999.
63. Dodds L, ed. *Drugs in Use*, 2nd edn. London: Pharmaceutical Press, 1996.
64. Greene R J, Harris N D. *Pathology and Therapeutics for Pharmacists*, 2nd edn. London: Pharmaceutical Press, 2000.
65. Miles C, Barratt C, Stone P. Development of a software package for performance indicator data for clinical pharmacy [poster]. European Conference on Clinical Pharmacy, 1988.
66. Batty R, Beech E F. Prescription monitoring interventions – is recording justified? *Hosp Pharm* 1994; 1: 100.
67. Batty R, Wind K. Monitoring packages for pharmacy interventions. *Hosp Pharm* 1999; 6: 176–178.
68. Campbell D. A clinical pharmacokinetics service. *Hosp Pharm* 1999; 6: 206–208.

7

Specialised hospital pharmaceutical services

UK Medicines Information Service

According to a strategy document recently published by the UK Medicines Information (MI) Service,[1] the service has two broad functions:

- to support medicines management within National Health Service (NHS) organisations by evaluating medicines, by producing guidelines and by providing training;
- to support the pharmaceutical care of individual patients.

The strategy document also defines the MI pharmacist's specialist skill – to link the provision of information with its clinical interpretation.

The MI Service is provided to most clients on a day-to-day basis by medicines information centres (formerly known as drug information centres) in district general hospitals (DGHs). These units, however, form part of a 'virtual organisation', or national network that enables access to a wide range of resources. In the following section, we discuss the way in which the service operates, and also how it is evolving to meet the changing needs of the users. Originally, the main clients were hospital doctors, nurses and clinical pharmacists. Increasingly, it is now realised that primary care health professionals need medicines and prescribing information, and nationally, the service is also responding to the emphasis on evidence-based practice from bodies such as the National Institute for Clinical Excellence (NICE; see Chapter 10). The organisation of the MI Service nationally is set out in Table 7.1, with brief details of the functions of each component.

In the past, information centres did not answer queries from patients. Increasingly, however, this is changing as it is now realised that patients and carers are entitled to information about their medicines, and patient helplines have been introduced at many centres. Also available to patients is the National Freephone Health Information Service and NHS Direct, whose numbers are listed inside the front cover of the *British National Formulary* (BNF).[2]

Table 7.1 Organisation of UK Medicines Information (MI) Service

UK Medicines Information Pharmacists Group	Coordinates MI Service nationally
	Plans development of UK MI Service
	Formulates practice standards for MI
	Provides new product evaluations
	Provides information technology, including website
	Publishes *Pharm-line*
	Organises training for MI pharmacists
	Publishes procedure manual for MI centres
	Liaises with primary care MI pharmacists
Regional centres	Provide extra resources for local centres
	Act as specialist centres
	Carry out audit and quality assurance of local centres
	Provide information network to local centres, e.g. early-warning systems
Local MI centres	Answer queries about individual patients' treatment, in both hospitals and primary care
	Prepare local formularies and newsletters
	Contribute to local policy making, drug and therapeutics committees and prescribing committees
	Patient helplines

The UK Medicines Information Pharmacists Group

The MI service is coordinated nationally by the UK Medicines Information Pharmacists Group (UKMIPG), formerly the UK Drug Information Pharmacists Group. The group has representatives from each of the English NHS regions or their equivalents, with one each from Northern Ireland, Scotland and Wales.[3] The UKMIPG has eight working groups, each undertaking specialised tasks, and reporting back to the parent group. These are listed in Table 7.2. It also maintains a website, whose address may be found inside the front cover of the BNF.

The new products assessment scheme organised by the UKMIPG represents one of its most important and developing roles.[4] The information is maintained in a database, and is circulated as hard copy to MI centres nationally. New drugs or chemical entities are assigned to one of the following:

- Stage one: includes new drugs in research, i.e. drugs that are in late phase II or phase III trials (see Chapter 2). The progress of these drugs is continuously tracked and reported throughout their trial stages, which may last for up to 5 years. During this period, MI pharmacists may receive queries about such drugs, and it also important at government level to be aware of possible resource implications in the future. A National Horizon Scanning Centre (NHSC) has been established to identify and monitor the development of new treatments, and both it and the Department of Health Pharmacy and Prescribing Branch receive information about drugs at this stage. The NHSC in turn liaises with NICE and the NHS Health Technology Appraisal programme.

- Stage two: includes up to 50 drugs that are considered by a UKMIPG prioritisation group to have greater potential, or to be nearing marketing. Such drugs are likely to be in the later stages of clinical trials or in preregistration trials. The information that these drugs are nearing release is of importance to a wider range of professionals, who may have to consider the practice and budgetary implications for their own field. These include senior pharmacy managers, prescribing advisers and drug and therapeutics committees. The information also flows to the National Prescribing Centre (NPC), which can estimate pharmacoeconomic and epidemiological data, which will be of value in later stages. Simister and Jackson[5] give further details of the collaboration between the UKMIPG and the NPC.

- Stage three: this comprises new drugs in clinical development. For several years, the UKMIPG has collaborated with NICE and the NPC with work on drugs at this stage, to assist in formulating the evaluations which enable NICE to make recommendations on the clinical use of a product.

- Stage four: this includes evaluations of drugs new to the market, and also of major new formulations and of new indications for existing drugs. The information can be accessed on the internet via the UKMIPG website under the title *New medicines on the market*.[6]

Table 7.2 UK Medicines Information Pharmacists Group (UKMIPG) working groups

New products
Education and training
Quality assurance of medicines information
Information technology
Primary care
Pharmaceutical industry liaison
Legal and ethical aspects of medicines information
Medicines information in Europe

The UKMIPG has an important role in the training of MI pharmacists, and in the maintenance of approved standards of practice within MI centres. This is partly achieved by organising courses for MI pharmacists, but probably the most important aspect is the publication of the *UK Drug Information Manual.*[7] This contains agreed standards for activities such as answering MI queries, education and training programmes and MI publications. It also includes assessors' packs for enquiry answering and MI publications. In addition, the manual covers legal and ethical considerations and gives a Code of Practice; it also lists resources, including books and journals, which should be available for an MI centre, and training material and exercises in various aspects of the work, from techniques in answering questions to evaluating published papers and drug advertisements.

The Information Technology (IT) working group of the UKMIPG is credited with the development of the excellent website which, as well as providing information about the UKMIPG itself, also provides links to local and regional MI centres, and to many fully evaluated MI internet sites. The group has also set up an e-mail discussion group for MI pharmacists. Further achievements have been the development of standards for computer facilities in MI centres, an internet guide for MI pharmacists and an IT strategy.

Perhaps the oldest persisting collaborative effort is the journal-abstracting service published as *Pharm-line*. With abstracts, newsletters and bulletins on pharmaceutical and medical topics written by MI specialists, this has evolved over the years from humble origins as a card index to its present CD-ROM format. It can also be searched on the internet.

Regional centres

Drug information services were originally organised on uniform lines throughout the UK, with 19 regional centres with a full range of facilities, and subregional centres located in large DGHs. Following the dismantling of the NHS regional structure, there have been some changes, but the organisation exists in an approximately similar form and the term 'regional centre' persists. These are listed, with contact telephone numbers, inside the front cover of the BNF. In addition to the facilities noted in Table 7.1, regional centres have been allocated the responsibility of acting as 'specialist centres' with extra resources to deal with queries on particular topics.[8, 9] These are listed in Table 7.3. Unless you are an MI specialist, it is probably preferable to direct queries to the local

Table 7.3 Specialist medicines information (MI) centres

Alternative medicine	Drugs in pregnancy
Community pharmacists' information	Drugs in psychiatry
Drugs in breast milk	Drugs in renal failure
Drugs in dentistry	Drug treatment of AIDS
Drugs in liver disease	Press index
Drugs in oncology	Toxicology and poisoning
Drugs in porphyria	Translation of German publications

AIDS, acquired immunodeficiency syndrome.

centre in the first instance rather than approaching the specialist centre direct.

The regional centre network operates an 'early-warning' grapevine system to alert MI pharmacists about impending media items on drug-related topics. This means that, with any luck, pharmacists should have some background information about an urgent drug recall in time to help the first anxious patients who have learned about it from the television news.

Medicines information centres

Local MI centres provide information passively, i.e. in response to users' queries, or actively, by publishing newsletters and bulletins. Although situated within hospitals, centres may provide both kinds of information to general medical practitioners and community pharmacists. The UKMIPG strategy referred to above[1] includes as one of its aims the goal of extending a full MI service to primary care. Quoting from the document, the intention is:

- to extend a full service to primary care, including a systematic risk assessment of drugs used in primary care;
- to provide routine dissemination of information on new medicines, key clinical trials and reviews of groups of medicines;
- to provide an enquiry service as for secondary care, with access to specialist services;
- to support community pharmacists across the range of their responsibilities;
- to provide specialist support for pharmaceutical advisers;
- to provide training and support for new nurse and other prescribers;
- to support prescribing committees.

The UKMIPG has published an implementation framework[10] that identifies key tasks that will achieve these ends. Both the strategy and the framework may be consulted on the UKMIPG website.[6]

It should not be assumed from this that primary care has no support at present. Some primary care groups/trusts employ MI pharmacists of their own, and many pharmaceutical advisers have come from an MI background. In 1999, Cairns and Lane[11] evaluated medicines information services available for primary care users in South Thames, where a pharmacist had been appointed to provide a service dedicated to primary care. This paper includes both an outline of current services and a 'wish list' of services which the users would value, ranging from community pharmacist research information to shared-care information and facilitation of a journal club, to quote but a few.

Medicines information centres: records and quality

As with all professional activities, it is important that MI procedures are developed and followed at all times. Each enquiry is recorded on a standard pro-forma and its receipt logged in a daybook, which is used subsequently to monitor progress. As a minimum the following details are recorded:

- name of hospital/MI centre;
- date and time;
- how soon the answer is needed;
- name, address and telephone number of enquirer;
- details of query;
- details of patient (name, sex, weight, age, diagnosis, treatment, allergies and any relevant laboratory data).

In most centres, additional data is recorded to provide costing information, either to be used in the pharmacy business plan or so that accurate costs for the service can be assigned to the directorates or care groups when service-level agreements are drafted. This data would include at least the speciality/directorate of the enquirer and the time taken to answer the query. As a quality index, the delay before answering is recorded, and the percentage of queries answered within the target time calculated. Reasons for delay should be noted, in order to plan improvements if necessary.

As with all pharmaceutical activities, quality will be achieved by meticulous management. The UKMIPG has agreed standards for MI enquiry-answering services. These were quoted in a paper by Kuczynska,[12] and are reproduced in Table 7.4.

Table 7.4 UK Medicines Information Pharmacists Group (UKMIPG) standards for medicines information (MI) enquiry-answering services

Service should be organised to permit the prompt handling of enquiries and all matters relating to the use of medicines

Centres should hold the minimum resources appropriate for the provision of the service

The service should meet the requirements of its users

Professional expertise and judgement should be used in processing MI requests. Enquiries must be handled in the accepted, logical manner

The Group has also formulated risk management plans based on quality assurance (QA) standards. Local MI centres can formulate their own risk management plans based on these. Kuczynska's paper[12] provides some examples of the required QA standards, of which full details will be found in the *UK Drug Information Manual*.[7] Pharmacy managers may also validate the effectiveness of their service by benchmarking it against that of similar providers. Such a scheme, operating in Lothian hospitals, is described in a paper by Irvine.[13]

Pharmacists must learn the correct way to explore queries, remembering that the question asked may not reflect the true nature of the problem. For example, a doctor may ask whether a particular drug causes jaundice, and fail to mention the several other drugs the patient is receiving, one of which happens to be chlorpromazine! It requires some skill and experience to deal quickly and accurately with MI queries, and students must have their work checked, as in dispensing. The quality and presentation of the answer must be first-class. Written replies should be well presented as letters on headed notepaper, and copies retained on file. The student must become familiar with the reference books and journals kept in the MI library, and with the local procedures for handling and filing data.

Completed MI queries are filed and cross-referenced with a card index or computer database using a key-word system. Thus, if the same or a related query occurs again, this record may provide a starting point for the second occasion, although clearly further research must be completed to ensure that the situation has not changed.

Proactive medicines information

Although a large part of MI work is answering queries, another aspect is the proactive provision of information by publishing bulletins and newsletters on selected topics. Certain bulletins are produced nationally

– for example, a modest subscription will purchase the *Drug and Therapeutics Bulletin*,[14] which is circulated to all prescribing doctors in England, Wales and Northern Ireland. The NPC publishes a regular bulletin on prescribing issues, the *MeReC Bulletin*,[15] which is circulated to general practitioners (GPs), primary care groups/trusts and pharmacists. There is also a quarterly, *MeReC Extra*, a concise and easy-to-read publication containing updates and reviews on current issues. *MeReC* publications are available on the NPC websites, for the NHSnet at nww.npc.ppa.nhs.uk, and on the internet at www.npc.co.uk. The Committee on Safety of Medicines and the Medicines Control Agency (MCA) jointly produce *Current Problems in Pharmacovigilance*, which is circulated to all doctors and pharmacists.

Local MI centres also produce newsletters and bulletins on various subjects targeted at local prescribers; a growth area in these cost-conscious days is comparative drug cost information. There are also links with health authority pharmaceutical advisers in many areas. This has led to bulletins being provided for GPs, sometimes based on Prescribing Analyses and Cost (PACT) data.

Information sources

Possibly the world's best-known source of drug information is *Martindale*,[16] which is produced, along with the other publications of the Pharmaceutical Press such as the BNF, within the Royal Pharmaceutical Society's headquarters. *Martindale* is also available on CD-ROM and as online and intranet versions, i.e. available to users through a local area network, through the Micromedex Healthcare Series of drug information databases. This series, available via the Pharmaceutical Press, includes a range of databases covering drug-related topics. The BNF is available on CD-ROM and online and also exists in a web-enabled version.[17] Intended for trusts, health authorities and primary care groups/trusts, this includes a local formulary editor, making it possible for users accessing it via an intranet to identify local formulary items. Links can also be created to local electronic prescribing software.

New technology has made available to MI pharmacists a wealth of data sources in addition to the ones discussed above. Daly and Lee[18] described some of the more important in an article in 1998, but rapid progress in expanding the range has been made since then. In particular, most major medical and pharmaceutical journals are now accessible online; their web addresses are quoted with the editorial details in the printed versions. The National Library of Medicine provides an online service, MEDLINE, which can be accessed as a link from the RPSGB website. This allows access to 11 million citations from medical and scientific journals, with links to further sites, many providing full text articles.

The RPSGB Information Centre is frequently consulted by members. Staff members are able to answer many queries and, in addition, books can be borrowed by post, photocopies of scientific papers obtained and, of course, the library is open for study to members. In addition, most large hospitals have a medical library, which should have a wide range of medical journals and specialist medical textbooks.

All large pharmaceutical companies have a medical information department, and this will provide detailed information on every aspect of the firm's products (although the restrictions of the marketing authorisation will limit giving out information about non-licensed indications). Pharmaceutical manufacturers are obliged by the Medicines Act 1968 to keep a register of adverse events reported or suspected about their products for the Committee on Safety of Medicines. This means that they have to follow up any adverse event enquiry with a request for further information from the doctor; this can be a source of aggravation for all concerned if the doctor is not willing, or is unable, to complete the necessary detailed questionnaire. Pharmacists should remember that doctors sometimes investigate suspected drug side-effects simply to eliminate them from the diagnosis, and lose all interest in the drug aspect when the true pathology of the symptoms has been revealed by other diagnostic procedures.

Medicines information: wider aspects

Drug usage review and clinical audit

This aspect of information work is achieving prominence with the emphasis on evidence-based medicine (EBM) and audit of clinical procedures that has resulted from the introduction of clinical governance throughout the NHS (see Chapter 10). Drug usage review is a process whereby prescribing habits are examined and advice formulated which, if followed, is intended to achieve both therapeutic benefits and cost-effective prescribing. Studies are usually undertaken on groups of patients or groups of drugs, rather than reviewing individual patients. An example might be the prescribing of perioperative prophylactic antibiotics, or postoperative analgesia. Hopefully, review of practice may enable a prescribing policy to be formulated, and then future studies may monitor compliance with the policy. Increasingly this is becoming a feature of clinical audit; pharmacies whose computers can record patient medication histories and access clinical data and laboratory test results are ideally placed to audit prescribing and make recommendations.

Evidence-based medicine

In a paper that forms part of a special feature on the subject, Wiffen[19] states that evidence-based medicine (EBM) involves finding and interpreting the best evidence available to answer a specific clinical question and implementing the findings. As a discipline, it has come into prominence with the advent of clinical governance, but practitioners have been following the concept ever since they began to formulate guidelines and develop formularies. Government funding has enabled various units primarily concerned with EBM to be established nationally. Wiffen lists these; they are outlined in Table 7.5. More details of the work of each will be found in his paper.[19]

In particular, the NHS Centre for Reviews and Dissemination (CRD) has been very active, producing a series of systematic reviews, some of which have been commissioned by NICE, and others by the NHS Research and Development Health Technology Assessment Programme. These are listed on the CRD website, which may be accessed via a link from the Royal Pharmaceutical Society of Great Britain (RPSGB) website. The CRD produces the monthly *Effective Health Care Bulletin,* aimed at decision-makers and distributed free to health authorities, trusts and to GPs. A complementary publication, *Effectiveness Matters,* is also widely distributed throughout the NHS. In addition to the centres listed, there is also a centre for evidence-based pharmacotherapy at Aston University, whose work was described in an article by Mason.[20]

The Health Technology Assessment programme was initiated as part of an NHS Research and Development Strategy.[21] Previously, a House of Lords committee[22] had investigated issues surrounding health service research and its funding, and had concluded that, at the time, large sums were sometimes spent on biomedical research with possibly little practical value, whereas little money was allocated to practice research or evidence-based practice. A detailed account of the work of the Health Technology Assessment programme may be read in a paper by Clark *et al.*[23] They emphasise that pharmacists could play a critical role, and indicate ways to achieve this aim.

Table 7.5 Evidence-based medicine groups in the UK

NHS Centre for Reviews and Dissemination (CRD), based at the University of York	CRD reports *Effectiveness Matters* reports *Effective Healthcare Bulletin* Electronic database: Database of reviews of effectiveness Electronic database: Economic evaluation database
Health Technology Assessment programme	Information for purchasers, providers and users of health services on the effectiveness and cost of interventions and medical services
Centres for Evidence-based Medicine (EBM)	Promote teaching, learning practice and evaluation of EBM and health care Conduct applied, patient-based and methodological research to generate new knowledge required for the practice of evidence-based health care Collaborate with other scientists in the creation of a graduate programme designed to train researchers in the techniques necessary to carry out randomised trials and systematic reviews
The Cochrane Library	Produces and maintains reviews through review groups covering specific topics, which are disseminated via the electronic Cochrane database

NHS, National Health Service.

Formularies

Local formularies are usually compiled and published by hospital MI centres, often drawing on specialist contributors from the consultant staff, or in collaboration with prescribing committees. Most hospitals have had formularies for many years, and now are often increasing their scope and target audience to include the GPs who refer their patients. Formularies vary from simple lists of drugs which may be prescribed to handbooks which contain monographs on the prescribing of the chosen drugs and include other information such as hospital prescribing policies, shared-care protocols and information about hospital departments. The intention of the formulary is not only to cut down the range of drugs in use, and hence the cost of stocking the pharmacy, but also to select agents that are proved to be both clinically and cost-effective, and to provide guidance for junior doctors. When local GPs are also involved and committed to its aims, a formulary may also contribute to the provision of 'seamless care'. Increasingly, primary care prescribers, with input from local prescribing committees and prescribing advisers, develop local practice formularies. These should be based on published guidelines and frameworks.

Developing a formulary is relatively straightforward but ensuring that its recommendations are put into practice is a separate problem. Slee and Farrar[24] survey the subject, and identify the problems to be overcome in their paper. The main ones they identify are:

- Hospital junior medical staff rotate between placements every 3–6 months.
- This requires repeated education of replacement staff, whose previous experience may lead them to ignore formulary recommendations.
- Feedback on prescribing practice is usually retrospective, and consequently relatively ineffective.
- Extra effort is required when drug recommendations are changed.

Slee and Farrar then outline the advantages of incorporating formulary management into the electronic prescribing system at Wirral Hospital. Their system permits only the prescribing of formulary drugs; it also includes prescribing protocols for certain clinical situations, and has overcome the problems listed above.

In primary care monitoring adherence to formulary recommendations can be achieved by analysing PACT data (see Chapter 3). In hospitals without electronic prescribing systems, formulary compliance may be monitored retrospectively by drug usage review, as discussed above. This remains the only method available where forms FP10(HP) are used for outpatient prescribing, since at present these are handwritten.

Pharmaceutical production in hospitals

Definition and scope

'Pharmaceutical production' is a term which encompasses both the manufacture and specialised dispensing of medicines for the patient. Manufacture is the preparation of pharmaceuticals by a bulk preparative method, i.e. not for an individual patient, whereas specialised dispensing uses similar techniques and facilities for preparing medicines for individual named patients.

Manufacture in hospitals used to be widespread and unregulated, but is now controlled by regulations imposed under the Medicines Act 1968. Manufacturing units must be licensed with the MCA and are inspected prior to granting a licence and routinely afterwards to ensure that they meet the standards required. These standards, as imposed on the pharmaceutical industry, are set out in the *Rules and Guidance for Pharmaceutical Manufacturers (The Orange Guide)*,[25] which includes the text of *The European Guide to Good Pharmaceutical Manufacturing Practice*. The costs of running a manufacturing unit are extremely high, so that there are now only a few within the hospital service. Not only do they have to comply with good manufacturing practice, but also with health and safety legislation such as the Control of Substances Hazardous to Health Regulations 1994.

Concurrently with the decline in hospital manufacturing units has emerged an increased need for preparations to be specially made for individual patients. These may include parenteral nutrition solutions, prepared intravenous (IV) additives and prepared cytotoxic injections. These may be prepared in pharmacies utilising exemptions from their manufacturing licensing regulations included under two sections of the Medicines Act 1968, sections 10 and 55. Section 10 gives exemption for pharmacists from the requirement to hold either a manufacturer's or a wholesale dealer's licence, providing that the preparative activity is carried out under the supervision of a pharmacist. Section 55 gives exemption for hospitals when the products are for the purpose of being administered in accordance with the directions of a doctor or dentist, and the activity takes place in the course of the business of the hospital. The MCA has issued guidance for hospitals on the interpretation of these regulations;[26] this guidance note can be downloaded from the MCA website (www.open.gov.uk/mca/mcahome.htm). In particular it gives guidance on quantities which can be prepared for stock using the facility of exemptions under the Act. It is, of course, inappropriate for preparations to be made in circumstances of lower quality, or with fewer controls, by utilising the exemptions of the Medicines Act. Quality controllers have drawn up nationally agreed guidelines setting out the standards to be followed in unlicensed units. Based on *Orange Guide* requirements, the guidelines[27] list the documentation required and also quote performance standards, including for the testing of filtered air supplies.

There is a NHS Pharmaceutical Production Committee with representatives from each of the former NHS regions and from Northern Ireland, Scotland and Wales. Amongst other activities, the committee acts as a liaison between government departments and agencies and

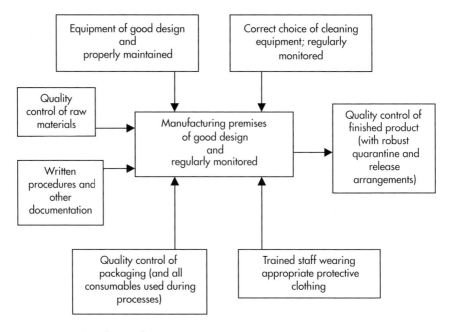

Figure 7.1 Good manufacturing practice.

production pharmacists; compiles resource and management information sources which are used to promote good practice, e.g. audit documents; and liaises with the NHS Pharmaceutical Quality Control Committee.[3] A joint working party of these groups and the UK Radiopharmacy Group is known as the Technical Specialist Education and Training Group. This Group identifies training needs and maintains a list of courses available in this field. It has produced a training manual for preregistration students gaining experience in technical services. This can be downloaded from the Group's website.[28]

Good manufacturing practice

The guidelines of the *Orange Guide* cover all aspects of the manufacturing process, as summarised by Baird (Figure 7.1).[29]

In addition to the controls on the manufacturing process, there are detailed requirements for the production and retention of documentation. This is not only to ensure that process controls are carried out, but also to enable the rapid tracing of the history of a batch or of an ingredient should a defect come to light at a later stage. The above factors apply equally to large- and small-scale operations such as extemporaneous dispensing. In the latter case, the environmental and documentary controls may not need to be so stringent, but the same principles must be followed. The end points are in fact the same, in that, as stated in the *Orange Guide*, 'there should be a comprehensive system . . . to provide assurance that products will be consistently of a quality appropriate for their intended use'.

Details of the requirements for premises used for pharmaceutical production are included in the *Orange Guide*.[25] In summary, the design should ensure protection of the product from contamination, and permit efficient cleaning. The standard of ventilation required as an adjunct to building design is described in the *Orange Guide*. Further information may be found in a textbook by Sharp,[30] which is directed at those responsible for the quality of manufactured medicines, and which should be read by anyone planning to work in this field.

Whatever the scale of the operation, all units should have in place a programme of both internal and external audit using audit standards approved by local QA. The auditor should evaluate every aspect of the operation. Findings should be discussed with local production managers, and action plans to remedy any deficiencies agreed and implemented.

Repackaging

A common manufacturing activity in hospitals is the repackaging of medicines. Special packs may be produced for one of several reasons, as shown in Table 7.6.

According to the MCA *Guidelines*,[26] small quantities of repackaged products can be prepared for stock without the need for an assembly licence. The guidance quotes 25 packs of a product as being the maximum to be prepared at a time, and this is not to be carried out more frequently than monthly. Any larger quantities must be prepared in licensed facilities. All repackaging operations should be fully documented and controlled in a similar manner to any other production

Table 7.6 Reasons for repackaging medicines

Suitable size of pack for issue to wards as stock
Suitable size and labelled pack for issue to patients on discharge or on a patient group direction
Item suitably labelled for a particular use, e.g. for bowel preparation before X-ray
Cardiopulmonary resuscitation kits
Anaphylactic shock kits (for immunisation clinics)

activity. To avoid cross-contamination of batches, it is important to account very accurately for stocks introduced into the repackaging area, and for all labels produced. Particularly stringent procedures are required for cleaning equipment and for operator protection from the dust from uncoated tablets, for which a dedicated facility should be maintained. For small units, this may be uneconomical, and such products should be purchased rather than handled locally.

Terminally sterilised products

In pharmacies, the two most frequently used processes for terminal sterilisation are autoclaving and dry heat. Soon after the Devonport incident, in which several patients died as a result of faulty sterilisation of IV fluids,[31] official guidance about running and maintaining sterilisers was issued as a Health Technical Memorandum (HTM). This has been updated since; the current edition, *HTM 2010*, was issued in 1994.[32] It covers all types of sterilisers used in health care premises (Table 7.7). *HTM 2010*[32] has five main parts, covering:

- management policy;
- design considerations;
- validation and verification;
- good practice policy;
- operational policy (with testing and validation protocols).

There is also a series of log books for recording maintenance procedures for the various types of steriliser. The HTM was reviewed by Shaw *et al.*; this article gives more details of the information included in the various sections.[33]

It is rarely economical for hospital production units to operate autoclaves since the capital outlay and running costs are very high. Most units purchase items requiring terminal sterilisation from another hospital or from a commercial source. For units which launder and process their own clean-room clothing, the local Central Sterilisation and Disinfection Unit will be able to sterilise the clean, appropriately packed garments in a porous load steriliser such as that used for surgeons' gowns. It should be noted that such autoclaves are *not* suitable for sterilising drugs.

Radiopharmaceuticals

Radiopharmaceuticals are prepared for patients usually for the diagnosis of, or sometimes for the treatment of, disease. Often prepared for

Table 7.7 Sterilisers used in health care premises

Porous load	Central sterilisation and disinfection departments
Unwrapped instrument and utensil	Clinics; doctors' surgeries
Fluid	Pharmacy production units
Dry heat	Central sterilisation and disinfection departments
	Pharmacy production units
Laboratory sterilisers	

individual patients, they may also be prepared in bulk for a series of patients. Their preparation must be to standards set out in the *Orange Guide*.[25] Many are given by injection, and therefore must be prepared as sterile products. There is the added complication, however, of the hazard of the radionuclide to the operator, and it is imperative to adhere strictly to local radiation protection rules, which will have been prepared by collaboration with the local physicist, and which have to comply with current legislation. Acknowledging the specialist nature of the work, there is a UK Radiopharmacy Group with 14 members representing former NHS regions. The group exists to advance current practices and standards and to supply advice and information.[3] It has a website giving information about its activities and publications.[34]

Radiopharmacy is governed by regulations covering every aspect of the work. These are outlined in a review by Maltby[35] which formed part of one of the regular features on radiopharmacy published in the *Hospital Pharmacist*. Later legislation, e.g. the Ionising Regulations (Medical Exposure) Regulations (IRMER) 1999 has come into force and was discussed at a UK Radiopharmacy Group workshop in 2000.[36]

QA is a particular problem with radiopharmaceuticals because of the short half-life of many of the preparations, and because of the potentially serious problems which could arise from defective products. Solanki[37] reviews the quality testing of radiopharmaceuticals, with illustrations of the clinical significance of quality aspects. A further article by Frier[38] discusses QA and lists the specifications with which radiopharmaceuticals are generally expected to comply. The MCA guidance gives advice on licensing such activities.

Centralised intravenous additive services

The recommendations of the Breckenridge Report on IV additives[39] led to an increasing proportion of drug additions to IV solutions being carried out in the pharmacy; dispensing operations were performed either in a laminar flow work station in a clean room, or in an isolator. Centralised intravenous additive (CIVA) services developed in a fairly haphazard way in response to local circumstances, and in some cases standards were less than ideal. Needle outlined the history of CIVA services and discussed the present situation in a review forming part of a special feature on CIVA services in the *Hospital Pharmacist*.[40]

In 1994, two children at a Manchester hospital died as a result of receiving infected total parenteral nutrition (TPN) solutions prepared in the hospital pharmacy.[41] Following this incident, a survey of hospital aseptic preparative services in 1994 led to the issue of a guidance document, often referred to as the Farwell document.[42] As well as summarising the various sources of guidance on standards available at the time, this document set out minimum standards for NHS pharmacy aseptic units. In a further study in 1996, MCA inspectors surveyed a 10% sample of unlicensed units, and found that there were still substandard facilities in use. The Chief Pharmaceutical Officer then instructed pharmacy managers to audit their aseptic facilities to assess the adequacy of standards, facilities, staffing and staff training, environmental and other quality control.[43, 44] Since then, many more managers have opted to license their units; some units have ceased to operate, opting to purchase a service from a licensed unit, and remaining unlicensed units have raised their standards.

Sterile dispensing may be undertaken on a one-off basis for an individual named patient, but some items are routinely prepared in most acute general hospitals. These are listed in Table 7.8.

The development of CIVA services has led to the formation of a special-interest group. The National Centralised Intravenous Additives Services Group has produced a manual intended to be used as a guide to the setting-up and operation of these services; it also contains IV additive stability data.[45] The group has a website with information about its activities and links to related sites.[46] The NHS Pharmaceutical Quality Control Committee has also produced a manual containing information and guidelines for all types of aseptic preparation services, including information on the provisions of the Medicines Act and exemptions.[47] A further text which should be available in all hospital aseptic units is the American *Handbook on Injectable Drugs*, which, in addition to information on product presentation and administration routes, also contains stability data for IV additives.[48]

With the increasing move towards treating patients at home, the need for domiciliary IV therapy has grown. TPN solutions, cytotoxic

Table 7.8 Centralised intravenous additive service (CIVAS): usual product range

Antibiotic infusions	AIDS in- and outpatients
	Cystic fibrosis patients
Continuous epidural syringes	
Cytotoxics and monoclonal antibodies	Oncology in- and outpatients
Patient-controlled analgesia	
Total parenteral nutrition infusions	Adults and neonates

AIDS, acquired immunodeficiency syndrome.

drugs, including acquired immunodeficiency syndrome (AIDS) therapy and antibiotics are now often prescribed for home use. These may be prepared in hospital departments or may be provided by specialist contractors after prescribing by general practitioners on FP10 forms.

Parenteral nutrition

Parenteral nutrition – often referred to as total parenteral nutrition (TPN) – is the administration of sterile nutrients to a patient intravenously. Patients' daily nutritional requirements are dependent on both their nutritional status and their medical condition. Because of this, prescribing for TPN is very specialised, and many hospitals have introduced multidisciplinary teams to guide prescribers by designing standard protocols. Pharmacists are usually members of these teams, since they can both give clinical advice on the choice of nutrients, and can also advise on the presentation of the infusion. Because of the complexity of the prescription, the daily requirements are likely to be formulated from several commercial products providing calories, lipids, vitamins and electrolytes. This could lead to the hazardous situation where the ward staff have to interpret and administer the prescription by setting up an IV drip with several bottles with additives running concurrently, possibly with different volumes and drip rates running in parallel. Current practice removes this hazard by assembling the daily requirements into a single, for adults usually 3-litre bag, by aseptic transfer within the pharmacy. This must be done under suitable conditions, i.e. in a laminar flow cabinet or isolator, and by trained staff. Some units purchase ready-mixed 3-litre bags, which have a reasonable shelf-life, from an outside source, and then tailor these to the patients' daily requirements of nutrients, vitamins and electrolytes by making additions locally, using agreed protocols to ensure stability of additives.

Delivery of TPN solutions to wards must ensure maintenance of the cold chain, e.g. by using cool boxes and minimising time in transit. Wards must have access to adequate facilities for storing TPN solutions, since the standard lockable ward drugs refrigerator is not large enough. For example, a surgical ward with three TPN patients might require storage for nine 3-litre bags to cover a bank-holiday weekend. It is unsatisfactory to stuff these IV solutions into the kitchen refrigerator, so dedicated refrigerated storage with regular temperature checks should be available, possibly located so that several wards can share it.

In hospitals with paediatric departments and special-care baby units, a substantial part of the workload will be preparing TPN for neonates. The same techniques are used, but in some ways the work is simpler since the majority of babies are fed intravenously because they are preterm; although small, their metabolic requirements do not vary so much from day to day as sick adults. A working party was commissioned in 2000 by the British Association for Parenteral and Enteral Nutrition (BAPEN) to report and formulate guidelines on TPN in children. The guidelines include information on pharmaceutical problems such as stability.[49, 50]

Cytotoxic or chemotherapy dispensing

This section must be read in conjunction with the section on dispensing chemotherapy prescriptions in Chapter 5.

In October 1999 the Secretary of State for Health identified the need to raise the quality of cancer services throughout the country. In 2000 a consultation exercise was introduced by a health circular[51] with the aim of establishing standards and performance indicators which could be applied to cancer services nationally. This was achieved with the publication of the *Manual of Cancer Services Standards* in 2000,[52] which can be downloaded from the Department of Health website.[53] The manual gives standards for services in a number of topics, and gives performance indicators by which these can be measured. The chemotherapy section is of particular importance to pharmacists, and establishes their role as part of the multidisciplinary team. In this section, the objectives are stated to be:

> To ensure that chemotherapy services are of a high standard through:
>
> - clearly defined leadership and organisational arrangements;
> - provision of dedicated and suitably equipped areas for the administration of chemotherapy;

- coordination and control over the use of specified chemotherapy regimens within a network [in this context, a network implies a cancer service which might be delivered in several hospitals sharing the same specialists or consultants];
- supervision of chemotherapy prescribing by appropriate specialists (clinicians and pharmacists);
- administration of chemotherapy by appropriately trained staff;
- use of guidelines for the prevention and treatment of side-effects and complications of chemotherapy;
- minimising delays in starting treatments;
- provision of facilities for aseptic reconstitution of cytotoxic agents;
- clear and comprehensive documentation of chemotherapy delivery.

Most drugs used in the treatment of malignant disease are cytotoxic. Their cytotoxic effect is not limited to abnormal cells, however, and may be a risk to persons handling them. Suitable precautions must be taken when handling such drugs, and it is recommended that the preparation of solutions for injection should be carried out in safety cabinets in the pharmacy rather than on the ward, and presented as filled syringes or IV bags. Because the product is for injection and needs to be sterile, such safety cabinets must give an environment similar to a standard laminar flow cabinet; these cannot be used, however, because of the risk of blowing cytotoxic material at the operator. It is important therefore to use isolator cabinets or specially designed vertical laminar flow cabinets in which bacterially filtered air passes vertically across the procedure area, and is refiltered on exit to remove any toxic particles. Information on cytotoxics dispensing is contained in *The Quality Assurance of Aseptic Preparation Services*.[27] A standard text which should be available for reference is *The Cytotoxics Handbook*.[54] There is a special interest group, the British Oncology Pharmacy Association (BOPA).

In recent years new therapeutic agents for cancer have included some which are monoclonal antibodies. These may pose different risks to both operator and patient, e.g. non-humanised antibodies might cause allergic reactions. Recognising this fact, the National CIVAS Group and BOPA have formulated a statement on handling monoclonal antibodies.[55]

A further aspect which must be addressed is the disposal of cytotoxic materials and syringes and other used items, both from the pharmacy and from wards and departments. Since few incinerators are licensed to operate at temperatures adequate to denature cytotoxics, it will usually be necessary to use a specialist waste disposal contractor.

Most units design specialised documentation for cytotoxic dispensing, often doubling as the agreed protocol for a given regimen. Such documentation may be computer-generated. Examples are illustrated in two articles by Lofthouse[56] and Sewell.[57]

Specials non-sterile dispensing

This is the dispensing of a non-sterile preparations for individual patients. (See also the section on dispensing extemporaneous preparations in Chapter 5.) A service specification for extemporaneous dispensing/compounding is appended to the RPSGB Code of Ethics.[58] There are four main elements in this process:

- To ensure that the preparation – although nominally non-sterile – has no undue contamination. Any dispensed item should be prepared under the best possible conditions. For many preparations, it is desirable to have closely controlled conditions. For critical items such as creams it may be desirable to have a clean preparation area with local environmental control such as air filtration.

- To ensure that there is no health and safety hazard in the preparation, it is necessary to protect the operator from hazards arising from the product, by the use of protective clothing – appropriate overalls and caps; gloves of suitable material and quality and eye protection to the appropriate British Standard; by enclosing weighing equipment in a purpose-designed unit to contain dust; and by the use of vertical laminar flow cabinets as for cytotoxics or enclosed safety cabinets. For some non-sterile highly active ingredients, incorporation into the vehicle inside a fume cupboard or extraction hood may be necessary, and for many pharmaceuticals, precautions must be taken because of their flammable nature. Large volumes must be stored in flammable stores away from occupied buildings, and up to 50 litres within metal flammables storage cupboards, isolated from combustible materials and oxidising agents, inside the building. Naked flames and sparks must be eliminated, i.e. no gas rings or jets, gas heaters, electrical relays in refrigerators, cigarettes and matches near the working area. Electrical fittings, including motors, should be spark-free. Hospitals are required to obtain a fire certificate under the provisions of the Fire Precautions Act 1971. The application, to the Chief Executive of the Fire Authority, requires that details of the quantities and method of storage of explosive and flammable materials are submitted; the application would usually be channelled through the hospital's fire officer, who should therefore be kept informed of any significant changes.

- To ensure that the formulation is appropriate, by consideration of the technical aspects of the formulation and by documentary control of the ingredients. If required to dispense an item extemporaneously, it is the responsibility of the pharmacist to ensure that the final product is efficacious. The formulation must in itself be stable, e.g. creams must not crack, and the active ingredients must be stable in the formulation for the required shelf-life. Checking these facets may be done by referring to standard publications like the *European Pharmacopoeia*[59] or the *Pharmaceutical Codex*,[60] or through a literature search – either directly or via the manufacturer of the main active ingredient. In some cases – perhaps a new indication for a drug – it may be necessary to do formulation studies locally.
- Finally, it is imperative to have full documentation on products dispensed extemporaneously. This should give the provenance of the formula and ingredients and the quantities used and their source, batch number and expiry date. The patient's name, hospital number or address and prescription details should also be recorded. Pharmacy personnel involved must also be recorded, including the name of the pharmacist taking overall responsibility for the preparation. Such records act not only as a safeguard against mishap, but also make it possible to supply exactly the same preparation should the patient return. The RPSGB Service Specification[58] states that extemporaneous dispensing records should be kept for a minimum of 2 years, but if possible for 5 years.

Quality assurance in hospitals

Definition and scope

The *Orange Guide*[25] has defined the principle of quality as follows:

> There should be a comprehensive system, so designed, implemented and controlled, and so furnished with personnel, equipment and other resources as to provide assurance that products will be consistently of a quality appropriate to their intended use. The attainment of this quality objective requires the involvement and commitment of all concerned, at all stages.

QA in hospitals is designed to apply this principle to the delivery of medicinal products to patients; the work may be divided as shown in Table 7.9.

There are two main reference texts which relate to QA in hospitals. The first is a series of documents on quality standards in the series

Table 7.9 Aspects of quality assurance in hospitals

Assurance of hospital manufacture
Assurance of dispensing
Assurance of storage and distribution of medicinal supplies, e.g. maintenance of cold chain
Assurance of medical gas supplies
Assurance of quality control accuracy

ISO9000 issued jointly by the British Standards Institute and the International Standards Organization. They are mandatory reading for any pharmacist wishing to plan or operate quality systems.

There is a specialist group, the NHS Pharmaceutical Quality Control Committee, with members representing the former NHS regions and from Northern Ireland, Scotland and Wales. Representatives from the MCA, the Medicines Inspectorate and the NHS Production Committee also attend meetings. The Committee achieves its objectives (quoting from an article in the *Hospital Pharmacist*[3]) by:

- operating a communications network at national and local levels;
- providing leadership, collective expert views and technical guidance;
- developing and promoting best practice;
- developing and operating educational programmes;
- supporting cost-effective procurement;
- coordinating resource-effective research and development;
- maximising efficient use of resources by sharing information.

Assurance of hospital manufacture

As the Medicines Act controls pharmaceutical manufacture in NHS trusts,[61] it follows that hospital QA closely follows the guidelines in the *Orange Guide*.[25] This should be studied for detailed recommendations; in summary there are four main sections.

Personnel and training

Staff structures must be planned to give proper professional control of all processes. A named pharmacist with appropriate qualifications and experience must be identified as production manager, with designated production staff reporting to him/her. Formal arrangements must be in place to obtain the services of a QA pharmacist. If the hospital does not have its own pharmacy QA laboratory, it must purchase a service, e.g. from another hospital. QA staff should not report to the production manager, but directly to senior pharmacy management, to enable independent action in the case of a dispute about quality standards. Although junior staff of all grades may be rotated through production areas to gain experience, there must be enough trained and experienced permanent staff to supervise them. It is imperative that personnel are adequately trained for their task, not only in specific skills, e.g. in operating equipment, but also in the underlying principles of good manufacturing practice. Quality controllers should be involved with production managers in the setting-up and monitoring of training programmes. High standards of personal and environmental cleanliness are necessary in all areas – not only in sterile and aseptic units. Appropriate and clean protective clothing should be worn properly, i.e. laboratory coats must be worn fastened, hats must cover all hair and masks cover mouth and nose. Staff should report any minor illness such as colds or skin lesions to their supervisor on arrival at work, as it may be inappropriate for them to carry out their normal duties. Eating, drinking and smoking are prohibited within production areas. It is important that staff from other departments, e.g. maintenance staff and cleaners, who may be unaware of or untrained in hygiene procedures, are not allowed unsupervised access to manufacturing areas.

Documentation

The production master document is an essential element in the assurance of quality of a product. It should include full details of the process, including equipment to be used and any safety precautions. There should be detailed specifications of starting materials, formulae, packaging materials, equipment, methods and labelling. It may be cross-referenced to standard procedures, e.g. a procedure for setting up, and subsequently dismantling and cleaning, a tablet counter or electric mixer. Master documents should be signed by the production pharmacist and approved by the QA pharmacist. Documents should not be amended; should changes be required, new documentation should be prepared. All documentation should be reviewed and updated regularly. These specifications must be supplemented by detailed worksheets to enable the recording for each batch of relevant data as the work proceeds. This will include raw material identification, weighings, methods to be used, personnel signatures, expiry dates, the identification number of the batch and samples of documents created such as labels or autoclave charts. Labels must be carefully accounted for, and the disposal of any spare labels must be witnessed. Batch worksheets are normally produced in hospitals by photocopying the master documentation. Any spare copies thus produced for future use must be logged, and stored securely. When later a master document is modified, obsolete worksheets can be traced and destroyed.

Premises and equipment

Even well-designed premises have to be monitored to ensure that environmental standards are maintained. This will include a regular programme of routine inspection of buildings and services, microbiological testing, e.g. settle plates for airborne contamination, control of cleaning procedures and control on the use of areas. Some checks are recorded on a daily basis. For example, manometers recording pressure differentials are checked before work starts in clean-room suites; results should be recorded graphically so that gradual performance failure can be detected before it becomes critical. Both portable and fixed equipment, e.g. ventilation installations, require microbiological monitoring, tests on performance and, in conjunction with engineering specialists, planned preventive maintenance (PPM). The latter is essential to ensure that no piece of equipment breaks down or becomes hazardous through insidious loss of performance e.g. gradual blockage of a filter. PPM should be organised with the hospital estates management department, who may choose to use specialised contractors for particular equipment.

Process and materials

The quality of processes and materials is closely linked with the use of adequate documentation. Each formula must be validated with a reference to its source, and starting materials defined unambiguously. Production runs must be preceded by the preparation of a trial batch. Any intermediate product of the manufacturing process must be fully labelled to avoid mistakes, and only one product should be processed in an area at any one time. When the product is finished, it should be removed immediately to a quarantine or bond store where it can be segregated from in-use stocks until final QA tests have been completed and its use authorised. The segregation of products which have been passed for use from those which have not is a vital part of QA. It may be achieved by the use of separate locked stores, or by well-controlled segregation within a store. Formal release for use should take place only after the reconciliation of all batch documentation with final control test results.

It is good practice for the person authorising the release of a product to be different from the one carrying out the analysis on it. Whilst awaiting release for use and afterwards, it is important that the product is kept in appropriate storage, e.g. refrigerator, Controlled Drugs cupboard.

All items – including containers and closures, consumables such as gloves and labels – used in the manufacturing process must be subject to QA. Service specifications must be drawn up and agreed with any external contractors who may provide a service, e.g. the provision of clean-room clothing. Such contractors must be monitored for compliance both when the contract is placed and regularly during its term. Specifications should be drawn up for all materials, and all deliveries received checked against this before use. Specifications may originate locally, or refer to standards such as the *British* or *European Pharmacopoeias*. The quality of materials produced locally, such as purified water, should be ensured by routine monitoring and sampling. Raw materials may be received from the manufacturer with a certificate of analysis confirming their compliance with specification. In these cases simple tests should be performed locally to confirm identity and eliminate any error through incorrect labelling.

Quality assurance of dispensing

Dispensing is not subject to controls under the Medicines Act 1968 comparable with those on manufacture. It is for each pharmacist to decide the risk inherent in each dispensing operation, and make suitable provision. In principle, many of the aspects of QA discussed above apply to dispensing, although the requirements may in some cases be less. Examples would be the provision of suitable premises, and the use of documentation for extemporaneous dispensing. Many of these points have been incorporated into the 'Service Specifications' section issued by the RPSGB in Part 3 of the Code of Ethics and Standards.[58] In hospitals it is common for raw materials used in dispensing to be controlled similarly to those used in manufacturing; equipment used in dispensing is also subjected to PPM and monitoring, e.g. dispensing balances are routinely tested for accuracy.

Quality assurance on storage and transportation of medicinal products

It is now recognised that these aspects of pharmaceutical practice should be audited by the QA service within hospitals. Recommendations setting

Table 7.10 Definitions of temperature for storage

Room temperature	15–30°C
Cool place	Below 15°C
Cold place	Below 8°C
Refrigerator	2–8°C
Freezer	Below –20°C

out standards of good practice have been drawn up by the MCA,[62] and regular audit of facilities should take place. Guidelines were also produced by quality controllers nationally[63] and are particularly concerned with storage temperature (Table 7.10).

Controlled-temperature storage facilities should be equipped with recording devices, and the storage temperatures should be monitored regularly by a named person. There should be a written procedure setting out the action to be taken when the temperature falls outside the specified range. Medicinal products such as vaccines, which require controlled-temperature storage, should be transported in such a way as to maintain the cold chain. The cold chain should be subject to regular audit. It should be noted that products should be protected from freezing which can, for example, irreversibly denature the protein in products such as vaccines, and render emulsions physically unstable.

Quality assurance of medical gases

Medical gases are supplied to hospitals either by bulk delivery of liquid oxygen into a local storage tank, each delivery being accompanied by a certificate of analysis by the supplier, or in cylinders. The quality of gases in cylinders is assured by the supplier, but there is a need for controls on the storage of the cylinders, which contain compressed or liquefied gas and therefore should be stored away from excessive heat. They should also be protected from impact or falling over, by using proper trolleys, and retaining chains or bars in cylinder stores. Individual gases may have specific storage requirements, e.g. Entonox, a mixture of nitrous oxide and oxygen, layers and separates out at temperatures below 10°C. There is a Code of Practice for the handling and storage of medical gas cylinders,[64] which contains, in addition, model procedures for every aspect of gas cylinder usage. It also contains what must surely be a complete bibliography of references on this subject, with 61 entries!

Wards and departments receive their medical gases either directly from cylinders, or from piped-gas installations drawing their supply from either a liquid oxygen storage tank or from a manifold holding several large cylinders of gas; the latter method is commonly used to supply nitrous oxide to operating theatres. In either case, the pipeline system itself is a potential source of problems. There is a guidance document, *HTM 2022* in three parts, covering the operational management of pipeline systems; design, installation, validation and verification; and management policy.[65–67] Guidance is necessary because there are many potential hazards in association with the use and maintenance of medical gas pipelines – the risk of an outlet being connected to the wrong manifold, or there being contamination with the wrong gas in the system. Other hazards are even more likely. These include particulate contamination from the pipework and excess moisture. Tests for identity and purity of medical gases from pipelines should be carried out by the Responsible Officer (engineer) assisted by the Suitably Qualified Person (SQP: pharmacist). In practice, the SQP, who is usually the quality controller, tends to do the testing witnessed by the engineer. See *HTM 2022* for descriptions of responsible officers and SQPs. Any engineering work carried out on the system is tightly controlled under a system of documentation known as a Permit to Work, also described in *HTM 2022*. A permit to work is invoked in critical situations where the cessation of supply to patients or machinery, e.g. medical gases or electricity, must be notified to, and agreed by, staff in several disciplines. Thus the medical gases Permit to Work involves doctors, nurses, engineers, fitters and pharmacists. This is intended to ensure that no patient comes to harm as a result of disconnecting a pipeline system, and that its integrity is tested before it is reinstated.

Good laboratory practice

Implicit in the provision of quality for pharmaceuticals is the assurance of quality of the quality control laboratory. In essence, the laboratory should act as though it were a minor production unit. Premises should be appropriate, and documentation should be kept not only for the analysis of production samples, but also for the control of reagents and analytical procedures. Laboratory procedures should reduce the risk of error from the mixing of products, or from inadequately monitored equipment. Many laboratories now take part in national and regional audits of accuracy, in which standardised samples are sent to all participating laboratories, and the results collated centrally.

References

1. UK Medicines Information. *Better Information for Managing Medicines: A Strategy for Pharmacy's Medicines Information Service* 2000. Available at www.ukmig.org.uk (accessed August 2001).
2. Mehta D K, ed. *British National Formulary*, published twice-yearly. London: British Medical Association/Royal Pharmaceutical Society of Great Britain.
3. Article. Specialist pharmacy groups in the NHS. *Hosp Pharm* 2000; 7: 260–262.
4. *Annual Report 1997/8 and 1998/9*. UK Drug Information Pharmacists Group. Available at www.ukmig.org.uk (accessed August 2001).
5. Simister K L, Jackson C W. Informing the effective introduction of new drugs into the National Health Service. *Pharm J* 1998; 261: 90–92.
6. UK Medicines Information Pharmacists Group website (2001). *New Medicines on the Market*. www.ukmi.nhs.uk (accessed 19 March 2002).
7. UK Medicines Information Pharmacists Group. *UK Drug Information Manual*, available from Dr A Judd, Director, Drug and Poisons Information Service, The General Infirmary, Great George Street, Leeds, LS1 3EX.
8. UK Medicines Information Pharmacists Group website. www.ukmi.nhs.uk (accessed 19 March 2002).
9. UK Drug Information Pharmacists Group website. *Annual Report* (1998/9). www.ukmi.nhs.uk (accessed 19 March 2002).
10. *Better Information for Managing Medicines: Implementation Framework*. UK Medicines Information 2000. Available at www.ukmig.org.uk (accessed August 2001).
11. Cairns C, Lane V. Drug information services for primary care. *Pharm J* 1999; 263: 251–255.
12. Kuczynska J. Quality assurance in drug information. *Hosp Pharm* 1998; 5: 210–212.
13. Irvine M K Å. Quality issues in drug information practice. *Hosp Pharm* 1997; 4: 263–265.
14. *Drug and Therapeutics Bulletin*, published monthly. Hertford: Which? Ltd.
15. *MeReC Bulletin*. Liverpool: National Prescribing Centre, The Infirmary, 70 Pembroke Place, Liverpool L69 3GF.
16. Sweetman S, ed. *Martindale: The complete drug reference*, 33rd edn. London: Pharmaceutical Press, 2002.
17. *The Web-enabled British National Formulary (WeBNF)*. London: Pharmaceutical Press.
18. Daly M, Lee A. Drug information: new technology in accessing and disseminating drug information. *Hosp Pharm* 1998; 5: 206–209.
19. Wiffen P. What is evidence-based medicine? *Pharm J* 1997; 258: 510–511.
20. Mason P. The Centre for Evidence-based Pharmacotherapy at Aston. *Pharm J* 1999; 263: 892–893.
21. Department of Health Research and Development Division. *Research for Health*. London: Department of Health, 1993.
22. House of Lords. *Priorities in Medical Research*. London: Her Majesty's Stationery Office, 1987.
23. Clark C M, Stevens A J H, Milne R I G. The Health Technology Assessment

Programme and its implications for clinical pharmacy. *Pharm J* 1997; 258: 275–277.

24. Slee A, Farrar K. Formulary management – effective computer management systems. *Pharm J* 1999; 262: 363–365.

25. Medicines Control Agency. *Rules and Guidance for Pharmaceutical Manufacturers and Distributors (The Orange Guide)*. London: Stationery Office, 1997.

26. Medicines Control Agency Guidance Note no. 14. *The Supply of Unlicensed Relevant Medicinal Products for Individual Patients*. London: Stationery Office, 2000.

27. Quality Control Sub-Committee of Regional Pharmaceutical Officers' Committee (1993). *The Quality Assurance of Aseptic Preparation Services: National Guidelines on the Design, Operation and Monitoring of Aseptic Preparation Services in NHS Hospitals.*

28. Technical Specialist Education and Training Group website (2002). www.tset.org.uk (accessed 4 February 2002).

29. Baird R M. Microbiological control of pharmaceuticals. *Pharm Int* 1986; 7: 255–258.

30. Sharp J. *Quality in the Manufacture of Medicines and other Healthcare Products*. London: Pharmaceutical Press, 2000.

31. Meers P D, Calder M W, Mazhar M M, Lawrie G M. Intravenous infusion of contaminated dextrose solution. The Devonport incident. *Lancet* 1973; 2: 1189–1192.

32. NHS Estates. *Health Technical Memorandum 2010: Sterilization*. London: Stationery Office, March 1994–March 2000.

33. Shaw R J S, Riley S J, Jones K P. Health Technical Memorandum 2010 – Sterilisation. *Hosp Pharm* 1996; 3: 95–96.

34. UK Radiopharmacy Group website (2002). www.ukrg.org.uk (accessed 4 February 2002).

35. Maltby P. The maze of regulations in radiopharmacy. *Hosp Pharm* 1999; 6: 42–54.

36. Meeting report. New legislation affecting radiopharmacy. *Hosp Pharm* 2000; 7: 99–102.

37. Solanki C. Quality testing of radiopharmaceuticals – clinical importance and methodology. *Hosp Pharm* 1998; 5: 12–14.

38. Frier M. Quality testing of radiopharmaceuticals. *Hosp Pharm* 2000; 7: 89–93.

39. Department of Health and Social Security Circular. *Report of the Working Party on the Addition of Drugs to Intravenous Infusion Fluids*. HC(76)9.

40. Needle R. The feasibility of centralised intravenous additive services. *Hosp Pharm* 1997; 4: 33–36.

41. News item. Two children die after receiving infected TPN solutions. *Pharm J* 1994; 252: 596.

42. Farwell J. *Aseptic Dispensing for NHS Patients*. London: Department of Health, 1994.

43. Department of Health. *Aseptic Dispensing in NHS Hospitals*. PL/CPhO(96)2.

44. NHS Executive. *Aseptic Dispensing in NHS Hospitals*. EL(96)95.

45. Needle R, Sizer T, eds. *The CIVAS Handbook*. London: Pharmaceutical Press, 1998.

46. National Centralised Intravenous Additives Services Group website (2002). www.civas.co.uk (accessed 4 February 2002).

47. Beaney A M, ed. NHS Pharmaceutical Quality Control Committee. *Quality Assurance of Aseptic Preparation Services*, 3rd edn. London: Pharmaceutical Press, 2001.

48. Trissel L A, ed. *Handbook on Injectable Drugs*, 11th edn. Washington, DC: American Society of Health-System Pharmacists, 2001.

49. News item. Paediatric PN: new guidelines. *Hosp Pharm* 2000; 7: 208.

50. British Association for Parenteral and Enteral Nutrition. *Current Perspectives on Paediatric Parenteral Nutrition*. Maidenhead: BAPEN. 2000. Available from P O Box 922, Maidenhead, Berks SL6 4SH.

51. NHS Executive. *Improving the Quality of Cancer Services*. HSC 2000/021.

52. NHS Executive. *Manual of Cancer Services Standards*. London: Stationery Office, December 2000.

53. Department of Health website (2002). www.doh.gov.uk/cancer (accessed 4 February 2002).

54. Allwood M C, Wright P. *The Cytotoxics Handbook*, 3rd edn. Abingdon: Radcliffe Medical Press, 1996.

55. National Centralised Intravenous Additive Service Group and British Oncology Pharmacy Association. Statement: monoclonal antibodies. *Hosp Pharm* 2001; 8: 153.

56. Lofthouse S. Why we overhauled our cytotoxic production worksheets and labels. *Hosp Pharm* 2001; 9: 25–26.

57. Sewell G. Introduction of chemotherapy software at Derriford Hospital. *Hosp Pharm* 1999; 6: 26–29.

58. Royal Pharmaceutical Society of Great Britain. *Medicines, Ethics and Practice: A Guide for Pharmacists*, published yearly. London: Royal Pharmaceutical Society of Great Britain.

59. European Pharmacopoeia Commission Council of Europe. European Department for the Quality of Medicines. *European Pharmacopoeia*, 4th edn. Brussels: Council of Europe, 2002.

60. Lund W, ed. *The Pharmaceutical Codex*, 12th edn. London: Pharmaceutical Press, 1994.

61. Department of Health and Social Security. *Application of the Medicines Act to Health Authorities*. London: Stationery Office. HSC(IS)128.

62. Taylor J. Recommendations on the control and monitoring of storage and transportation temperatures of medicinal products. *Pharm J* 2001; 267: 128–131.

63. Regional Quality Control Sub-committee of Regional Pharmaceutical Officers. *Storage and Distribution of Medicinal Products in Health Authority Premises: Guidelines on the Safe Storage of Medicines*. 1993.

64. Health Equipment Information no. 163. *Code of Practice: Safety and Care in the Storage, Handling and Use of Medical Gas Cylinders on Health Authority Premises*. London: Department of Health and Social Security, NHS Procurement Directorate, 1987.

65. NHS Estates Health Technical Memorandum no. 2022. *Medical Gas Pipeline Systems: Operational Management.* London: Stationery Office, 1997.
66. NHS Estates Health Technical Memorandum no. 2022. *Medical Gas Pipeline Systems: Design, Installation, Validation and Verification.* London, Stationery Office, 1997.
67. NHS Estates Health Technical Memorandum no. 2022. *Medical Gas Pipeline Systems: Management Policy.* London: Her Majesty's Stationery Office, 1994.

8

The pharmacist as a health care professional

Introduction: the profession of pharmacy

Over the years, much thought and debate has been devoted to defining the true professional role of the pharmacist, and deciding what special aspects only the pharmacist can contribute to the health care team. When professional practice consisted purely of compounding and dispensing, the role of the pharmacist was clearly understood by both the public and fellow health care professionals. Latterly the traditional skills have become less important to most pharmacists – although their spirit lives on in modern pharmaceutical production and formulation techniques – and new areas of practice such as clinical pharmacy and medicines management have been developed. The changing face of the profession and health care generally and the need for rigorous standards of practice have been acknowledged by the development of a new Code of Practice and Standards of Professional Performance. The new Code was adopted at the May 2001 Annual General Meeting of the Royal Pharmaceutical Society of Great Britain (RPSGB), and is published as Part One of the *Medicines, Ethics and Practice* guide (MEP).[1] Part Two sets out standards of professional performance, and Part Three includes service specifications agreed by the Council of the RPSGB. Some specifications relate to topics included in the Code, and others are additional.

In this chapter, we look in detail at some important practice activities, and discuss aspects that go towards the delivery of a high-quality service. We also consider the interface with other health care providers such as doctors and nurses, and delineate some of the professional responsibilities which pharmacists have in dealing with other members of the health care team.

Professional indemnity insurance

It will be seen from the 'Standards of Professional Performance' that pharmacists should arrange indemnity insurance to cover their professional activities. Proprietor pharmacists' professional insurance comes automatically with membership of the National Pharmaceutical Association

(NPA) through the Chemists' Defence Association.[2] Also included in membership is insurance against those hazards unconnected with dispensing – for example, damage to property or accidents on the premises which may befall customers and staff – known as public liability, through an associated organisation, the Pharmacy Mutual Insurance Company Ltd, an NPA-affiliated company; their insurance schemes are available to any pharmacist, whether a member of the NPA or not.

Hospital pharmacists are advised to arrange for their own insurance cover rather than relying on the support of their employers in the event of a patient complaining or suing for damages. In this way they will ensure that they receive timely advice about how to handle statements and investigations into incidents, and will be sure of legal representation to protect their personal interests and professional reputation in any legal proceedings, including inquests, which may have to apportion blame, and hence damages, between several members of the staff. Membership of the Guild of Healthcare Pharmacists confers a certain amount of protection of members' interests, but many hospital pharmacists supplement this with specific professional indemnity insurance arranged through an insurance broker.

Indemnity of National Health Service (NHS) hospital doctors is now provided by their employing authority. Claims involving litigation are handled by the NHS Litigation Authority. Its activities have been the subject of a recent audit by the National Audit Office,[3] which reported that the system was excessively bureaucratic, with claimants frequently awarded less in damages than the legal costs incurred. An overhaul of the system is to be undertaken,[4] with a White Paper setting out proposed reforms to be published in early 2002.

Relationships with other professions

Doctors and pharmacists

When receiving a prescription, the first step is to ensure that it has been written by a registered medical practitioner who is entitled to prescribe in the UK. Pharmacists are required to be on their guard against forged prescriptions, and the MEP guide[1] has a section on detecting forgeries. Failure to observe the precautions listed has led to admonition by the Statutory Committee for a pharmacist who had been convicted on six counts of dispensing forged prescriptions.[5] Dispensing forged prescriptions for Prescription Only Medicines (POMs) is an offence under Section 58(2)(a) of the Medicines Act 1968. In 1986,[6] Law Lords upheld a High Court decision to uphold a conviction of this nature, even though the defendants, who had supplied Physeptone, Ritalin and Valium tablets on forged prescriptions, had no idea that they had been duped (*Pharmaceutical Society* v *Storkwain Ltd*: further information will be found in Appelbe and Wingfield[7]). After this case, a modification of the POM order was made to enable a pharmacist to be protected from prosecution (or, at least, from automatically being found guilty), who 'having exercised all due diligence, believes on reasonable grounds that the prescription is genuine'.[8]

There are four categories of medical registration: full, provisional, limited and visiting European Union (EU) practitioner. Full details will be found *in Dale and Appelbe's Pharmacy Law and Ethics*.[7] General practitioners are always fully registered; this is true also of general practice trainee doctors. In most cases, the doctor and his/her writing will be known to the pharmacist; otherwise some steps must be taken to check validity, particularly in the case of drugs liable to abuse. The simplest check is to telephone the surgery and make sure that the patient has been seen on the relevant date and was in fact prescribed the items in question. The telephone number of the surgery should be checked from the directory, and not read off the prescription; there have been cases where numbers printed on headed notepaper have turned out to be a payphone down the road.

In hospitals, provisionally registered doctors work as house officers on medical and surgical units, since 6 months' experience in each is a requirement for full registration. Most prescriptions for hospital in-patients are written by house officers or senior house officers. (Medical students may not legally prescribe POMs or initiate any treatment: see Chapter 6 for details.)

Doctors with limited registration may work in any hospital speciality, since they have an overseas qualification, and are usually in the UK to gain specialised experience or a higher qualification. Provisionally registered doctors and those with limited registration do not usually write FP10(HP) prescriptions for hospital outpatients, since they are permitted to do so only if outpatient prescribing is a normal part of their duties, and this would only rarely be the case. Enquiry as to the status of an individual may be made by telephone, either to the hospital medical staffing department or to the registration authority, i.e. the Registrar of the General Medical Council.

On occasion, doctors, because of misdemeanour, lose their right to prescribe and possess controlled drugs. The Department of Health from time to time sends out circulars listing the names of doctors and dentists (and also pharmacists!) prohibited from exercising their powers in relation to controlled drugs.

Dealing with queries

The final professional responsibility for dispensing the prescription, including whether a decision should be made *not* to dispense, lies with the pharmacist. Thus he/she has a duty to clarify and confirm with the prescriber any unusual prescription and, in particular, any dose in excess of that usually recommended. This duty was established in law by the Migril case, in which a pharmacist's failure to query an excessive dose resulted in his being held liable for 45% of the resultant damages. It is, of course, easier to approach doctors with queries if the parties are on friendly terms and have established a good working relationship already. Most young doctors now have had experience during their hospital years of working with ward pharmacists and have come to expect, and welcome, pharmacists' help in prescribing appropriately; hopefully this cooperative attitude can be maintained, but it will be only if the pharmacist exercises discretion. For example, it is important to avoid interrupting busy doctors with trivial queries that could be resolved by discussion with a more experienced pharmacist colleague. Likewise, one must avoid embarrassing prescribers by discussing possible errors in front of patients, nurses or their senior colleagues. In hospitals, where prescription queries are sometimes communicated in writing, the style must be concise, accurate and professional in appearance. An envelope should be used if the subject matter is better kept confidential for any reason. Notes should be on presentable stationery, legible, dated and signed. Abbreviations should be used judiciously, particularly when writing to doctors whose first language is not English; I have known the last paragraph of a long note to be overlooked because the recipient did not know the meaning of 'PTO'.

Agreed amendments to prescriptions must be confirmed in writing by the prescriber as soon as possible to protect the interests of all parties. FP10 prescription forms are retained by the Prescription Pricing Authority for at least 6 months after pricing and, in the event of a serious mishap that requires investigation, may be produced for evidence. FP10(HP) forms are returned to the issuing trust and should be retained so that they are available for financial audit. Although not specifically mentioned in the Health Circular[9] that gives guidance on the recommended periods for retention of hospital documents, it is recommended that audit documents should generally be retained for 2 years, and this could be taken to apply also to FP10(HP) forms.

Pharmacists and nurses

Nurses working in the community may be attached to a general practitioner's surgery, or have as a practice base primary care group/trust-managed premises such as a health centre or clinic. Some community nurses work out of hospitals, providing a liaison role between inpatient care and care in the community. Macmillan cancer nurses are an example. The role of community nurses has expanded in recent years with the advent of nurse prescribing (see Chapter 1) and various other initiatives, e.g. nurse practitioners may run specialist clinics such as diabetic and asthma monitoring within surgery premises, much as their hospital colleagues do. In addition, nurses may undertake home visits to monitor elderly patients, and many are attached to the community psychiatric service.

In addition to qualified nurses, pharmacists will encounter student nurses who are in training in both community settings and hospitals. In most areas, student nurses wear a national uniform, and pharmacists should learn how to distinguish them from qualified staff. Student nurses have no statutory rights to order ward stock drugs as do registered nurses; however, they may perform these duties under supervision if so authorised. Hospitals vary in the range of delegated duties that are permitted to student nurses, and local procedures must be studied for guidance. The ordering and receipt of Controlled Drugs are usually restricted to registered nurses on the permanent staff, i.e. not agency nurses. More details of the organisation of the ward nursing team will be found in Chapter 12.

Nurses are probably the client group most eager to receive advice about handling, storing, administering and disposing of unwanted drugs. They are highly trained to be responsible in their attitudes to treatment and they see the action of drugs first hand, and are thus able to impart much information as well. In addition, nurse managers often need advice about the implementation of drugs legislation, which will require cooperation in the design of ordering and prescribing documents, drug storage facilities on wards, and procedures for drug administration, including self-medication schemes.

Pharmacists and police officers

There are a number of aspects of pharmacy practice that may result in contact with police officers. Officers of the Drugs Squad may be involved with cases of drug abuse and thefts of drugs, and of course local chemist inspection police officers have duties regarding Controlled Drugs and may be requested to witness the destruction of unwanted Controlled Drugs. A move to coordinate the work of such officers has recently been made by the formation of a professional organisation, the National Association of Chemist Inspection Officers. The association is to establish its own section on the European Police internet (EpiCentre), which can be used securely by police personnel to act as a noticeboard to report details of current trends and problems.[10]

If a pharmacist believes that a drugs-related crime has occurred, it should be reported in the first instance to the local police, who will refer the matter to the Drugs Squad if they think it appropriate. In hospitals, contacts with the police are usually made via hospital managers.

On occasions, police officers may approach pharmacists during an investigation to seek information about suspects who may be patients. This may pose an ethical dilemma for the pharmacist, who has a professional duty not to reveal confidential information about patients. In the section on confidentiality in the 'Standards of Professional Performance' in Part Two of the MEP,[1] it states that an exception may be made in the case of a police officer or NHS Fraud Investigation Officer who provides in writing confirmation that disclosure is necessary to assist in the prevention, detection or prosecution of serious crime. The contents of hospital case records may only be made available as evidence if a court directs that they are to be produced; if this happens, they are delivered to the court by a trust officer (usually a patient services manager), who retains the document in his/her possession. Patient prescription record details may be revealed to the police only on the production of a warrant. This would not, of course, preclude giving pharmaceutical advice or dispensing the occasional prescription written by a police surgeon for a patient who is taken ill while in police custody.

By arrangement with the Local Pharmaceutical Committee, police stations hold a list of the names and addresses of community pharmacists who are willing to dispense urgent prescriptions outside normal hours. Dispensing such prescriptions attracts an extra fee. For details, including the prescription endorsements needed to claim, refer to the *Drug Tariff* Part IIIA para 2 section G.[11] To safeguard the pharmacist returning at night to a lonely premises, a police escort may be provided if deemed advisable.

Pharmacists and excise officers

Excise officers have the right to enter at all reasonable hours premises where methylated spirits, rectified spirit and other forms of ethyl alcohol including potable, i.e. drinkable, varieties, are stored, sold or used. They may require certain records of use to be made, and subsequently monitor them, and also check stores to see that permitted quantities are not being exceeded. Isopropyl alcohol may be used without formality, as it is not included in the regulations governing the use of methylated spirits. Hospitals may purchase spirits such as brandy and gin without paying excise duty so long as they are used for medicinal purposes only; records of issues must be maintained in a format agreed by the excise officer to show that use is *bona fide*.

Stills must be registered with the local excise office, which will have been notified of the purchase by the supplier. There is a standard form, which must be completed by the pharmacist in charge; even stills permanently incorporated in apparatus such as instrument-washing machines must be declared. Excise officers inspect stills from time to time and may check that the effluent is indeed distilled water. When old stills are taken out of use, the local excise officer must be notified, and may insist on witnessing the breaking-up of the equipment.

Professional practice standards

Disclosure of information

The importance of maintaining confidentiality of any information, both medical and otherwise, about patients and their families cannot be emphasised too strongly. All pharmacists must familiarise themselves with the standards set for confidentiality in Part Two of the MEP.[1] Written information should be accessible to staff only on a 'need-to-know' basis and gossip about patients and their affairs is forbidden. In hospitals, revealing the contents of a patient's case record, including details of his/her medication, to an unauthorised person is a disciplinary offence which may result in dismissal; some trusts require their staff to sign a confidentiality agreement on appointment. In our own experience, a pharmacy technician was disciplined for discussing a patient's prescription in the hospital staff dining room when a relative overheard the discussion.

In 1996, the NHS Executive issued guidance on the protection and use of patient information,[12] and directed health authorities[13] to put into place policies and procedures to ensure that patients were made personally aware of the purposes to which information about them may be put, as well as ways in which they can exercise choice. Some changes in the use of data for commercial research purposes have followed. For many years, it has been the practice to sell anonymised prescription data to specialist companies who market the resulting statistics on drug usage to pharmaceutical companies. In 1999 a prescribing database compiler challenged in the High Court an earlier ruling that the sale of such information was a breach of confidentiality. The High Court upheld the earlier decision, and subsequently both the RPSGB and the NPA advised members to cease data sales.[14–16]

Patients often ask pharmacists about the nature of their own illness and treatment. Such enquiries must be handled with tact and discretion since doctors may not reveal the full diagnosis, or the unfavourable future course of the disease process, to patients if they do not consider it to be in their best interest at that time. It is as well to attempt to find out what the patient already knows, and build on that. A complete refusal to discuss the illness may well make the patient fear the worst.

Data Protection Act 1998

The Data Protection Act 1984 was replaced on 1 March 2000 by the Data Protection Act 1998. Unlike the earlier legislation, the new Act covers all types of data retrieval systems, including paper records. Guidance for health authorities and health care professionals has been published by the NHS Executive.[17,18] Information relating to any living persons who may be identified by details held in the filing system or by information which may come into the possession of the data controller is subject to the provisions of the Act, and such systems must by law be registered with the Data Protection Commissioner (formerly the Data Protection Registrar). The Access to Health Records Act 1990 gave patients the right to see those parts of their own records which were compiled after 1 November 1991, however they had been compiled and filed. However, the Data Protection Act 1998 permits patients to have access to their records whenever they were compiled, subject only to specified exemptions. Records kept by any health professional are included; the Act thus applies to patient medication records (PMRs). The implications of the new Act for pharmacists were summarised in an article by Wingfield.[19] They include principles which must be followed in how personal data is processed, the uses to which it may be put, the length of time it may be retained and security that must be adopted. Doctors and pharmacy employees whose names appear in computer-produced statistics count as data subjects; the Act does not only relate to patients' records.

Patient medication records

Records must be kept of medicines supplied on private prescriptions, the emergency supply of drugs previously obtained on a doctor's prescription, and should be kept for those prescribed by the pharmacist in response to symptoms described by the patient ('counter prescribing'). In 1997 the law was amended to permit the use of electronic records. Full details of the current requirements may be found in the 'General Legal Requirements' section of the MEP.[1]

In addition, most pharmacies keep PMRs – a file recording both prescription and over-the-counter drugs supplied. There are specifications for PMRs in Part Three of the MEP.[1] In theory, such a complete medication profile should make it easy to anticipate interactions between prescription and non-prescription drugs, and to keep track of involved treatment regimens. In practice, since patients are free to go to any pharmacy, there is no guarantee that the record is complete. It has been suggested that patients should register with a pharmacy as they do their doctor, but the idea has never gained much support. Pharmacy contractors may now receive a fee for maintaining patient medication records for:

- those who are exempt from prescription charges: men and women aged 60 or over;
- others whom the pharmacists considers may have difficulty in understanding the nature and dosage of the drug supplied and the times at which it is to be taken.

To be eligible, pharmacists must have successfully completed an appropriate distance learning course. Further details about maintaining the records, and of qualifying training schemes, will be found in the *Drug Tariff*, Part XIV B.[11]

Procedures for maintaining safety standards

Pharmacists need to be aware of a number of methods which have been devised over the years to protect the public from harm arising from defective drugs, faulty medical equipment and unwanted chemicals. The defects may have arisen because of design faults, or from errors during manufacture. Additionally, materials may become potentially hazardous because they have outlived their usefulness and have been left around in inappropriate conditions to act as a trap for the unwary.

Table 8.1 Adverse incident and defect reporting

Medicinal products Drugs/ingredients Diagnostics Contraceptives Contact lens fluids	Medicines Control Agency www.mca.gov.uk
Medical devices Sterile disposables Medical and laboratory equipment Orthotic and prosthetic appliances Laboratory chemicals and reagents Enteral feeds Medical textiles	Medical Devices Agency www.medical-devices.gov.uk
Non-medical equipment and plant Engineering plant/services Lifts Fire equipment Sterilisers/autoclaves Medical gas/vacuum installations Communications equipment Fume cupboards Microbiological safety cabinets Ventilation systems	NHS Estates www.nhsestates.gov.uk
Foods	Local authority environmental health department

Defective products: reporting procedure

Health workers have a professional responsibility to consider, and if necessary to act upon, the possibility that a defect that they may encounter in the course of their work, or an accident or untoward incident, may have the potential for causing harm not just to one person, but on a national or regional scale. A system has been devised for reporting accidents and defects with plant, equipment, buildings, drugs and other supplies which enables problems to be investigated, and, if necessary, reported to other users. The scheme is set out in a Medicines Control Agency (MCA) booklet (the Red Book)[20] and in a Medical Devices Agency (MDA) document.[21] Defects in medicinal products are referred to the MCA Defective Medicines Report Centre, which forms part of the European Rapid Alert System, which disseminates information on drug quality issues within EU member states. For defects in other items, such as installed plant and equipment, and contact details, refer to Table 8.1.

In the managed service, each NHS trust is responsible for ensuring that staff know about the procedure, and for carrying it out. The notification of incidents in particular categories will be delegated to certain officers, e.g. drug defects would probably be the responsibility of a senior pharmacy manager, medical equipment that of the supplies manager and building and engineering items that of the estates manager. Reports from community pharmacists would be channelled via their health authority or primary care trust. This avoids duplication, and also ensures that adequate local action can be taken to quarantine suspect items pending investigation. The local procedure should also ensure effective communication between departmental managers and quality control staff. Defects in hospital-produced items must also be reported to the quality control pharmacist. In the case of serious accidents and incidents, it may be necessary to inform the Health and Safety Executive as well.

Drug alerts and hazard notices

A national notification network exists to alert health workers about defects and hazards. Drug defects, recalls or product withdrawals are notified by the Defect Reporting Centre of the MCA to the senior pharmacy managers and pharmaceutical advisers using a cascade system, which will have previously set up a contingency plan which can initiate an urgent recall day or night.

Drug alerts are classified into four categories,[22] listed in Table 8.2. The MDA issues:

- hazard notices;
- device alerts (formerly called advisory notices);
- safety notices;
- implantable pacemaker/ICD technical notes.

When trusts and health authorities receive hazard notices, the staff responsible take action in a similar manner as a drug alert. Past issues may be accessed on the MDA website.[23]

Decontamination of medical devices

Considerable attention has been paid to the decontamination of medical devices and equipment in recent years. Validated procedures are required to be in place to ensure that equipment is effectively decontaminated both between use on patients, and to protect staff when it is repaired and serviced. There have been health circulars on the subject[24, 25] of the

Table 8.2 Classification of drug alerts

Class 1 – Action now (including out-of-hours)
Wrong product (label and contents are different products)
Correct product but wrong strength, with serious medical consequences
Microbial contamination of parenteral or ophthalmic product
Chemical contamination, with serious medical consequences
Mix-up of some products ('rogues') with more than one container
Wrong active ingredient in a multicomponent product with serious medical
  consequences

Class 2 – Action within 48 hours (excluding any in Class 1)
Mislabelling: wrong or missing text or figures/wrong or missing batch number or
  expiry date
Missing or incorrect information – leaflets or inserts
Microbial contamination of non-parenteral, non-ophthalmic sterile product, with
  medical consequences
Chemical/physical contamination (significant impurities, cross-contamination,
  particulates)
Mix-up of products in containers ('rogues')
Non-compliance with specification (e.g. assay, stability, fill or weight)
Insecure closure with serious medical consequences (e.g. cytotoxics, child-resistant
  potent)

Class 3 – Confirmation if manufacturer has decided to recall (Action within 5 days)
Faulty packaging
Faulty closure
Contamination: microbial spoilage/dirt or detritus/particulate matter/single 'rogue'
  tablet

Class 4 – Caution in use (Action within 48 hours)
To include low hazard defects where the fault is readily visible and there is a low
  incidence in the batch concerned

---

decontamination of medical devices, and there is also a Controls Assurance Standard,[26] which gives a bibliography of available guidance and defines the organisational requirements for effective management and also sets out an action plan.

Unwanted medicines

From time to time, patients or their relatives return partly used courses of treatment to pharmacies. Drugs returned in this way are not suitable for reissue to other patients since their quality cannot be guaranteed: their storage history, shelf-life, cleanliness and, quite often, identity are unknown. The Part Three: 'Service Specifications' section of the MEP[1] states that 'Medicines returned to a pharmacy from a patient's home, a nursing or residential home must not be supplied to any other patient'.

Upon admission to hospital, patients are requested to bring with them all current treatment so that it may be identified. As recommended in the Duthie guidelines,[27] the admitting nurse or a pharmacist should determine whether the patient has brought in any medicines. If so, an appropriate designated person (admitting doctor, nurse, care team or pharmacist) should decide what is to be done with them. Such drugs are legally the patient's property, and they may only be destroyed or confiscated with the consent of the patient. If this is not forthcoming, even after adequate counselling, the drugs must be returned to the patient, however unwise this may seem. In default, the patient may claim financial compensation. (For unwanted Controlled Drugs in hospitals, see Chapter 6.) In certain cases, with due safeguards, if prescribed by the hospital doctor, they may be used for that patient's treatment while in hospital, e.g. in the case of a non-formulary drug not stocked by the pharmacy (see also Chapter 6). Under no circumstances may they be used to treat another patient.

Hospital wards return to the pharmacy unfinished courses of treatment dispensed for individual inpatients when the treatment has been changed or the patient is discharged or dies. In 1986, the RPSGB Hospital Pharmacists' Group issued guidelines on the reuse of medicines that are still applicable.[28] The guidelines aim to minimise waste while not compromising patient safety:

- Any time-expired medicines must be destroyed.
- All other medicines should be examined by a pharmacist, to assess their suitability for being returned to stock.
- Medicines should only be considered for reuse where any necessary storage conditions have been fulfilled and the condition of the pack and its contents are judged to be satisfactory.

It should be noted that the cost of examining returned drugs, and making the necessary adjustments to the stock levels in computerised pharmacies, may well exceed the value of the stock saved.

Disposal of clinical waste

Pharmacists should be aware of the need to dispose of waste materials which may be potentially harmful, with due precautions for the safety of persons and the protection of the environment. The passing of the Environmental Protection Act (EPA) 1990 made the requirements for

Table 8.3 Clinical waste categories

Group A	All human tissue, including blood-soiled surgical dressings, swabs and other soiled waste from treatment areas
Group B	Discarded syringe needles, cartridges, broken glass and any other contaminated disposable sharp items
Group C	Microbiological cultures and waste from pathological laboratories
Group D	Pharmaceutical products and chemical wastes

Table 8.4 Colour coding for waste containers

Yellow	Group A waste, infectious waste for incineration
Yellow and black stripes	Non-infectious waste
Light blue	Potentially infectious waste for autoclaving before disposal
Black	Non-clinical or household waste

disposing of hazardous materials much more stringent than hitherto. The Health Services Advisory Committee has produced guidance on the disposal of clinical waste.[29] It sets out categories of clinical waste, with the main ones of concern to pharmacists summarised in Table 8.3.

There is a Controls Assurance Standard for waste disposal[30] that contains a bibliography of legislation and official guidance. It is an audit document, which defines standards for both organisational and management requirements for efficient waste management within health care organisations. It also contains information about defined quality standards for items such as waste containers. There is a nationally agreed colour code for waste containers, and this is set out in Table 8.4.

As few hospitals have incinerators capable of operating at the temperatures prescribed by the disposal regulations, arrangements must be made with a licensed waste contractor. The local waste disposal authority (WDA) is not responsible for removing unwanted stock free of charge from pharmacies, although they will offer advice, and may offer a disposal service for a fee. POMs are designated as 'special waste' and some WDAs require these to be individually itemised on consignment notes. Waste carriers have a duty under the EPA to be registered with the Environment Agency for the collection, transportation and disposal of waste. A certificate of registration is issued by the Agency, which includes the date on which the carrier's registration expires. It is the organisation's responsibility to verify that the carrier holds a valid certificate prior to waste being removed from the site. There are several references about pharmaceutical waste in the MEP.[1] The NPA Information Department has a directory of waste disposal contractors.

Patients or carers may be advised to dispose of very small quantities of unwanted oral medicines by flushing them down the lavatory, but this method is not suitable for anything more than a minimal quantity (the RPSGB has suggested a maximum of 50 tablets), since the water and sewerage authorities have very strict regulations precluding the disposal of drugs and chemicals via the public water and sewage services (other than in sewage!). It is good practice for unwanted pharmaceuticals to be returned to a pharmacy for disposal. Since 1993, funds have been made available to health authorities to cover the provision of waste containers, the transport of waste to disposal sites and the costs of disposal.

Any organisation involved with clinical waste is required by the guidelines and the Controls Assurance Standard to have a clinical waste policy. Since pharmaceutical waste is classified as clinical waste, carefully thought-out procedures are needed in hospitals to deal with it, whether originating from wards or from within the pharmacy department. Used pharmaceutical containers are classified as clinical waste. Hospitals must either apply for a licence to operate as a waste disposal carrier themselves, or use a licensed contractor. In practice, most use a contractor to remove all categories of clinical waste from the site. Monitored procedures should be in place to cover the training of staff, the packaging of waste, safe transit to the collection point, security while awaiting collection, proper disposal of sharps and procedures to deal with spillages and needlestick injuries.

Cytotoxic waste is a special category; few hospitals have incinerators complying with both the regulations for emissions and the high temperatures required for cytotoxic residues, and so a specialist contractor is usually employed.

When it is necessary to dispose of large amounts of toxic chemicals, drugs or organic solvents, the advice of the local environmental health department or WDA should be sought. Some authorities run a poisonous waste disposal service which, for a fee, will collect. Alternatively, there are private contractors who will dispose of items at a fee per cubic foot of space needed.

Disposal of unwanted medicines (DUMP) campaigns

Pharmacists are sometimes asked to participate in campaigns intended to safeguard the public from the dangers of hoarding old drugs in the home. The new regulations have made the disposal of the medicines collected virtually impossible, since POMs are sure to be included, and their classification as 'special waste' (see above) means that they should itemised and listed – this is clearly impossible if identity is uncertain. Recently a ruling has been made that an exception to this requirement may be made for items handed-in in DUMP campaigns. Pharmacists should note that unwanted stocks from pharmacies must not be included with DUMP materials.

Pharmacists may be approached by well-meaning charity workers who suggest sending unwanted drugs to underprivileged countries. Pharmacists should only participate in schemes which conform with World Health Organization guidelines,[31] a copy of which may be obtained from the RPSGB Professional Standards Directorate. In outline, schemes may be acceptable if:

- No obsolete drugs are included.
- Only those drugs which are estimated to have a shelf-life of at least 1 year after arrival in the recipient country are collected.
- No medicine supplied to or returned by an individual patient is included.
- A specific list of which medicines are needed is provided.
- Arrangements are made for the safe and secure supervision of collection and sorting of unwanted medicines and subsequent disposal of medicines not required.[1]

Schemes which involve volunteers calling at houses to ask for unwanted drugs are liable to abuse, and, in many cases, it would of course be illegal to take possession of drugs prescribed for another person.

Mercury spillage

Mercury is used in a number of departments in hospitals and clinics, e.g. it is used in dental amalgam, in thermometers and sphygmomanometers and also to weight some types of enteral feeding tube. Inhalation of the vapour if mercury escapes is potentially dangerous, and absorption can occur through the skin. Spillage of even small quantities must be properly dealt with. Particularly dangerous is a spill on to carpet, which cannot be effectively decontaminated. Vacuum cleaners should not be used since they themselves may then contaminate the environment. These and other essential facts are included in a paper by Anderton,[32] on which a local procedure could be based.

Poisoning

From time to time pharmacists in both community and hospital practice have to deal with a patient who is believed to have been poisoned, or to give advice about the identity of drugs or potentially toxic ingredients of ingested or absorbed materials. Accidental poisoning usually occurs either in young children or in occupational exposure in adults; deliberate poisoning is mainly seen in adults. Administration of noxious substances is sometimes a feature of child abuse, and this possibility should be borne in mind. Pharmacists must familiarise themselves with the section on emergency treatment of poisoning in the *British National Formulary* (BNF)[33] which sets out the basic principles and lists the telephone numbers of the national poisons centres. Some people will seek advice because they are not sure whether they, or their child, have taken a toxic dose or eaten a poisonous plant or fungus. If there is any real chance that they have, they should be referred to a casualty department, without delaying for first-aid measures of any kind, other than placing an unconscious patient in the recovery position to protect the airway. If the patient has any obvious symptoms, particularly impairment of consciousness, an ambulance should be called by calling 999. An article by Morley *et al.*[34] in the *Pharmaceutical Journal* included a study of a suspected poisoned child and gives an excellent account of how to handle this type of problem. The authors emphasise the need to calm the patient or parent to make it easier to get a reliable history, and suggest that it may aid the hospital if the tablets can be identified by comparison or from knowledge of the patient's previous prescriptions. Any referral note accompanying the patient to hospital should include this information. It is reassuring to learn from these authors that only one in 10 000 poisoning cases in children results in death.

Identification of poisons

A frequent request in hospital practice is for identification of tablets that are believed to have been taken as an overdose (recorded in case notes as 'O/D'). The label may be useful, but patients commonly transfer and mix contents, so this cannot be relied upon. There are various published tablet and capsule identification guides, but the preferred one is TICTAC, a computer-aided identification system available via regional and district drug information centres and poisons information centres.

Reference to the local poisons centre is the first step when household, gardening or farm products are involved. In addition, the National

Poisons Information Service maintains a clinical toxicology database called TOXBASE that gives information about routine diagnosis, treatment and management of patients exposed to drugs and chemicals. This may be accessed on the internet: the web address is given in the BNF.[33]

Treatment of poisoning

Treatment is usually symptomatic and supportive. The principles are set out in the BNF. A few poisons have specific treatments or antidotes, and pharmacists who supply accident and emergency departments must liaise with the consultant in charge to agree which agents should be stocked. It is as well to ensure that they are not inadvertently removed from stock lists by inexperienced staff who may not appreciate that they are needed even though they are only infrequently, if ever, used.

Although stated by the BNF to be of limited value, in certain cases removal of poisons from the stomach to minimise absorption, by either gastric lavage, or emesis using ipecacuanha is attempted. The only appropriate preparation is ipecacuanha emetic mixture, paediatric BP (equivalent to ipecacuanha syrup USP).

References

1. Royal Pharmaceutical Society of Great Britain. *Medicines, Ethics and Practice: A Guide for Pharmacists*, published yearly. London: Royal Pharmaceutical Society of Great Britain.
2. National Pharmaceutical Association website (2001). www.npa.co.uk (accessed 12 July 2001).
3. National Audit Office. *Handling Negligence Claims in England*. London: Stationery Office, 2001.
4. News item. Overhaul for NHS clinical negligence scheme announced. *Pharm J* 2001; 267: 43.
5. News item. Dispensing of forged scripts leads to admonition. *Pharm J* 1989; 243: 304.
6. News item. Law Lords ruling on pharmacists' liability for script forgeries. *Pharm J* 1986; 236: 829.
7. Appelbe G E, Wingfield J. *Dale and Appelbe's Pharmacy Law and Ethics*, 7th edn. London: Pharmaceutical Press, 2001.
8. Harrison I. Dispensing private prescriptions. *Pharm J* 1991; 247: 189.
9. NHS Executive. *For the Record: Managing Records in NHS Trusts and Health Authorities*. HSC 1999/053.
10. News item. Police launch National Association of Chemist Inspection Officers. *Pharm J* 2001; 266: 700.
11. Department of Health and National Assembly for Wales. *Drug Tariff*, published monthly. London: Stationery Office.
12. NHS Executive. *The Protection and Use of Patient Information*. London: Stationery Office, 1996.

13. NHS Executive. *The Protection and Use of Patient Information.* HSG(96)18/LASSL(96)5.
14. News item. Prescription data sale ruled unlawful. *Pharm J* 1999; 262: 794.
15. News item. Society and NPA advise halt to data sales. *Pharm J* 1999; 262: 794.
16. Editorial. Confidentiality of prescribing information. *Pharm J* 1999; 262: 793.
17. NHS Executive. *Data Protection Act 1998: Protection and Use of Patient Data.* HSC 2000/009.
18. NHS Executive. *Data Protection Act 1998: Protection and Use of Patient Information.* London: Stationery Office, 2000.
19. Wingfield J. The Data Protection Act 1998. *Pharm J* 2000; 265: 131.
20. Medicines Control Agency. *Guidance on Reporting Accidents with, and Defects in, Medicinal Products.* London: MCA, 1999.
21. Medical Devices Agency. *Reporting Adverse Incidents.* MDA SN 2001 (01).
22. Medicines Control Agency. *Personal Communication to North East Thames RHA Principal Pharmacist, Technical Services* dated 9 September 1991.
23. Medical Devices Agency website (2001). www.medical-devices.gov.uk (accessed 23 July 2001).
24. NHS Executive. *Controls Assurance in Infection Control: Decontamination of Medical Devices.* HSC 1999/179.
25. NHS Executive. *Decontamination of Medical Devices.* HSC 2000/032.
26. NHS Executive Controls Assurance Standard. *Medical Devices Management.* London: Stationery Office, 2000.
27. Department of Health. *Guidelines on the Safe and Secure Handling of Medicines: A Report to the Secretary of State for Social Services* (Duthie Guidelines). London: Her Majesty's Stationery Office, 1988.
28. RPSGB Hospital Pharmacists' Group. Guidance on the re-use of medicines. *Pharm J* 1986; 236: 812.
29. Health Services Advisory Committee. *Safe Disposal of Clinical Waste.* London: Stationery Office, 1999.
30. NHS Executive Controls Assurance Standard. *Waste Disposal.* London: Stationery Office, 2000.
31. WHO Department of Essential Drugs and Other Medicines. *Guidelines for Drug Donations*, 2nd edn. Geneva: World Health Organization, 1999.
32. Anderton D. The hazards of mercury spillage. *Pharm J* 1986; 237: 294–295.
33. Mehta D K, ed. *British National Formulary*, published twice-yearly. London: British Medical Association/Royal Pharmaceutical Society of Great Britain.
34. Morley A, Blenkinsopp J, Nicholls J R, Nicholls J L. Case studies in community pharmacy: acute poisoning. *Pharm J* 1986; 236: 619–620.

Part Two

Management of resources, quality and audit

9

Human resource management

Employment law

The appointment and employment of staff are subject to regulations introduced by numerous Acts of Parliament over the last 20 years or so. The legislation is aimed to protect both the individual employee and the employer, and also aims to reduce disruption caused by industrial disputes. The regulations are wide-ranging, and must be appreciated by all pharmacists, who are potential employers as well as employees. As legislation is subject to change, it is wise always to check the current position. Some of the more important current legislation is summarised in Table 9.1, and an overview of terms of employment is included in an article by Hodgkiss in *Tomorrow's Pharmacist*.[1] A summary of law for retailers is included in the annual *Chemist and Druggist Directory*.[2] Copies of unreferenced legislation can be accessed through the Stationery Office,[3] which has the responsibility for printing Acts of Parliament.

Discrimination in employment

It is illegal to discriminate against employees or potential employees because of their race, sex or colour. The 1986 Sex Discrimination Act[4] extended and consolidated previous legislation, including small firms or partnerships with five personnel or fewer within the legislation for the

Table 9.1 Important employment legislation

Equal Pay Act 1970
Health and Safety at Work etc. Act 1974
Race Relations Act 1976
Employment Protection (Consolidation) Act 1978
Employment Acts 1980, 1982, 1988 and 1990
Social Security and Housing Benefits Act 1982
Sex Discrimination Acts 1975 and 1986
Disability Discrimination Act 1995
Employment Rights Act 1996

first time. Discrimination because of marital status is also illegal. The laws apply not only to the filling of posts, but also to ancillary provisions such as retirement age and holiday entitlement. To be illegal, discrimination need not be openly applied, e.g. by advertising for a male or female employee; it occurs if any action or statement has led to it happening, e.g. by imposing conditions which may be discriminatory, such as minimum height. All job advertisements must indicate specifically equal opportunities, as must the conditions of employment. Equal pay for similar jobs was imposed by the Equal Pay Act of 1970.

Discrimination against a person because of race, nationality or colour is prohibited by the Race Relations Act 1976.[5] Its interpretation is similar to the Sex Discrimination Act in that it is not necessary to be overtly discriminatory to be in breach of the Act. Complaints of discrimination may be heard by an industrial tribunal (see below). In response to this legislation, many employers, including health authorities (HAs), have set their own detailed policies. In contrast with many regulations introduced by other Acts, those relating to discrimination apply to all personnel, including those working part-time for only a few hours. Issues relating to discrimination, and in particular those impinging on disability, are reviewed in an article by Elson.[6]

Appointing and dismissing staff

Contracts

A contract of employment exists as soon as an employee has taken up a post by starting work. At this stage the contract is usually based on verbal agreements, but under the Employment Protection (Consolidation) Act 1978 a written contract must be provided within 13 weeks of commencing work.[7] This must cover the main conditions of employment and include notes on disciplinary and grievance procedures as well as pay, hours, holidays, sick pay and length of notice. Many of these conditions are regulated by legislation. The 1978 Act does not cover staff who work for less than 16 hours per week unless they have worked for 8 hours or more for a period of 5 years. After 4 weeks' employment the employee is entitled to be given a minimum period of notice of termination of employment dependent on the length of service. The hospital service – in common with many employers – often sets periods of notice in excess of the statutory minimum.

Dismissal

A number of Employment Protection Acts impose several restrictions on the dismissal of staff. Primarily, all employees have the right not to be unfairly dismissed, either overtly or covertly. Particular problems in the dismissal of part-time staff are included in an employment law update in the *Pharmaceutical Journal* in August 2000.[8] Dismissal would be held to have occurred if:

- an employee's contract was not renewed upon expiry;
- an employee resigned because of conduct by the employer ('constructive dismissal');
- an employer did not allow a member of staff to return after an allowed absence, e.g. maternity leave.

If employees consider that they have been unfairly dismissed, they may, in certain cases, appeal to an industrial tribunal.

Industrial tribunals

Industrial tribunals were set up to give an independent judgement on matters of interpretation of employment legislation. They have similar status to courts of law in that their decisions are legally binding. They are administered independently, and each tribunal is chaired by an experienced lawyer with the additional two members being nominated by the local trade unions and employers' organisations. Tribunals are not bound by the same laws of evidence as courts of law, e.g. hearsay evidence is acceptable. Many hearings are very informal, with appellants arguing their own case against their previous employer, but in complex matters, or if large organisations are involved, the parties to the dispute may have legal representation. The tribunal may uphold the employer's decision to dismiss, but if it considers that the dismissal was unfair, it may make an order requesting the employee's reinstatement or re-engagement. Conversely, if it finds that a completely unwarranted claim has been brought, the tribunal may penalise the appellant.

Because of the risk of being found liable for unfair dismissal, many employers have a detailed disciplinary policy. While protecting the employee from unfair dismissal, this allows the employer or manager to dismiss when necessary, following a set, publicised procedure. All employees should receive, and read, their employer's disciplinary policy which, although varying in details, normally allows for a series of warnings to be given to the employee before dismissal can take place, e.g. for persistent absence. Such warnings must be confirmed in writing, and the employee must be given the opportunity to be accompanied by a friend or a representative (legal or trade union) at disciplinary interviews. If the offence is serious or criminal, e.g. theft, there are usually provisions for instant, or summary, dismissal. The problems in so doing, however, are considerable, and if a serious offence is suspected it is often wise to suspend the employee on full pay whilst investigations are completed. It should be noted that suspension in itself is *not* a disciplinary procedure, and may be used in other circumstances for the protection of the employee.

Health and welfare

There is considerable legislation designed to improve the health and welfare of people at work. Some important aspects will be summarised below.

Health and Safety at Work, etc. Act 1974

This was introduced as a consolidation act to bring all the previous legislation, developed since the Industrial Revolution, under one Act of Parliament. This included all the earlier Factories Acts, Clean Air Acts, Shops, Offices and Railway Premises Acts, etc. It is an 'enabling act', allowing future governments to bring in regulations on health and safety without needing additional legislation. The Act set up a Health and Safety Executive to enforce the legislation through health and safety inspectors, and encompassed previously exempt employers such as HAs and general practitioners. Non-industrial workplaces, and certain areas of health premises such as the kitchens, are inspected by local authority environmental health inspectors. Inspectors have considerable powers, and can issue improvement orders should they consider that some part of a premises or a procedure is unsafe. In extreme cases they can order the closure of all or part of a factory or workplace. They are also called in to investigate any serious accidents or incidents occurring at work. Information booklets on the Act and its interpretation are published by the Stationery Office and are available through the Health and Safety Executive website.[9]

There are two provisions of the Act which are particularly important to pharmacists. The first of these is the duty of each employer to ensure the health and safety at work of his/her employees and also anyone affected by his/her business. Not only the employees, but also any visitors or members of the public are protected from dangerous working conditions. These might range from a loose floor tile in a shop to emission of a noxious substance from the workplace. Lack of reasonable compliance is a criminal offence. Any accident or dangerous occurrence must be recorded (written notes should be made within 24 hours of the incident to be valid as evidence later), and in some instances reported to the Health and Safety Executive. It is prudent for all employers to set out a written statement of their health and safety policy, which should be read by all employees; in fact, for businesses employing more than five staff, it is a requirement of the Act. Additionally, procedures should be written for any hazardous machinery or process.

The second important provision of the Act is the imposition of a duty of care upon the individual. Thus, each person must take reasonable care that he/she does not endanger the health or safety of him/herself or any other person. So if, for example, an accident happens because someone left an electric flex trailing across a floor, the person so doing would be liable under the Act. It is also an offence for a person not to follow the health and safety policy at his/her workplace, e.g. by not wearing protective gloves or mask. Because this aspect of the Act is aimed at the individual, it covers all persons, including locums.

Control of Substances Hazardous to Health (COSHH) Regulations 1988

These Regulations, made under the Health and Safety at Work Act, came into force on 1 October 1989. They require employers to identify potentially hazardous substances to which their workforce or other persons present in the workplace may be exposed, to assess the risk arising from exposure and, if necessary, to take steps to control the risk. Health and Safety Executive area offices can supply, free of charge, a range of leaflets for employers explaining the actions required under the regulations. Virtually all substances which may be hazardous to health are covered, and employers must make a systematic assessment of all work which is liable to expose the employee to hazardous solids, liquids, dusts, fumes, vapours, gases or microorganisms. Only substances which are covered by their own specific laws, e.g. radioactive materials, are excluded. After the identification of hazardous materials, the risks to health must be assessed and action taken to remove or reduce the risks. This might be by excluding the hazardous substance by substituting something less dangerous, or by supplying protective clothing or improving ventilation systems. Suppliers of hazardous substances are required by law to provide information necessary for safe use; pharmacists must be aware of their own responsibilities to their clients, and must ensure that safety information is available.

The normal range of medicines handled by a pharmacy is unlikely to pose any health hazards to the pharmacy staff (potential adverse effects in patients treated by the drugs are not covered by these regulations). The commonest exceptions are cytotoxic drugs, and procedures must be written to cover safe handling and disposal of these and any equipment contaminated in use, e.g. syringes. Another problem material, widely used in hospitals, is glutaraldehyde disinfectant. This should be eliminated where feasible, and where its use is deemed essential, procedures for its use should be drawn up. These must include the use of effective protective clothing, including rubber gloves and goggles to British Standard 2092 protection grade 1CD (Grade 1 impact/chemical/dust). Suitable lidded containers, or purpose-designed equipment, must be used to minimise the users' exposure to the very irritant fumes.

The Reporting of Injuries, Diseases and Dangerous Occurrences Regulations (RIDDOR) 1995

These Regulations require the notification by employers of certain diseases related to work, to the Health and Safety Executive in the case of factories, building sites and hospitals, and to the environmental health department of the local authority for offices, shops and restaurants. All workers, including trainees and self-employed people, e.g. locums, are covered, but self-employed people are responsible for making their own reports. There is a special form (F2508A) for reporting, or reports may be made through the dedicated website of the Incident Contact Centre, introduced in 2001;[10] further information is available from Health and Safety Executive area offices. In addition to a list of specific diseases relating to a number of industrial processes, any injury resulting from an accident at work which is serious, or which causes incapacity for more than 3 consecutive days, including days off and weekends, has to be reported. Hardly any of the listed diseases are related to health care. The notable exceptions are bone cancer and blood dyscrasias arising in persons exposed to ionising radiations, and tuberculosis or hepatitis arising in persons working with infected humans or exposed to their secretions or blood.

Statutory Sick Pay (SSP)

This scheme was introduced by the Social Security and Housing Benefits Act 1982, and means that employers have a duty to pay staff during sickness absence. The details of the scheme are particularly complicated, and are best studied from the most up-to-date leaflets published by the Department of Social Security (DSS). From April 1986 – as amended by subsequent regulations – employers are required to pay SSP to an employee for up to 28 weeks in any tax-year, and the employee's sickness record is transferable between jobs. Specimen record forms for sickness history are produced by the Department of Health (DoH). The rate of pay depends on the employee's earnings, and the amount paid is reclaimable by the employer as a deduction from their monthly payment of pay-as-you-earn (PAYE) tax and National Insurance contributions. The statutory sum payable has no effect on any other scheme for payment during sickness negotiated between employer and employee, e.g. the National Health Service (NHS) pays employees full pay for a period related to their length of service, but a new employee not yet eligible for this would still get the SSP allowance.

Maternity pay and leave

Like SSP, the detailed regulations on the payment of allowances and leave entitlement during a woman's absence due to pregnancy are complicated and subject to change. In essence, a pregnant woman may take leave for up to a stated maximum period of absence, and retain the right to return to her job. During the leave, statutory payments are allowable – statutory maternity pay – and these have been integrated into arrangements similar to those for SSP. Leaflets giving details are available from DSS offices, but several points relating to maternity leave need highlighting. Pregnant workers are entitled to the following:

- a minimum of 18 weeks' continuous maternity leave;
- paid time off for antenatal examinations;
- protection from dismissal during the pregnancy and maternity leave, except in exceptional circumstances, which are wholly unconnected with the pregnancy;
- the preservation of contractual rights during the period of maternity leave;
- pay at a rate not less than the appropriate sick pay during the period of maternity;
- 18 weeks' maternity leave (ordinary leave), irrespective of length of service and number of hours worked. Ordinary leave may commence at any time the woman wishes after the 11th week before the expected week of childbirth;

- additional leave for women who have accrued 2 years' service at the 11th week before the expected week of childbirth.

As in the case of SSP, certain occupational maternity leave schemes offer employees more than the statutory minimum. Thus, the Whitley Council scheme, to which most hospital staff are entitled, entitles the woman to 8 weeks' leave on full pay, 10 weeks at half-pay, with the option of taking further unpaid leave up to a total absence from work of 52 weeks.

Staff recruitment and training

Recruitment

The first step in the recruitment of staff is not the placing of an advertisement; before that stage is reached, an assessment must be made of the post to be filled. Often, recruitment is to fill an established post made vacant by a resignation, and in such cases the good manager will consider whether it is appropriate to replace with the same grade of staff, or even if a replacement is strictly necessary. Factors considered will range from the effectiveness of the post to future requirements, and may include an analysis of the reasons for resignation of the previous post-holder. As an example, following the resignation of a pharmacy technician a range of questions should be asked to confirm the need for replacement. Some of these are illustrated in Table 9.2.

Once a decision has been reached in principle to proceed with recruitment, the next stage is to consider the job content of the new post in detail. Even if there is to be a straight replacement, it would be extremely unusual if there had not been some changes in the post from the time of the previous appointment. These can be included in a job description or specification. It is good practice to give each employee a job description that details his/her post to supplement the contract of employment. In public employment, where it is common for a personnel

Table 9.2 Example questions to be asked before replacing a member of staff

Why did he/she leave?
Was he/she bored in the post?
Was he/she overstretched in the post?
Could the job be done effectively by a less well-trained person?
Should the job be carried out by a pharmacist?
Were the hours of work correct?

officer to be employed with a specific brief to prevent discrimination, managers are usually required to draw up a person specification which will be used later, during the selection stages, as an aid to appointing the most suitable candidate, and also to demonstrate that there has been no unfair bias or discrimination during the selection process. The specification lists the personal attributes required of the post-holder. These would include qualifications and skills needed, experience and personal factors, e.g. a good telephone manner, ability to work while standing up for long periods. They must not, of course, be discriminatory in any way. It is usual to score each item on the list considering whether the attribute is essential, important or merely desirable. In theory, every candidate who matches the specification should be given the opportunity of an interview; in addition, any registered disabled candidates should be included in the list. In practice, during periods of high unemployment, this may pose difficulties. When the interview stage of the selection procedure is reached, the questions must be designed to measure the candidates' performance against each item on the specification, and a score chart kept for reference, in the event of a later challenge to the fairness of the selection process. Obviously, all candidates must be asked the same questions.

Having defined the post for which one wishes to recruit, one can now proceed with advertising for applicants. The first step is to select the medium most likely to reach the required personnel. For pharmacists, the *Pharmaceutical Journal* has comprehensive cover of the target group, so would normally be the first choice. Additionally, for pharmacy technicians one might use the *Chemist and Druggist* or local newspapers. The choice will partially depend on past success rates using each medium. For unqualified staff one would use local newspapers or job centres. Advertising is expensive and not always the best means of recruitment. Other methods might include circulation of local schools or careers offices for trainee posts, and internal circulation, possibly using a staff bulletin, if there may be local candidates. If any staff redundancies are pending, e.g. if a hospital faces a planned closure, local policy may require that preference be given to staff whose jobs are at risk. If accusations of unfairness and discrimination are to be avoided, all posts must be advertised by some means, and recruitment to vacancies must never be just by word-of-mouth or personal recommendation.

The advertisement must encourage suitable applicants and tell them how to apply, and give sufficient information to discourage unsuitable candidates. It is good practice to include a closing date for the receipt of applications so that further stages in the recruitment process can be planned from the beginning. Advertisements should contain the minimum number of words to achieve enquiries; details of the post, its base or the employer should be sent out as further information to interested candidates, as soon as they make contact. This may be a few paragraphs for junior appointments, but may be an information folder for senior posts. Essential facts are details of the post (including job description), management responsibilities and staffing, details of the employer, and geographical information. It may be useful at this stage to give the date of the interview, if known, both to aid candidates to prepare and to avoid last-minute withdrawals. The issue of further information not only gives the employer the opportunity to extol the virtues of the post, but also protects him/her from a multitude of telephone enquiries about standard conditions of the post, e.g. salary, base and holidays. Prospective candidates who make preinterview contact will additionally be better informed so that such a contact – either an informal visit or telephoned enquiry – may provide a useful aid to selection. With the further particulars, many employers send an application form.

If a number of applications is expected for a post, it is useful to have a standard application form. This ensures that all applicants give the same minimum information, and aids the objective of shortlisting candidates for interview. The form must include all the questions that need to be asked. There may be a case for having differing designs, e.g. a short form for posts requiring no formal qualifications, and another with sections for details of educational achievements. It is usual to ask the candidate to supply the names of persons who are willing to supply a reference. For senior posts it may be useful to ask candidates to submit their own application and career history (or curriculum vitae or CV) in order to assess their ability to produce reports.

Selection

Once applications have been received, the critical process of selection may start. The main method of selection is normally the interview. From the applications it is necessary to identify candidates who meet a majority of the requirements defined in the person specification. This process – 'shortlisting' – can be as difficult and important as the final interview; all forms of discrimination must be avoided. To help in this process, and to act as an extra check against discrimination, it is usual to involve an independent assessor both at this stage and at the final interview. For junior posts this may be a local colleague or personnel officer, but for senior posts, it is normal to invite at least one assessor from outside the employing authority. The assessor may be a professional, e.g. pharmacist, or an independent manager, or both. No matter how junior the post, it is bad practice to appoint or interview without having advice from a second person, and can lead to problems in later claims of discrimination or bias. Once candidates for interview have been shortlisted, their references are sent for. This will introduce a time delay, as it is best not to interview until these have been received. However, with the objective of avoiding discrimination, some personnel officers now advocate a policy of not viewing the references until after the selection process has been completed. Prospective candidates should note that it is courteous to ask potential referees whether they are willing to be named.

Selection interviews must be well-planned in advance. They may be supplemented by other methods of selection such as aptitude tests, e.g. typing or shorthand tests for secretaries. Some important points – surprisingly often forgotten – are:

- Ensure that both the members of the interviewing panel and the candidates know the place and time of the interview together with any supplementary information, e.g. bringing certificates of registration.
- Ensure that the panel has received in plenty of time all information about the candidates (applications) and the post (job description and person specification).
- Ensure that any receptionist who meets the candidates knows the arrangements, and is briefed to put them at their ease.
- Structure the interview so that the candidate is given a chance to settle down and take in the surroundings, relevant questions are asked of him/her, the candidate has a chance to ask further questions, and leaves knowing when to expect to hear the result.

A useful review of the selection interview process is to consider the interview from the position of the candidate. In fact, at the beginning of their career most pharmacists will have more experience from this perspective! A review of important points for interviewees is included in *Tomorrow's Pharmacist*,[11] and a more thorough, but eminently readable approach is covered in a book by Eggert.[12]

Before the job is offered formally to the preferred candidate, it is important to check that favourable references have been received, and that any other conditions, e.g. satisfactory medical examination, have been completed. Ensure that a written offer of the post is sent, and do not expect the appointee to hand in notice to his/her current employer until this has been received.

Staff development

Staff development should commence the day a person takes up his/her post, and should be a continuing task of the manager thereafter. The first element concerns new staff, who should start a planned programme of induction from their first day. At its simplest this will include meeting other members of staff, learning departmental procedures and completing any personnel documentation. This should then be complemented over the first few weeks or months by a planned introduction to the job and its relevance to the organisation. At the end of this programme, an interview should be held between manager and the individual to appraise how he/she is doing. This should be the first of a series of regular appraisal interviews held by a manager with all his/her immediate subordinates.

Appraisal

This is a management technique that has been in use for many years, but because early schemes encountered problems, it has been widely used only in some industries. Many of the early schemes were criticised because appraisal seemed to be used purely as a method of censuring an employee. Appraisal should be much more constructive than that, and it is to take advantage of the constructive aspects that many employers are now implementing appraisal schemes. The main objectives of appraisal are summarised in Table 9.3.

Appraisal was first formally introduced to pharmacy by the Royal Pharmaceutical Society's scheme for preregistration graduates. The design of this scheme encourages good techniques for the appraisal interview in that the employee (in this case, the preregistration graduate) is forewarned of the content of the interview, has considered his/her own progress by means of the checklist, and signs it with the manager as an agreement of performance achieved and action required, and finally, a set period is given until the next review. Similar schemes have been introduced for managers in the NHS but these cannot use the detailed

Table 9.3 Main objectives of appraisal

Assessment of performance, identifying strengths and weaknesses
Identification of training needs
Identification and consideration of career development potential

preprinted questions that can be used for a closed group of trainees. For managers, there is often a greater element of performance review, although it is important that the individual's training and developmental needs are not forgotten because of this.

Performance review

An important element of the NHS schemes is performance review based on the concept of management by objectives. This technique has been in and out of favour for many years, but the concept is simple in that all managers can be assessed on their performance in achieving (or otherwise) previously agreed objectives. These will vary considerably in scope depending on the level of the manager. For example, a business manager may be required to save 1% of his/her overall budget in a 12-month period, whereas a clinical pharmacy manager may wish to introduce a pharmacist visiting service to a ward or to an off-site hospital. In practice the use of management by objectives requires considerable managerial skill. For success, it is important that objectives are set by the agreement of both manager and subordinate, and also that the objectives set should reflect the objectives agreed by the manager. In other words, a pyramidal scheme should operate, e.g. if the business manager's task is to save 1%, this may be passed to operational managers like the pharmacy manager to save 1% in their turn. Objectives must be set with a defined time scale, and their achievement must be measurable. It is no use having a vague objective such as 'to improve the ward pharmacy service'. Such objectives could lead to dispute between manager and appraisee as to whether improvement has been achieved. A much clearer objective would be 'to ensure that each ward receives a daily visit from a ward pharmacist'. In summary, used properly as a part of appraisal and performance review, management by objectives can improve communications between manager and staff whilst aiding the development of the service.

Competencies

As a development of appraisal systems, many organisations are now using the concept of competence to practise to judge performance. The National Council for Vocational Qualifications has been established for many years, and categorises levels of competence within bandings relating to factors such as necessity to interpret information, or routine application of simple skills/knowledge. Within the NHS, various technical grades are now being trained under the National Vocational Qualification (NVQ) scheme using competencies, e.g. operating department assistants. It is governmental strategy that the concept is eventually introduced to all grades. Pharmacy technician training has been incorporated into this scheme for some years. Because competency-based training is a measure of performance, much of the assessment is carried out in the workplace, and there is a need to ensure that workplace supervisors of trainees are themselves trained in assessment techniques. The Royal Pharmaceutical Society of Great Britain (RPSGB) arranges a series of tutorials for preregistration tutors in this, and they must attend regular (currently 5-yearly) updates. Although starting with preregistration pharmacy students, it can be expected that the concepts of competency-based assessment will soon extend into other areas of pharmacy, including postqualification assessment and development.

Identification of training needs

As part of any appraisal/review process, it is important to identify any training needs of the individual. These may be specific to that individual, or may relate to a group of staff. The introduction of a computer system at a department would lead to a group need of all staff to learn how to use the dispensing programs, but might have an individual need for the dispensary manager to learn how to set up programs for warning labels for dispensing. Many training needs can be met from within the resources of the organisation, e.g. the needs of a new member of staff or one given new duties will often best be met by utilising existing expertise within the department. The choice should be influenced by the training objective identified, and not by an impending convenient study day, even though these may play a useful part in achieving certain objectives – especially if they arise from previously identified needs of a similar group of staff. Then it may be most efficient to run a study day or seminar as part of a formal training programme: in the hospital service this might be at district or regional level.

For professional staff, an identified need for an individual might include some element of further education; the person should then be encouraged to carry out a course of study. This may be completely or partly sponsored by the employer, and may include time off work for attendance at sessions. Not only are courses expensive, but also in giving time off, an employer is in effect spending that person's salary for the day; that sum is further enhanced if a locum is needed. If all the costs of

Table 9.4 Examples of postqualification courses available

Certificate in Pharmacy Practice
Clinical Pharmacy Diploma
Master of Science (MSc) in Clinical Pharmacy
Master of Science (MSc) in Biopharmacy
Master of Science (MSc) in Pharmacology
Master of Business Administration (MBA)
Diploma in Management Studies (DMS)
Member of the College of Pharmacy Practice (MCPP) by studying for College
   examinations, or by submitting a Practice Portfolio
Management courses at various levels organised by employers or local colleges
Study days organised by RPSGB membership groups
Study days organised by College of Pharmacy Practice, UK Clinical Pharmacy
   Association, etc.

RPSGB, Royal Pharmaceutical Society of Great Britain.

a day-release scheme, e.g. for student pharmacy technicians, are taken into account, the total can be surprisingly high in relation to the employee's nominal salary. A decision on whether to utilise a formal course must therefore take into account cost-effectiveness as well as a detailed consideration of the courses available. Some of these are listed in Table 9.4, but note also that the *Pharmaceutical Journal* contains continually updated information on further education ranging from lectures to formal courses.

The National Pharmaceutical Association (NPA) has an active training department which organises events ranging from half-day seminars to correspondence courses for dispensing assistants. The Centre for Postgraduate Pharmacy Education bases much of its programme on subjects that have been identified nationally as being of general developmental need for community pharmacists, e.g. human immunodeficiency virus (HIV)/acquired immunodeficiency syndrome (AIDS); care of the elderly. It is useful to review the course immediately the employee returns to work, and even more important to follow this up at periodic intervals (probably as part of the appraisal process) to confirm that the original training objectives have been achieved.

Education and training

Education is an essential component of the career of any professional. The main elements are those arising from an identified training need of current or potential employment, and those arising from the need to keep professional knowledge maintained at a level to ensure competence to practise. The requirement to keep up to date is incorporated in the Code of Ethics.[14] The relevance of training needs arising from employment is described in earlier sections of this chapter; professional continuing education will be explored further here.

Continuing education

The role of the RPSGB

The RPSGB is recognised as the leading body for strategy relating to continuing education for pharmacists as it is the registration body, and represents all pharmacists. Policy matters are decided by the full Council of the Society, and support is provided by the Education Division of the RPSGB. A link with practising pharmacists is provided by the Postgraduate Education Committee (PEC) whose membership consists of practitioners from all aspects of practice, as well as members of Council and the Head of the Education Division. The PEC reports to the Education Committee, which is a formal subcommittee of Council, and which advises Council on all educational matters, including undergraduate education, and formally reports matters discussed by the PEC. The RPSGB set up a working party which reported on a strategy for postgraduate education and training in 1989.[13] Arising from this, Council approved PEC recommendations to introduce a National Syllabus for Continuing Education in Pharmacy. The syllabus, which is set out in the *Medicines, Ethics and Practice* guide,[14] consists of a core syllabus together with sectorial syllabuses for the main areas of pharmacy practice, i.e. academic, agricultural, community, industry, hospital and veterinary. The core syllabus is intended to apply to all pharmacists, and contains a description of a knowledge base together with a section listing skills required. The syllabuses will be revised annually, and it is expected that each pharmacist will maintain his/her education to meet the core syllabus and appropriate sectorial one(s). The RPSGB Council has also approved a recommendation that it expects all practising pharmacists to undertake a minimum of 30 hours' continuing education each year. This can comprise self-directed study (including reading journals such as the *Pharmaceutical Journal*), as well as attendance at formal courses. It is particularly recommended that a pharmacist should join other pharmacists for continuing education on at least one occasion per year. This is to encourage the benefits of discussing problems with peers. The 30 hours' requirement is voluntary, but strongly recommended, and failure to undertake this would most likely be seen to be relevant in any breach of the Code of Ethics.[14] To widen the opportunities for self-directed learning, the *Pharmaceutical Journal* publishes regular material for continuing education.

Standing Committee on Education and Training and Standing Committee for Pharmacy Postgraduate Education

Under the NHS Act of 1948, continuing education of professionals providing contractor services was regulated and funded under Section 63. The principles of this legislation have been maintained in that a separate allocation is made for the education of doctors and pharmacists. In 1991, the government announced the setting-up of a new system to control this education and, arising from this, a new Standing Committee for Pharmacy Postgraduate Education (SCOPE) was formed. The remit of this committee is quite broad, encompassing preregistration training, community and hospital pharmacist training. It was asked initially, however, to concentrate on community pharmacists as there were perceived difficulties in this area, such as variation in access to courses and variable uptake. To enable this, a Centre for Pharmacy Postgraduate Education (CPPE) was formed and a Director of Continuing Education appointed. This paralleled arrangements in Scotland, Wales and Northern Ireland. The CPPE, funded by the DoH, is currently based in Manchester, and is linked with the University Department of Pharmacy. A network of local tutors has been appointed across England to implement courses designed by the Centre, and to link with and encourage local pharmacists to participate in continuing education. Details of these tutors, including contact points, is published regularly in the *Pharmaceutical Journal*, or through direct mailing to all pharmacists. They organise a series of courses which is partly set nationally, and partly according to local needs ascertained by the tutor. The courses are organised to be available during weekdays, during weekday evenings or at weekends to enable as many people as possible to attend. These courses are backed up by a range of distance learning material available through the CPPE. The educational material and courses are published by a direct mailing to every pharmacist.

The College of Pharmacy Practice

The College of Pharmacy Practice (CPP – not to be confused with CPPE, see above!) was set up by the RPSGB as an independent body to further the pharmaceutical profession and the professional development of pharmacists. In 1986 it became a fully autonomous organisation with its own governors and Board of Management. Its objectives are to encourage high standards in the practice of pharmacy through continuing education and research.[15] As part of the objectives, it encourages professional development by accepting practitioner members by examination, and by supporting and organising study days and courses. Members of the CPP agree to undertake a minimum of 20 hours' annual continuing education at approved courses or by approved study. This requirement is mandatory, unlike the RPSGB recommendation, and an annual return giving details is required from each member. Pharmacists who wish to support the ideals of the College without undertaking the formal examination may become associate members. Associates must commit themselves to the continuing education requirement.

The College's mission statement[16] is: 'To promote professional and personal development, through education, examination, practice and research, benefiting patients and health care provision'. Members of the College receive a variety of benefits from their association:

- a personal voluntary commitment to continuing professional development (CPD);
- a high-quality annual professional development programme;
- the CPD portfolio;
- membership by either the examination or practice route;
- reports of study days and seminars;
- guides to developments in pharmacy practice;
- Credit for Learning;
- involvement in a progressive college concerned with professional development and the future of the profession.

In 2001 the College announced the establishment of its first faculty. It defined this as 'a distinct group within the College who work in a specific and identifiable area of practice which is normally recognised by the profession as requiring its practitioners to be educated, trained and experienced in such a manner as to be, or eventually be, specialists in that area'. The first faculty was that of Prescribing and Medicines Management.

Continuing professional development

The RPSGB is gradually moving to a system of CPD to ensure the competence of the profession. In the Code of Ethics[14] the need for pharmacists to maintain competence and effectiveness as a practitioner is stressed. The section on 'Good practice for ensuring professional competence' in *Medicines, Ethics and Practice*[14] recommends the concept of CPD to enable this and gives guidance on how to meet the needs. Further advice is given by Hancox in *Tomorrow's Pharmacist*.[17] This concept is likely to become most important for practitioners over the next few years, and ongoing updates published in the *Pharmaceutical Journal* will need to be followed closely. An article by Farhan is a good introduction to the process and the parallel debate about its introduction.[18]

Departmental management

This chapter has so far been primarily about personnel management. However important, this is only one aspect of management skills. These can be studied in depth by reading books which are readily available in libraries or bookshops, or by attendance at management courses.

Communication

Effective communications are important for the progress of any organisation. Communications can vary from interpersonal skills in a person-to-person exchange to more formal written-message transmission. Communication failure is, unfortunately, common. Examples can be seen or heard daily in almost any situation: 'what I meant was . . .', 'I thought you meant . . .', etc. Often caused by a lack of understanding of the communication process, communication is not simply passing a message by voice or script; it also relates to the reception and understanding of that message. There are five essential elements to communication:

- the sender;
- the message itself;
- the receiver;
- feedback;
- interference.

Pharmacy practice gives good examples of the problems that can occur:

- There is often a difference in intellectual ability between sender and receiver, e.g. pharmacist and patient.
- There is almost certainly a difference in education.
- The receiver may not be at his/her most receptive, e.g. because he/she is in a hurry, or worried.
- The environment may be antagonistic to effective communication, e.g. a noisy shop.
- The patient may not wish to indicate that he/she did not understand in front of other patients or staff.

If one additionally considers the scenario that the pharmacist does not know how much the patient knows about the illness, and does not wish to worry him/her unduly, or lessen confidence in the prescriber, the need for careful effective communication, and the barriers that may exist, cannot be stressed enough. The problems mentioned above arise at all levels of communication, including the pharmacist who leaves an incomplete message for a prescriber, thus necessitating further communication, and the manager who sends out an ambiguous memorandum. Always consider your messages from the viewpoint of the recipient and make sure that he/she will find them clear and complete. A useful paper on communicating with patients has been published by Wisner.[19]

Authority

Authority is a concept which has two equally important meanings in management terms. Firstly, 'he/she has the authority to do something'; secondly, 'he/she is an authority on this subject'. The second concept, referred to in textbooks as sapiential or knowledge-based authority, is often confused with the first in a professional environment, but this is not always the case. In a democratic society authority is derived from nomination and election by the group affected. Although the seemingly tortuous hierarchy of the NHS organisation, mentioned in Chapter 12, appears little related to the presence of a hospital departmental manager, the theoretical links are reinforced by the rights of every voter to raise through his/her Member of Parliament matters of concern at operational level. The situation is similar in industry where shareholders have similar rights. A small pharmacy with a proprietor pharmacist has in effect one shareholder! In practice, of course, it is not possible for a few elected persons to run a large organisation on their own. To enable it to function they must delegate some of their authority.

Delegation

Delegation takes place when a manager gives authority to a subordinate to carry out some of his or her, i.e. the manager's duties. It is important in delegating that the task is well defined, and that authority is delegated. For example, it is no use a pharmacy manager delegating management of the equipment budget to a pharmacist whilst still asking for all orders to be approved by the manager. The task must be clearly stated to the subordinate, together with any restrictions, e.g. no expenditure to exceed £400, and the necessary authority given. This will be done by informing the rest of the department, or the finance department. It should be noted that delegation of authority does not absolve the manager from responsibility, which cannot be delegated. Thus, if the pharmacist makes a mistake in his/her management of the equipment budget, it is still the responsibility of the manager. It is as a result of this principle, which holds in public administration, that occasionally politicians or chair of large companies resign because of errors made by very junior members of their department. Many managers are poor at delegation either because they fear that their subordinates may make a mistake, or because they do not wish to 'give away' their own job. The former fear should be negated if the manager has a good system of monitoring performance. This will be enhanced if there is an active and effective system of performance review, and can be ensured if monitoring tasks are built into the delegation. In the example above, the manager might ask for a monthly report on expenditure. The second fear is often related to managers getting 'bogged down' in day-to-day matters, and paying insufficient attention to their role in planning and forecasting.

Planning

At whatever level one is working, there is a need to plan and forecast. For a senior manager, these tasks may take up a large proportion of one's time, but even a pharmacist or technician with no theoretical management responsibilities will need to spend some time on them on occasions. The planning might be as simple as deciding whether to leave a problem until the next day, but at whatever level, it is important that planning is done efficiently. Most pharmacists will have worked in the dispensary where the manager allowed work to accumulate so that there was a last-minute rush to complete. The need for planning at all levels becomes more obvious if a system of management by objectives is in operation. Monthly, weekly and even daily objectives must be interwoven with operational achievement. In order to achieve this planned workload, most managers – even at a senior level – utilise a more or less formal written plan of action.

An adjunct to planning is forecasting. It is no use planning to visit extra wards on a day when one might forecast extra work, e.g. the day before a bank holiday. The senior manager has a wealth of statistics available to aid forecasting, e.g. the number and type of patient attendances, but at all levels it is perhaps true that managers do not devote enough time to forecasting the effects on their service of anticipated developments, as well as to the effect on others of their own plans.

References

1. Hodgkiss K. Terms of employment. In: Mason P, ed. *Tomorrow's Pharmacist*. London: Royal Pharmaceutical Society of Great Britain, 1999: 55–57.
2. Law for retailers. *Chemist and Druggist Directory 2001*. Tonbridge, Kent: United Business Media: 396–405.
3. Her Majesty's Stationery Office website (2001). www.hmso.gov.uk (accessed November 2001).
4. Sex Discrimination Act 1986. London: Her Majesty's Stationery Office.
5. Race Relations Act 1976. London: Her Majesty's Stationery Office.
6. Elson V. Pharmacy and the Disability Discrimination Act. *Pharm J* 1999; 263: 716–717.
7. The Employment Protection (Consolidation) Act 1978. London: Her Majesty's Stationery Office.
8. Hibbs M. Part-time workers and the disciplinary process. *Pharm J* 2000; 265: 245–247.
9. Health and Safety Executive website (2001). www.hse.gov.uk (accessed August 2001).
10. Health and Safety Executive RIDDOR Incident Contact Centre website (2001). www.riddor.gov.uk (accessed August 2001).
11. Benson A. Success at interviews. In: Mason P, ed. *Tomorrow's Pharmacist*. London: Royal Pharmaceutical Society of Great Britain, 1999: 52–54.
12. Eggert M. The perfect interview. London: Random House Business Books, 1999.
13. Working Party Report. A strategy for postgraduate education and training. *Pharm J* 1989; 243: 142.
14. Royal Pharmaceutical Society of Great Britain. *Medicines, Ethics and Practice, A Guide for Pharmacists*, published yearly. London: Royal Pharmaceutical Society of Great Britain.
15. Mitchell R, Veitch B. Continuing professional development – a role for the College of Pharmacy Practice. *Pharm J* 1992; 249: E8.
16. The College of Pharmacy Practice website (2001). www.collpharm.org.uk (accessed October 2001).
17. Hancox D. Continuing professional development. In: Mason P, ed. *Tomorrow's Pharmacist*. London: Royal Pharmaceutical Society of Great Britain, 1999: 61–63.
18. Farhan F. A review of pharmacy continuing professional development *Pharm J* 2001; 267: 613–615.
19. Wisner K. How to communicate effectively with patient. In: Mason P, ed. *Tomorrow's Pharmacist*. London: Royal Pharmaceutical Society of Great Britain, 1999: 64–66.

10

Quality management in health care

For many years, most flourishing private enterprises have founded their business success on the concept of total quality management. Rather than leaving the quality of their operations to chance, they have adopted a systematic approach to maintaining quality at every level of the organisation. In such organisations, every member of staff knows that he/she has a role to play, and the whole culture of the workforce and its attitudes is directed towards identifying and meeting the needs of its customers. The company benefits in a variety of ways. The most obvious one is that it gets and keeps plenty of customers, but in addition, the operation will be cost effective, as every activity will have been planned to be as efficient as possible, and money wasted in correcting errors will be saved.

The National Health Service (NHS) has been slow to adopt these concepts. Rather than having to seek customers, it has traditionally been a demand-led service, and in the past there have been few incentives to improve performance and, it has to be said, little interest in doing so. Too often, services were started up and organised to suit the interests or perceived training needs of the providers of the service, rather than being tailored to the needs of the clients. The emphasis began to change with the publication of Sir Roy Griffith's 1983 report into the NHS,[1] which for the first time made quality a priority for services to patients. Local initiatives stemming from this included surveys of patients' views on the service, the provision of information to patients and staff training in quality. Many health authorities (now trusts) established directors of quality, usually senior nurses with a remit to improve the quality of direct services to patients. The Griffith report also emphasised the importance of ensuring value for money, which has led to the scrutiny of many traditional ways of providing services, with the result that many support services formerly carried out at excessive cost by directly employed labour are now contracted out.

Government's commitment to quality management in the NHS was reinforced by the White Paper *Working for Patients*[2] and, later, quality featured as a topic in the management review programme then being established. For the first time with the White Paper, doctors were specifically included in the drive towards quality management. *Working for Patients* was followed by a series of working papers which translated the ideas in the paper into operational format; working paper number six required authorities to introduce a programme of medical audit – 'the systematic and critical analysis of the quality of medical care, including procedures for diagnosis and treatment, the use of resources and the resulting outcome and quality of life of the patient'. Later, clinical audit programmes took the place of purely medical audit. The term 'clinical audit' has come to imply a more comprehensive approach to audit, with the contributions of non-medical interventions such as physiotherapy and even broader aspects of treatment being included as well.

The purpose of audit is to identify opportunities, and to implement improvements in the quality of medical care, medical training and continuing education, and the effective use of resources. The definition and objectives stated could, with a minimum of adaptation, equally well be taken to apply to pharmaceutical services, although it is important to remember that patients are not the only clients. Where pharmacies form part of a large organisation, clients of a clinical pharmacy service may include doctors, nurses and other health care professionals, while finance managers and management accountants may receive a service which enables them to operate effectively, e.g. to pass invoices for payment and make accurate budget forecasts.

Different methods of quality management exist; whatever method is used, it is important that review of quality forms a continuous process in each organisation – the so-called quality cycle is illustrated in Figure 10.1. Unfamiliar terms will be discussed later in the chapter.

It is important to remember that the success of each process has to be evaluated in the light of its outcome; the criteria adopted to measure standards must reflect this. Thus, in another field of endeavour, the quality of a concert would be better judged by the length of the applause or the number of encores than by recording the percentage attendance of the musicians at the rehearsals or the cost of hiring the music! A common professional misconception is to set standards without involving the customer.

Quality standards imposed by government

Audit Commission

The NHS and Community Care Act 1990 transferred the responsibility for the external audit of health authorities from the Department of

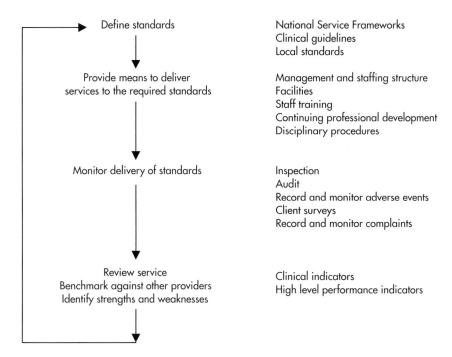

Define standards — National Service Frameworks / Clinical guidelines / Local standards

Provide means to deliver services to the required standards — Management and staffing structure / Facilities / Staff training / Continuing professional development / Disciplinary procedures

Monitor delivery of standards — Inspection / Audit / Record and monitor adverse events / Client surveys / Record and monitor complaints

Review service / Benchmark against other providers / Identify strengths and weaknesses — Clinical indicators / High level performance indicators

Figure 10.1 The quality cycle.

Health (DoH) to the Audit Commission, which had been set up in 1983 to audit local government. The government's objective, quoted from *Working for Patients*,[2] was 'that there should be more commitment to value for money studies, which should cover a wide range of NHS activity, by an audit body that is demonstrably independent of the health authorities and FPCs [Family Practitioner Committees: the predecessors of the health authorities (HAs)] and of the Health Departments'. There is inevitably overlap with quality issues. The Commission addresses on average three topics in areas of high spending each year, and makes an in-depth study followed by recommendations on improved management practices to government. Subjects have included pathology services, day-case surgery, estate management, sterile services and prescription fraud. The main features of each survey are to look for improvements in management and at financial and quality control aspects of the service delivered so that users know what they are getting and how much it costs. This leads to the emergence of a national picture against which local managers can judge their own operations.

Table 10.1 Legislating for quality in the National Health Service (NHS)

1997	*The New NHS: Modern, Dependable* (White Paper)[3]	National Service Frameworks and guidelines for treatment Commission for Health Improvement (CHI) National Institute for Clinical Excellence (NICE)
1998	National Frameworks introduced (HSC 1998/074)[7]	Frameworks to be set according to priorities set in *Saving Lives: Our Healthier Nation* White Paper[8]
1998	*A First Class Service: Quality in the NHS* consultation document. Health Improvement Programmes launched by HSC 1998/167[23]	National Performance Assessment Framework announced Clinical governance to be introduced Three-year rolling plans to be drawn up between HAs, local authorities, PCGs and trusts
1999	*Clinical Governance: Quality in the New NHS* report[12]	Identifies key areas for change: A new culture in NHS organisations Inequity and variability Involvement of users and carers Sharing of good practice Detecting and dealing with poor performance and adverse effects
1999	The NHS Performance Assessment Framework Improving quality and performance in the NHS: clinical indicators and high level performance indicators	Measures to include quality and efficiency, including introduction of high level performance indicators To be used to review and compare performance between trusts and HAs

HAs, health authorities; PCGs, primary care groups.

The New NHS: Modern, Dependable

Since it came into office in 1996, the government has undertaken a programme of change intended to reform the management of the NHS and to raise standards. In 1997, the White Paper *The New NHS: Modern, Dependable*,[3] discussed more fully in Chapter 12, set out the proposed new legislation. A timetable of key events is set out in Table 10.1, and the following sections will discuss each in more detail.

Amongst its six key principles, the White Paper included three that were directly connected with quality:

- to renew the NHS as a national service. Patients would get fair access to consistently high-quality, prompt and accessible services right across the country;

- to drive efficiency through a more rigorous approach to performance;
- to shift the focus of care towards excellence. Quality was to become the driving force for decision making.

Some inequalities in health care to support the case for change were cited – the death rate for coronary heart disease in people younger than 65 is almost three times higher in Manchester than in West Surrey, and the percentage of drugs prescribed generically varies from below 50% to over 70%, to quote two examples.

The New NHS[3] announced a number of legislative changes intended to drive quality, which have subsequently been enacted. In addition to far-reaching management changes (the abolition of fund-holding general practitioners, the formation of primary care groups (PCGs), etc.), these were:

- the development of national standards and guidelines for services and treatments. These were to be issued as National Service Frameworks;
- the formation of a new statutory body, the National Institute for Clinical Excellence (NICE), which would provide guidance for the NHS and patients on medicines, clinical procedures and medical equipment, by assessing evidence on clinical and cost-effectiveness;
- the concept that local service agreements between HAs, PCGs and trusts should reflect national standards;
- a new NHS Charter to replace the existing Patient's Charter;
- a new statutory body to be formed to monitor NHS care and address shortcomings – the Commission for Health Improvement (CHI).

Under the previous regulations, NHS trusts' statutory responsibilities were mainly financial: in simple terms, they had to provide services without overspending. In the new order, they have additionally a new duty of quality of care. This is to be achieved by introducing the system known as clinical governance.

In 1997 Greg Dyke was commissioned by the Secretary of State for Health to develop proposals for the content, style and format of the new NHS Charter, which the government had pledged to introduce to replace the existing Patient's Charter. After undertaking a detailed investigation and consultation exercise, Dyke produced a report.[4] He considered, in common with many NHS staff, that the Patient's Charter had in fact done little to drive up standards. One reason was that it had been imposed by government with little opportunity for local input to adapt

262 Quality management in health care

monitoring requirements to local circumstances. In many cases it was resented by the very staff whose performance it was supposed to be improving. The Patient's Charter also had had little impact on primary care services. For these reasons and a number of others, Dyke concluded that simply to replace it with a new charter was unlikely to produce better results. He proposed instead that there should be local charter standards. This approach seems now to have been adopted as government policy since it has been recommended throughout the public service.[5] Dyke recommended that a number of pilot schemes should be set up to test the theory of local charters and to provide appropriate templates which could then be used by other NHS organisations to develop their own charters. He further proposed that these pilots should be undertaken in typical NHS trusts and PCGs, rather than those 'at the cutting edge of innovations'.

In spite of the changes discussed above, a number of the former Patient's Charter standards, with some additional ones, have in fact been included in a patient information booklet, recently published by the DoH.[6] Although the book contains a number of references to pharmacists as providers of advice on minor illnesses, there are no standards set for any pharmaceutical service.

National Service Frameworks

The New NHS set out a package of measures to drive up quality in the NHS, including the introduction of National Service Frameworks. In 1998, a circular[7] gave more detail about the programme for developing frameworks, and confirmed that their implementation would be linked with Health Improvement Programmes (see below). National frameworks would:

- set national standards and define service models for a defined service or care group; these will be underpinned by a clear statement of the evidence base, drawing on existing research evidence, or commissioning further work as necessary. They will be drawn up by experts in the field;
- put in place strategies to support implementation. HAs will implement strategies through their Health Improvement Programmes, in conjunction with their partners in providing health care, i.e. NHS trusts and PCGs/primary care trusts;
- establish performance measures against which progress with an agreed timescale will be measured, using the existing NHS performance management framework.

The frameworks were initially to cover mental health and coronary heart disease, cancer and paediatric intensive care. Further frameworks were to be added according to priorities set in the White Paper *Saving Lives: Our Healthier Nation,*[8] and more have been developed subsequently.

As expected, the coronary heart disease framework was soon issued, under the cover of a health circular[9] which introduced a raft of measures, including amongst others:

- research and development to be commissioned;
- clinical decision support systems, including clinical guidelines, clinical audit methodologies and appraisal, to be commissioned through NICE;
- the development of clinical governance in every NHS organisation, backed up by lifelong learning and rigorous professional self-regulation.

Cross-referenced to a series of papers, there were also strategies to allocate resources, and to ensure a quality workforce – *Working Together*[10] – and references to the NHS information strategy – *Information for Health*[11] – and partnerships with local authorities – *Partnership in Action.*

In December 2000, a Performance Management Framework for Medicines Management in Hospitals was published. Initially, it was to be used as a self-assessment tool for NHS trust hospitals, but the information so gathered is to be collated by regional offices, which will take the lead in sharing data and stimulating development work as deemed necessary. In the future, Audit Commission review of medicines management is proposed.

There are six domains for assessment within the framework:

- senior management, i.e. board-level downwards – awareness and involvement;
- information and financial issues;
- medicines policy management, including the introduction of new drugs;
- procurement of medicines;
- the primary and secondary care interface;
- influencing prescribers.

Clinical governance

The term 'clinical governance' describes the system of quality management that will enable NHS organisations to deliver their new duty to provide quality care. It has been defined as 'a framework through which NHS organisations are accountable for continuously improving the quality of their services and safeguarding high standards of care by creating an environment in which excellence in clinical care will flourish'. Quoting from *The New NHS*:[3]

A quality organisation will ensure that:

- quality improvement processes (e.g. clinical audit) are in place and integrated with the quality programme for the organisation as a whole;
- leadership skills are developed at clinical team level;
- evidence-based practice is in day-to-day use with the infrastructure to support it;
- good practice, ideas and innovations (which have been evaluated) are systematically disseminated within and outside the organisation;
- clinical risk reduction programmes of high standard are in place;
- adverse events are detected and openly investigated, and the lessons learned promptly applied;
- lessons for clinical practice are systematically learned from complaints made by patients;
- problems of poor clinical performance are recognised at an early stage and dealt with to prevent harm to patients;
- all professional development programmes reflect the principles of clinical governance;
- the quality of data collected to monitor clinical care is itself of a high standard.

A 1999 circular[12] directed HAs and trusts to implement structures to put clinical governance into place, by identifying lead clinicians and by setting up appropriate structures for overseeing the process. It further states that there must be an integrated planning process for quality at local level, to be achieved by Health Improvement Programmes in which HAs, trusts and local authorities collaborate to plan for local needs (see below). This mammoth circular amounts to a treatise devoted to the means and aims of achieving clinical governance. It sets out the key responsibilities for NHS organisations at all levels, and also sets out a vision for the next 5 years. It does not refer to individual professions or their potential contributions at this stage, but should be used as an introduction to the subject by anyone planning or reengineering a service.

The Royal Pharmaceutical Society of Great Britain (RPSGB) has developed a policy on clinical governance,[13] which forms part of the Pharmacy in a New Age initiative. This makes a number of recommendations about the application of clinical governance principles to the profession of pharmacy. In particular, it addresses the problem of establishing a framework of accountability for clinical governance in community pharmacy. Hospital and primary care pharmacists also have to consider their role within their organisation. The *Hospital Pharmacist* organised a conference on clinical governance. Its proceedings were reported,[14] and these papers would make a useful starting point for further reading on the subject.

In 2001 the Hospital Pharmacists Group of the RPSGB issued a statement on clinical governance for pharmacists in the managed service.[15] This sets out the pharmacist's role in key areas:

- the supply, storage and administration of medicines;
- prescribing support;
- error management;
- continuity of care.

In each case it refers to policy documents and published standards, such as Controls Assurance Standards and the Performance Management Framework for medicines management in hospitals, and demonstrates how each area ties in with the terminology and overall clinical governance strategy of the organisation.

National Institute for Clinical Excellence

NICE was set up as a special health authority on 1 April 1999. It has three main functions:[16]

- appraisal of new and existing health technologies;
- development of clinical guidelines;
- promotion of clinical audit and confidential enquiries. (An example of a previous confidential enquiry is the Confidential Enquiry into Peri-operative Deaths (CEPOD), where anonymised data have been collected from hospitals all round the UK in an attempt to identify causes of mortality and morbidity arising from surgery.)

Some input is made by a NICE Partners' Council, which includes representatives from stakeholders – health professions, health care industry, patients and carers. The main function of the Council is to review annually the Institute's work and to contribute to it.

Clinical guidelines already exist for the management of many conditions. However, in some cases they have proliferated, and their status and quality have been in doubt. NICE will produce its own clinical guidelines; these will be based on a rigorous review of the available evidence, including existing guidelines, and will address both clinical and cost-effectiveness of interventions.

The results of NICE reviews of drugs and procedures are issued in the form of Health Technology Appraisals. These cover:

- pharmaceuticals (around 40 new and existing medicines to be evaluated each year);
- devices;
- diagnostics;
- procedures;
- health promotion.

As well as making recommendations to support the practice of evidence-based medicine, technology appraisals include rapid audit tools to enable the monitoring of the implementation of their guidance. In August 1999, NICE's initial work programme was announced.[17] Possible topics for assessment were to include both new and existing health interventions and clinical practice. Of the original 23 topics, 15 were related to drug therapy, but a range of other clinical interventions was included, e.g. an evaluation of hip prostheses and developing basic standards for hearing-aid provision. Reviews of some new drugs were included, e.g. the taxanes' paclitaxel and docetaxel, and others were in fields where there were many competing agents on the market, e.g. proton pump inhibitors for dyspepsia. NICE may consider treatments before they have received marketing authorisation, but does not issue its final guidance until this process had been completed. According to NICE's Chairman, it is not intended that the guidance produced should restrict the availability of treatment for individual patients;[18] it is still possible for health professionals to exercise their own judgement. Whether this freedom will continue with government requirements to control costs and standards remains to be seen.

A number of Technology Appraisal Guidances are now available, issued and sequentially numbered in a manner similar to health circulars. The role of NICE was reinforced when it was announced that, from January 2002, primary care commissioning organisations will be given 3 months to provide funding for treatments recommended in technology appraisal guidance.[19]

Commission for Health Improvement

The CHI was set up in 1999 as a statutory body to oversee the introduction of clinical governance throughout the NHS. It operates in a similar way to the Audit Commission, but concerns itself with clinical rather than financial performance. The CHI undertakes reviews of NHS organisations, e.g. trusts. Such reviews, which take about 6 months, examine clinical governance management structures, and the provision and quality of services, monitoring the implementation of National Service Frameworks and guidelines. The review will seek evidence that guidelines and technology appraisal recommendations have been implemented. Examples might be:

- appropriate medicines have been included in local formularies;
- guidelines have been adopted as a model of practice, unless there is a valid local reason for their non-adoption;
- there has been adequate training and provision of information;
- plans to implement guidelines have been included in local health improvement programmes;
- guidelines are followed in daily practice.

Data, e.g. prescribing statistics, must be made available to the review team to provide evidence of change. Where service failures have occurred, the CHI will be involved in any disciplinary process.

In the future, the CHI may become involved in the regulation of professionals; in *The New NHS* White Paper,[3] the government revealed that it planned to take a more active role in the regulation of the professions. It stated that, while individual professions would retain responsibility for self-regulation, the government would work to ensure that the systems in place are open, responsive and publicly accountable.

National Performance Assessment Framework

The NHS Performance Assessment Framework was launched in 1999.[20] It is to be developed to establish clinical indicators (CIs) and high level performance indicators (HLPIs) for six dimensions:

- health improvement, reflecting social and environmental factors, e.g. changes in rates of premature death, reflecting social and economic factors as well as health care;
- fair access to NHS services for the population as a whole, including groups with specialised needs;
- effective delivery of appropriate health care, e.g. the extent to which health care provision is clinically effective and evidence-based;
- efficiency in the use of resources;
- patient and carer experience, e.g. reduced waiting times for operations;

- health outcomes of NHS care, e.g. success in increasing survival rates and reducing events such as second heart attacks in patients treated for coronary heart disease.

It is planned that together the CIs and HLPIs will enable and encourage benchmarking, i.e. the comparison of the quality of services between providers across the NHS. A separate circular[21] introduced CIs and HLPIs, based on retrospective data. HAs, PCGs and trusts were directed:

- to compare their local services across the headings given above with similar health care providers, and to identify areas for improvement;
- to share information about achieving good results and to take forward benchmarking;
- to assist in work to take forward clinical governance and to fulfil the new duty of quality;
- to strengthen the emphasis on quality and outcomes in local Health Improvement Programmes and local service and accountability agreements;
- to involve the users of local services by incorporating the indicators into arrangements for public accountability, and to provide information about the performance of local health services to patients and the public;
- to secure improvements in the quality and accuracy of data collected routinely within the NHS.

This circular was reviewed by Bower,[22] who discussed the HLPI on cost-effective prescribing, mainly in primary care. It required statistics on combination products, modified-release products, drugs of 'limited clinical value' and inhaled corticosteroids. Bower explains how the comparisons were to be calculated, using a formula intended to offset factors such as the age of the local population. There was a separate HLPI for generic prescribing rates in primary care, and a CI for the prescribing of benzodiazepines in the HLPI for mental health in primary care. As the system progresses, and more frameworks are developed, further HLPIs will be issued. Particularly in PCGs and trusts, pharmacists may expect to contribute to initiatives to improve performance. Bower cites some possible examples for pharmaceutical involvement – there are HLPIs on hospital discharge, delayed discharge for people aged 75 and over, adverse events and complications of treatment, all of which could have a pharmacy component.

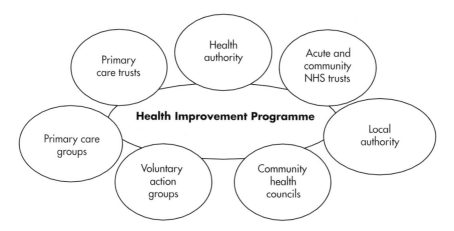

Figure 10.2 The Health Improvement Programme planning partnership. NHS, National Health Service.

By mid 2001, it had become apparent that the performance indicators in the earlier Performance Management Framework were of variable quality. Accordingly, a consultation exercise was undertaken to develop more useful indicators. At the time of writing, the outcome of this exercise is awaited.

Health Improvement Programmes

One of the declared aims of the White Paper *The New NHS*[3] was to foster working in partnership, and to break organisational barriers by forging stronger links between health care providers and local authorities, which manage social services provision. This aim was realised with the publication of a circular launching Health Improvement Programmes.[23] These locally produced plans supersede earlier planning arrangements. Figure 10.2 illustrates the various organisations that may make an input to the planning process in each HA area.

Health Improvement Programmes differ from the earlier planning process because of the wide range of local organisations and authorities concerned in developing the plans, tailored to local circumstances. The programmes, published annually, have to follow a 3-year rolling planning cycle, and to respond to national planning guidance and targets. They are widely distributed among health and social care providers, and may also be consulted in public libraries.

National Controls Assurance Documents

In addition to the frameworks and guidelines discussed above, the NHS Executive has developed a series of Controls Assurance Documents that are to be used to audit the effectiveness and efficiency of certain non-clinical services. Each document lists the statutes and key references that define best practice in this field. There is one on medicines management within hospitals,[24] which provides an audit tool to monitor compliance with the Duthie guidelines[25] and subsequent guidance and standards on many aspects of hospital pharmacy practice. At the time of writing, there are several other Controls Assurance Documents that are relevant to pharmacy, and more may be added in due course. There is one on medical records, covering management and disposal;[26] this should be read in conjunction with a circular on the same subject.[27] There is another document on medical devices management, which seeks to ensure that all risks associated with the acquisition and use of medical devices are minimised.[28] Emergency preparedness, covering the planning and preparing for major incidents and emergency situations, is included in the series.[29] Finally, there is a standard on waste management.[30]

Accreditation by independent bodies

Accreditation first developed in the USA in 1919. Since then, only health care providers who achieve accreditation can treat patients funded by private insurance schemes and the two state-run schemes Medicare and Medicaid. In the USA the main accreditation body is the Joint Commission for the Accreditation of Health Organizations (JCAHO). This publishes standards for service delivery across the organisations; detailed standards for pharmacy are published jointly with the American Society of Health System Pharmacists. JCAHO was originally set up for secondary care organisations, but has recently expanded to include standards for home care. Accreditation was introduced in Canada in 1959, in Australia in 1974 and in New Zealand in 1989. In each case, the accreditation programme is run by an organisation which is independent of central and local government and which is non-profit-making. The standards are published in the form of a manual, and reflect the current professional standards in the relevant health care service. The standards are reviewed and updated regularly.

The accreditation process is designed to improve the quality of practice; it is intended to be educational rather than disciplinary. At the outset, the institution applies to be considered for accreditation. Staff members are issued with the manuals setting out the nationally agreed standards, and may then receive training and guidance in the form of workshops or seminars, often with input from the professional staff of the accreditation body. The date of the survey will be set; usually about 12 months is allowed for preparation. When the survey takes place, a multidisciplinary team of specially trained surveyors, usually including a doctor, a nurse and an administrator, spends 3–5 days at the institution, visiting each department and scoring the 'required characteristics' set out under each standard. If the surveyors conclude that the institution is substantially compliant with the standards, they will recommend accreditation. In the USA, the process has to be repeated every 3 years.

In the UK, there has been no comparable requirement to achieve overall accreditation, and it seems unlikely that there would be a place for it now in the light of the government's quality initiative. There are, however, standards to which individual departments or businesses may aspire, and these are discussed below.

British Standards Institute

The British Standards (BS) Institute is an independent, but government-funded body. It is responsible for setting and publishing BSs for components of technical processes in many engineering and scientific fields. It also acts as an inspection, testing and accreditation body, and additionally has an important educational role, running courses and seminars for managers and organisations that are working towards accreditation. There are standards for many items of hospital equipment, e.g. pharmaceutical containers and closures, and medicine measures. These are identified by a number and dates, the first date being the original, and any others being updates, e.g. BS 4230: 1967 (1992), *Metal collapsible tubes for eye ointments*. The Institute interprets international standards for use in the UK, and also represents the UK view on standards in Europe and internationally. The International Organization for Standardization (ISO) is a worldwide federation of national standards bodies. Its work of setting standards is done by ISO technical committees, on which international governmental and non-governmental organisations develop standards in liaison with ISO representatives. When the BS Institute adopts an ISO standard, it may have both a BS number and the equivalent ISO number, but new standards are known only by ISO numbers.

There is a BS relating to quality management; it was originally designated BS 5750 (ISO 9000). Issued in several parts, each dealt with a different aspect of quality management. ISO 9000 – 1 gave an overview of the series, and stated that, in an organisation with a quality management system of the required standard, to quote:

> All employees, including the newly-hired, part-time and temporary employees, should be trained so that they understand the objectives of the organisation and the commitment required to achieve these objectives. The policy should be expressed in language that is easy to understand, and the objectives should be achievable, planned and periodically reviewed; management should continuously demonstrate visible commitment to the quality policy by activities which may include, but not be limited to, the following:
>
> - ensuring that the organisation's personnel understand and implement the quality policy;
> - ensuring that the organisation's personnel have quality objectives consistent with the organisation's overall objectives;
> - initiating, managing and following up on the implementation of the quality policy, including implementation and maintenance of the quality system;
> - not accepting deviations from the quality policy in any part or aspect of the organisation;
> - providing adequate resources and training to support quality system development and implementation.

ISO 9000 is currently under review, and henceforth will be designated ISO 9001 (2000). When complete, it will comprise the following main sections:

- quality management system;
- management responsibility;
- resource management: people and physical;
- product realisation: processes needed to provide product or service;
- measurement, analysis and improvement.

In addition to its usual role in accrediting organisations to this standard, the BS Institute is also offering 'conversion courses' for organisations already accredited under the earlier standard.

Investors in People awards

Investors in People is a national standard which was set up by the government in 1993. It establishes a standard for good practice for improving an organisation's performance through its people, by integrating human resources strategy with business strategy. The emphasis is on developing a planned approach to setting and communicating business goals through all levels in the organisation, and then to develop the members of the workforce so that they are both motivated and able to achieve the objectives. This philosophy is, of course, very similar to that expressed in the ISO discussed above, but the difference is that the ISO standard is more wide-ranging in that it sets standards for every aspect of the organisation's operation, rather than focusing on human resources.

The award is administered by a company, Investors in People UK, whose board of directors includes representatives from business, training, employee and government interests. It has links with the technician education councils. Organisations work towards the standard by a pathway similar to the accreditation process discussed above. The process is explained in detail in an Investors in People publication.[31] Once an organisation considers that it is ready, an assessor visits and undertakes an audit of a series of 23 assessment indicators. Written evidence of commitment to training will be inspected, e.g. statements in job descriptions, training and development plans, and also employees will be interviewed to assess aspects such as the effectiveness of induction programmes and equal opportunities policies. If the organisation is deemed to have met the standard, a recommendation for recognition as an Investor in People is made to a panel of business people. If they are satisfied with the evidence, the organisation will be officially recognised, and will be entitled to display the Investors in People official logo on their premises and business stationery. The assessment process follows a continuous cycle: once recognition has been achieved, the organisation is reassessed either every 3 years, or every 12–15 months, according to the nature of the operation.

Quality from within the organisation

Professional audit

The profession of pharmacy has a good history of active promotion of high-quality practice. In 1992, the Council of the RPSGB decided to promote professional audit of pharmacy practice as a way of improving standards. A working party report on the subject stated: 'The principal objective of professional audit is the continuing improvement of professional performance and patient care, in community and hospital pharmacy and at the interface between them. The process must therefore be designed to create change and must be cyclical'.[32] The process outlined in the report is analogous to the accreditation process, the essential difference being that no outside body is involved in the assessments. Since then, parallel initiatives have been the development of stated standards for professional practice set out as in the 'Practice Guidance' section of the *Medicines, Ethics and Practice* (MEP) guide,[33] the requirement to participate in professional audit set out in the section on good practice for ensuring professional competence of the MEP, and in manufacturing units the need to comply with the current standards of good pharmaceutical manufacturing practice.

Since the RPSGB Council embraced the policy of professional self-audit, it has undertaken several initiatives to bring the concept to the attention of the members. One of these was the appointment of an Audit Development Fellow based at the Society's headquarters, with additional audit contacts in Wales and Scotland.

Professional audit received a further stimulus with the launching of a professional audit distance learning course for pharmacists. *Moving to Audit* is available free of charge; details may be found in the MEP guide.[33] This package, which was originally distributed to all pharmacies in the UK in 1993, encourages pharmacists to complete a series of audit challenges – practical audits of practice in community and hospital settings. These could then be submitted for anonymous peer review. A recent addition to the range of self-audit tools is a CD-ROM *Audit to Excellence*, available from the Audit Division of the RPSGB. This contains model standards for self-audit in community pharmacy, audit templates and an audit handbook.

Quality circles

All the methods described so far have a common feature, i.e. the quality standards are determined by people largely outside the actual workforce. There is always the risk that the people on the job will not identify themselves with the quality management effort, and it will founder from lack of commitment from the operatives. At the very least, managers must make positive steps to sell the quality concept to the workers so that they experience some ownership of the problems. One way of achieving this is by setting up quality circles. These are non-hierarchical groups which meet on a regular basis to identify quality-related problems and to come up with possible solutions. They may be formed from within a department, e.g. in a large pharmacy there might be representatives from the various sections – but not usually the managers. The meetings should have some structure, and there must be some formal system of two-way communication between the group and management at a level that has the power to implement change.

It should be noted that some companies which have tried the quality circle approach have in recent years abandoned it following the realisation that it does not necessarily produce results. The difficulty with this approach is that junior staff members have no authority to commit resources to solve problems, and also their priorities may be different from those of the organisation. This can lead to frustration for the managers, who are being pressed to divert their energies into projects which form no part of their personal objectives, and for the circle members who think that their problems and ideas are being under-valued. A more effective method may be to involve each top manager in the organisation in the quality management programme by making him/her head up an initiative that runs through the organisation at all levels. Thus, the chief executive of one company headed up a project to improve communications at all levels both within the company and with customers. This project was one of his key objectives and was the subject of performance review – a good incentive to produce results! Identify-ing quality topics at top management or board-level ensures that resources will be committed and that the outcome is aligned with the objectives of the organisation; this is the underlying principle of clinical governance.

In another model, quality circles may be formed within an organis-ation with representatives of services that interface, to look at processes that have multidisciplinary input. An example might be the admission procedure for patients coming in for planned surgery, which could involve the bed manager, pathology services, an anaesthetist's review, the portering service and the nursing staff on the ward.

Suggestion schemes

These are seen as a way of motivating staff and getting 'grass-roots' opinion about problems that may be totally unperceived by top manage-ment. However, they may backfire badly if no action is seen to result from ideas that the staff see as perfectly reasonable, but which unfortu-nately do not relate to the main aims of the organisation. At the very least, staff who identify problems should receive the courtesy of a reply from their managers. The author visited a hospital in Texas where the succinctly named 'yak'n flak' scheme was much prized by the staff – they were encouraged to highlight their grievances, which went straight to top management and always produced a reply, and usually some action.

References

1. Department of Health and Social Security. *National Health Service Management Enquiry*. London: Her Majesty's Stationery Office, 1983.
2. Department of Health. White Paper. *Working for Patients*. London: Her Majesty's Stationery Office, 1989.
3. Department of Health. White Paper. *The New NHS: Modern, Dependable*. London: Stationery Office, 1997.
4. Dyke G. *The New NHS Charter – A Different Approach*. London: Stationery Office, 1998.
5. Department of Health. White Paper. *Service First – The New Charter Programme*. London: Stationery Office, 1998.
6. Department of Health. *Getting the Most from your National Health Service: Your Guide to the NHS*. London: Department of Health, 2001.
7. NHS Executive. *National Service Frameworks*. HSC 1998/074.
8. Department of Health. White Paper. *Saving Lives: Our Healthier Nation*. London: Stationery Office, 1999.
9. NHS Executive. *National Service Framework for Coronary Heart Disease: Emerging Findings Report*. HSC 1998/218.
10. Department of Health. *Working Together: Securing a Quality Workforce for the NHS*. London: Stationery Office, 1999.
11. Department of Health. *Information for Health*. London: Stationery Office, 1999.
12. NHS Executive. *Clinical Governance: Quality in the New NHS*. HSC 1999/065.
13. Royal Pharmaceutical Society of Great Britain. *Achieving Excellence in Pharmacy Through Clinical Governance*. London: Royal Pharmaceutical Society of Great Britain.
14. Clinical governance conference report. *Hosp Pharm* 1999; 6: 288–297.
15. Hospital Pharmacists Group of the Royal Pharmaceutical Society of Great Britain. Statement on clinical governance for pharmacists in the managed services. *Hosp Pharm* 2001; 8: 198.
16. News item. NICE launched by Health Secretary. *Pharm J* 1999; 262: 490.
17. NHS Executive. *NICE: Initial Work Programme*. HSC 1999/176.
18. News item. NICE – no restriction to treatment of patients as individuals. *Pharm J* 1999; 263: 225.
19. News item. NICE's advice to be made compulsory. *Pharm J* 2001; 267: 807.
20. NHS Executive. *The NHS Performance Assessment Framework*. HSC 1999/078.
21. NHS Executive. *Improving Quality and Performance in the New NHS: Clinical Indicators and High Level Performance Indicators*. HSC 1999/139.
22. Bower A C. Review of circulars and official publications. *Hosp Pharm* 1999; 6: 222–223.
23. NHS Executive. *Health Improvement Programmes*. HSC 1998/167.
24. NHS Executive – Controls Assurance Standard. *Medicines Management (Safe and Secure Handling.)*. London: Stationery Office, 2000.
25. Department of Health. *Guidelines for the Safe and Secure Handling of Medicines* (Duthie Guidelines). London: Department of Health, 1988.

26. NHS Executive. *Controls Assurance Standard. Records Management.* London: Stationery Office, 1999.

27. NHS Executive. *For the Record: Managing Records in NHS Trusts and Health Authorities.* HSC 1999/053.

28. NHS Executive. *Controls Assurance Standard. Medical Devices Management.* London: Stationery Office, 2000.

29. NHS Executive. *Controls Assurance Standard. Emergency Preparedness.* London: Stationery Office, 2000.

30. NHS Executive. *Controls Assurance Standard. Waste Management.* London: Stationery Office, 2000.

31. *The Investors in People Standard.* London: Investors in People UK, 1998.

32. Working Party Report. Audit in pharmacy. *Pharm J* 1992; 248: 208.

33. Royal Pharmaceutical Society of Great Britain. *Medicines, Ethics and Practice: A Guide for Pharmacists*, published yearly. London: Royal Pharmaceutical Society of Great Britain.

11

Finance, information and procurement

National Health Service (NHS) funding

Source of NHS funds

In the year 2000–01, expenditure on the NHS for England was forecast to be £44 485 million.[1] This had risen over a 10-year period from a sum in 1991 of £23 632 million. By far the greatest proportion of this expenditure is funded through general taxation, and this makes expenditure on health a highly political item. Allocations for Wales, Scotland and Northern Ireland are made separately. The NHS allocation for each of the home countries is negotiated with the Treasury by the appropriate organisation, e.g. the National Assembly for Wales or the Department of Health for England, whereas the Scottish Parliament has the authority to set its own budget for health.

The previous method of allocation was to set the budget on an annual basis, but this led to problems in not being able to plan expenditure further than 1 year, so in 2000 the Chancellor of the Exchequer amended the process to set an ongoing budget for 3–5 years. The allocation is made in the Comprehensive Spending Review announced by the Chancellor of Exchequer – the most recent was in summer 2000. This review makes allocations to all major spending departments such as Education, Health and Defence out of the total sum for government spending agreed in advance by the Treasury. As major departments will all be competing for a larger share than the others, final decisions are made taking into account political factors such as impending elections and public awareness of the topic. In recent years, it is perceived that health has been relatively successful, but it has become increasingly clear that, with developments in technology, the global sum will never be enough.

Cash allocation to the NHS

The global sum agreed for the NHS is treated in different ways. The majority is allocated to health authorities (HAs), but a sum is retained centrally to pay for the cost of the Department of Health (DoH) and also for any services purchased centrally such as through special HAs (e.g. National Blood Authority). For 2001–02 the sum allocated to HAs was £41 465 million, and this was distributed according to a circular, HSC 2000/034.[2]

The money allocated to HAs is cash-limited. This means that the authority has an obligation to stay within the allocation. Most of the sum allocated is spent by NHS trusts on hospital and community health services (HCHS) but the allocated sum also pays, through primary care groups/primary care trusts (PCGs/PCTs), for primary care contractors, including general practitioners (GPs) and pharmacists. In theory there-fore total government expenditure on the NHS is controlled, but success-ive governments have found this difficult and have tried a variety of measures to impose controls. The basic problem is in restricting primary care spending, in particular, where there is a narrow margin between rationing treatments and controlling expenditure. Recent recommen-dations from the National Institute for Clinical Excellence (NICE) indi-cate increasing controls through this route on the availability of high-cost drugs.[3] Recommendations in a consultation document *Shift-ing the Balance of Power*[4] indicate that base allocations will in future go directly to PCTs, with only special allocations being held at HA level. Many elements of HA funding, as described below, are, however, unlikely to change significantly.

Health authority finance

Cash limits

The allocation of finance to the NHS has been discussed above. The greater proportion of the total is subject to 'cash limits'. Each HA is required by law to ensure that spending does not exceed this limit. Prior to the introduction of cash limits, Parliament was asked to vote supple-mentary sums throughout the year to cover the costs of services. Now, once the cash limit has been set, the onus is on authorities to keep spending within that figure. The use of cash limits has enabled govern-ments to keep closer control on public expenditure, but in times of high inflation it can also be used to reduce public spending. If an authority's allocation for a year is assessed on an estimated 5% inflation, then any increase of expenditure above that figure will have to be found locally, either by increased efficiency or by a reduction in services. In simple terms, this describes the effects of the cash limit for the NHS.

Capital and revenue

Cash given to HAs is divided into three categories: capital, revenue and special allocations. The last of these is of relatively minor importance, but the others include the vast majority of an authority's allocation. Capital is money allocated to finance the acquisition and maintenance of assets, e.g. new building work and major equipment. Capital schemes are increasingly funded by the use of private finance (see below). Revenue is the money required to finance the running expenses of health services, and includes major items like salaries and wages, drugs and catering.

Private finance

The use of private finance is a means of meeting the costs of a public sector capital project (such as the construction or refurbishment of a hospital) using funding provided wholly or partly by the private sector. Its objective is to speed up the availability of new buildings/facilities by adding private finance to the limited amount of government finance. The Private Finance Initiative (PFI) was launched in the early 1990s and is now seen as part of the broader initiative called Public Private Partnerships (PPP) in which joint working and joint investment between the public and private sectors are promoted. Full details of the scheme can be found on the DoH website.[5]

The introduction of the PFI has meant that all significant capital investment proposals in the NHS have to be considered for PFI procurement. Schemes have to be approved by the Treasury, and detailed criteria have to be met. The two main criteria are to achieve value for money and to transfer risk from the public to the private sector whilst maintaining NHS control on service outcomes. A simple example might be the arrangement that a private company will fund the construction of a new facility and the NHS will pay a rental to that company over a significant number of years.

Distribution of allocation to health authorities

When the NHS was formed in 1948, financial allocations were made on the basis of historical expenditure. Over the years, however, it was perceived that this basis did not reflect the current requirements of different parts of the country, so methods have been introduced to rectify this. The first significant change was introduced by a Resource Allocation Working

Party (RAWP) in 1976.[6] This proposed an allocation formula based on several criteria, including population size, morbidity (sickness rates) and age/sex ratios of the population. Regional health authorities (RHAs) at the time were to be given a target allocation as part of the global sum. As this would have resulted in significant changes to the allocation for several regions, some through cuts and others with increased funding, it was realised that any change had to be gradual. It was not practical to reduce immediately allocations by factors of around 10% in order to give this money to 'underprovided' regions. Not only would the patients of the reducing regions be at risk of inadequate provision of services, but also the recipients of the new money would not have the organisation in place to spend it appropriately. Changes were therefore to be effected by small variations over several years, by targeting inflationary increases and by making additional allocations to 'underprovided' regions. By the mid-1980s the four Thames regions were the only ones nationally still receiving an allocation over their target.

RAWP allocations were made to RHAs, but most regions used a similar formula to reallocate resources within their region. Although the RAWP formula did much to reduce perceived inequalities in health service funding, its use was subject to much debate. As a result of the changes of policy which led to the 1990 NHS and Community Care Act,[7] the government decided that future allocations would be made on a weighted capitation basis. Although the detail methodology varies with political expediency, the principles are similar to that originating in RAWP. A formula is used which includes factors such as age of the population, morbidity and the cost of providing services. Currently, allocations are made to HAs against a formula based on historical allocation, inflation and any new money allocated. This is then adjusted by comparing the authority's financial allocation against that predicted by the formula using the capitation indicators.[2]

The internal market

As a new means of trying to control the rising expenditure on health, the government introduced the concept of an internal market in the 1990 NHS and Community Care Act. In this, the allocation received by an HA was the sum available to purchase, i.e. commission, services and treatment for HA residents. This sum was paid to providers of health services including NHS trusts, either against contracts agreed in advance between the HA and the provider, or against specific invoices raised for a service or treatment provided. Any one HA (commissioner) might have contracts with several providers, especially in highly populated areas when the numbers may be in dozens. Conversely, NHS trusts may have income from several HAs, especially if they have specialist services, when the number again may counted in dozens.

The original scheme encouraged competition between trusts on a cost basis, but recent government policies have removed a substantial element of this factor. In effect, contracting has been abolished, and whilst income will still come from a variety of commissioners, the choice of provider is considered to be more of a quality and collaborative decision than one made competitively through costs. Contracts have been replaced by service-level agreements, and these are gradually being set up between PCGs and PCTs and NHS trusts as HAs take on a more strategic role.

Control of finance within NHS trusts

Financial management: budgets

Once a unit has firmed up its income for a year it has to plan its expenditure. It does this by allocating budgets for goods and services. Historically, allocation of funds within units was through budgets given to a budget manager to control, e.g. to a function such as pharmacy, or to a facility such as operating theatres. The main problem with this method of allocation was that the budget manager often did not control the workload and hence the expenditure. For example, although a pharmacy manager would have a considerable influence over drugs expenditure, the final decision to prescribe was generally made by a clinician. To overcome this problem, most trusts are now devolving budgetary control to service groups, directorates or divisions (see Chapter 12) which will further divide up the allocation between their constituent clinical directorates. Taking the example of a surgical directorate, the clinical director would manage within the budget a range of services across the trust. These are illustrated in Table 11.1.

Control through clinical directors gives better utilisation of resources, since the users will have an interest in using their funds wisely. It is easier, for example, for a clinical director to see the benefits of introducing a new expensive drug which might save money by reducing the length of inpatient stay, or avoiding the need for surgery. There are difficulties, however, in providing the detailed management information (including budgetary information) to make this an easy process. Problems may also arise if changes are introduced which lead to

Table 11.1 Services included within a surgical directorate budget

Nursing staff of the surgical wards and departments
Operating theatre staff and overheads
Drugs supplied to in- and outpatients
Medical and surgical equipment and other supplies
Departmental costs of facilities (pharmacy, radiology, pathology, hotel services)
Administration and management costs

additional costs for another director. This might occur if a director ceased to use a facility where previously the overheads were apportioned between several directorates, leaving the residual costs to be shared as an extra cost to the remaining users.

The development of service groups and directorates has led to the requirement for the management of services such as pharmacy to be reformed in line with the local structure, and this has led to a variety of pharmacy organisational models. A common factor is the provision of pharmacists targeted to each directorate or service group.

It is the budget-holder's responsibility to ensure that expenditure does not exceed the allocation, and this can only be achieved with accurate and up-to-date information on expenditure. This is provided by the finance department in the form of regular – usually monthly – statements which analyse expenditure under various headings. Examples of the sub-headings which are usually included for pharmacy managers are illustrated in Table 11.2.

Financial management: audit

All legally constituted organisations have an obligation to protect the interests of their owners, whether these are shareholders or, in the case of the NHS, the general public. Financially these obligations are met by the publication of annual accounts which are approved by independent auditors. Auditors' duties include ensuring that the financial rules of the organisation have been followed; that expenditure has been on authorised items and that supporting paperwork is available for inspection; and that income and expenditure records balance. These principles are equally relevant for small organisations such as an independent retailer, or even in voluntary work for clubs and societies.

Within the NHS audit is carried out at two levels. Internally, the director of finance of each authority or trust is responsible for ensuring that there are appropriate and effective audit procedures. Such internal

Table 11.2 Possible elements of a pharmacy manager's budget

Staff, analysed by grade and unit
Equipment and the cost of its maintenance
Laboratory chemicals
Consumables, e.g. sterile disposables
Containers
Travelling expenses
Training expenses

audit may be carried out by employees of the organisation or by external contractors, and usually includes audit studies of parts of the organisation, as well as carrying out an overview of the accounts. Studies are often targeted at financial areas of risk, and might include checking controls on goods (including drugs) to ensure that there is no theft, and monitoring systems, to ensure that money is paid to suppliers only when evidence of receipt of goods or services is available. From these examples it will be seen that pharmacy departments often work closely – and usually in cooperation – with internal auditors who, in addition, can often give useful advice when new procedures are implemented.

As well as internal audit controls, the annual accounts of the authority/trust are subject to external audit by auditors appointed by the Secretary of State. This function was given to the Audit Commission by the 1990 NHS Act. The Audit Commission is an independent body originally set up to audit the accounts of local authorities; it is funded by fees paid by its clients. It is prudent for all organisations, and a requirement for legal entities, that there are written procedures to be followed for the control of money and goods. In the NHS these are called 'standing orders' (SOs) and 'standing financial instructions' (SFIs), and they must be formally approved by the authority or trust board. They will be based on model documents set out in two health circulars.[8,9]

SOs cover all aspects of business, ranging from the membership of the authority or trust board and the frequency of its meetings to detailed instructions relating to tendering for the supply of goods or services. SFIs give more details on financial controls, such as the method of accounting and cheque signatories and limits. They will include rules on the handling of departmental/sectional budgets, including those on transfer of money allocated for one purpose to another (also called virement). All employees are bound by these rules, and everyone should be aware of their contents – especially in pharmacy, which handles goods and originates expenditure.

Table 11.3 Examples of activities for computer audit

Password access, strictly applied, should be in place for all systems which control money or patients' records

There may be different levels of password access for different users

Passwords should be hard to guess, i.e. Not proper names, and should preferably be a mixture of alphanumeric symbols

Passwords should be changed regularly; good systems will enforce a regular change

Back-up copies of programs and data should be available and kept in a secure but distant location (in case of fire or theft)

Back-up copies must be made regularly, at least daily, for operational data, and copies rotated with those in safe storage

If the computer is used for stock control, then regular physical counts of stock should be made; these may be initiated randomly by some systems

---

Computer audit

The use of computers is an increasingly important area for audit control. Computer procedures are gradually taking over in many areas, and these must be adequately controlled to ensure information security and procedural integrity. Commercially supplied systems may include adequate controls, but it is the responsibility of the purchaser to ensure that these are comprehensive, and are properly implemented. Locally written programs should be produced with audit in mind. Examples of computer fraud are given regularly in the national press through (usually) publication of the details of criminal trials, and the authors are aware of instances where advanced pharmacy systems have been entered ('hacked' into) by unauthorised persons. Such fraud can result in the misappropriation of goods or money, or in access to information protected under the Data Protection Act 1998. The Royal Pharmaceutical Society of Great Britain (RPSGB) publishes practice guidance in the *Medicines, Ethics and Practice* guide,[10] but as all pharmacists will have dealings with computer systems, through which they may potentially lose money or break patient confidentiality, it is worth stressing some key points (Table 11.3).

Computing and information technology

Computers in pharmacy

The use of computers in pharmacy has evolved over more than a decade; the origins were often simple dispensary labelling systems. As hardware

Table 11.4 Key priorities from the Royal Pharmaceutical Society strategy for information technology

Management of prescribed medicines
Management of long-term conditions
Management of common ailments
Promotion and support of healthy lifestyles
Advice and support for other health care professionals

has developed and become more powerful, then pharmacy systems have become more comprehensive, both in the community and in hospitals. The authors remember their first district hospital system, in the early 1980s, which was a minisystem with two 28 megabyte Winchester-type hard-disk drives maintained in an air-conditioned room. Compare the memory capacity of today's 'notebooks' and 'laptops'! As computer technology has advanced, it has become more important that systems are introduced which are capable of networking with the other information systems in use within the organisation; therefore system specification has become more important.

There are many suppliers of computer systems for pharmacies, as can be seen from the advertisements in journals. Most systems now have the facility to include clinical information such as drug interactions and warning labels, and have the ability to hold patient medication records and to carry out stock control and ordering. Integration with other systems is increasingly important, and the development of such links will be discussed later. As these developments occur, it becomes more difficult for pharmacists to compare systems that are on the market. As part of the Pharmacy in a New Age initiative, the RPSGB set up a focus group – the Information Technology and Management Focus Group – which reported its findings in 1997.[11] Key points from the strategy are included in Table 11.4. In addition, information relating to pharmacy computer system specifications is updated and summarised in the *Medicines, Ethics and Practice* guide[10] sent yearly to all members.

Like those in community pharmacy, many hospital systems have evolved from labelling and simple stock control software. There are, however, now additional requirements to integrate with other hospital systems, and potentially with primary care systems. This causes major problems in both system specification and intersystem communication. Although to a large extent pharmacy systems have been developed in isolation, there is an increasing need for compatibility. In the 1980s the NHS Management Executive (NHSME) addressed the problem of 'stand-alone' systems by introducing the concept of the Common Basic Specification (CBS). The CBS was to be produced as a high-level system specification intended to define in generic terms the complete activity of the NHS, and the need for transfer of data. One of the first to be produced was a hospital pharmacy project. This work is described in an article by Bailey et al.[12] This is a useful reference to the problems of producing practical specifications. In 1992 the NHSME agreed that the hospital pharmacy CBS should be one of four that would be used to take this one step further. The concept of the CBS has now been abandoned by the NHS, but the original work is available to interested parties – such as computer suppliers.

It is important to realise that many specifications such as the CBS define the desired outcome and not necessarily how to achieve it. For example, patient medication details could be held by a stand-alone pharmacy computer, or by a hospital information system which is networked with a smaller pharmacy system.

The NHS information strategy

In 1998, the government, responding to concerns about piecemeal implementation of information technology and in many cases wasted money on unsuccessful systems, introduced *Information for Health*[13] – a new national information management and technology strategy for the NHS. This announced the formation of a new special HA to oversee the delivery of the elements of the strategy. This, the NHS Information Authority, is monitored and controlled by the Information Policy Unit of the DoH. Key elements of the strategy are listed in Table 11.5, and significant issues discussed in later paragraphs.

Many elements of this strategy are in progress, but the timetable has slipped in several areas so that implementation will occur over a longer period. Some of the problems in implementation are discussed in an article by Whitfield.[14] An updated response to the strategy was

Table 11.5 Key issues included in *Information for Health*[13]

Electronic patient record and electronic health record
NHS-wide network, including electronic transfer of records between GPs
New resources, including the establishment of NHS Information Authority
Access of patients to easy information, e.g. through NHS Direct

NHS, National Health Service; GPs, general practitioners.

Table 11.6 Targets included in *Building the Information Core*[15]

March 2001	95% of GP practices and 25% of trust clinical staff with NHSnet connections and using National Electronic Library of Health
March 2002	Desktop connections for NHS clinical staff for e-mail and browsing
March 2003	National standards for e-mail and browsing completed, and all NHS staff with desktop access
March 2004	Major national payroll and human resource systems implemented
March 2005	Electronic booking systems in place, electronic transfer of records in primary care, and substantial electronic patient records and first-generation electronic health records in place

GP, general practitioner.

published in 2001 in response to the issue of the *NHS Plan*.[15] This repeats many of the original targets, but intends to accelerate the spread of information technology across the NHS by, for example, ensuring that all staff have access to NHSnet and the internet by March 2003. Some of the targets included are listed in Table 11.6.

NHS networks

Over the early years of the introduction of information technology within the NHS, systems were developed very much in isolation. The development of a system was generally funded on immediate needs rather than as part of an ongoing strategy. For example, in the 1980s–1990s hospital pharmacy systems became a priority because of the information they could provide on drugs expenditure and use – a key financial issue for most hospitals. They usually did not connect with other hospital systems, e.g. pathology or patient administration systems, and communication outside the organisation – to other hospitals or primary care systems – was almost non-existent. One of the inhibitions to this exchange of data was the lack of a system for such communication, so in its 1998 paper *Information for Health*,[13] the government proposed the development of a national system of communications, known as NHSnet. The purpose of this data-networking system is to enable easy and secure communications between all parts of the NHS, whether between individuals, NHS trusts or HAs/health boards. The system also provides for communication to parties outside the NHS through a secure gateway or 'firewall' to the internet, so that the NHS can access the information available there. Similar developments are in progress in Scotland.

Electronic health records

One of the key points of *Information for Health*[13] is the introduction of the electronic patient record (EPR) and subsequently the electronic health record (EHR). The EPR aims to describe and make accessible to all health professionals an element of care for an individual, e.g. an operation, whereas the EHR describes the lifelong health history of an individual. The aim is to replace all current manual health records produced by each hospital and, using a unique identifier, link data from individual, the EPR, into the lifelong summary of health experience, the EHR. The use of such technology will facilitate the swift availability of care records to wherever a clinician is meeting a patient. Its use in the wider professional arena, e.g. by pharmacists, is still subject to debate.

Electronic information

As information technology develops, so access to information becomes more significant. There are three initiatives which are fundamental: the use of the internet; the National Electronic Library for Health; and NHS Direct.

The internet has revolutionised information access, and it is now quite common for patients to have 'surfed the net' before they visit their doctor. This can mean that they are well informed about treatment options, and this may influence the outcome of treatment. However, many doctors have concerns about this because the information gained by the patient often does not come from evaluated and recognised information sources. Treatments may not be proven, and may well not be available in this country. Nevertheless, the informed patient is a theme of both government policy and medical thinking, so that the use of the net in this way must be harnessed for improved outcomes. The role of the internet in consumer self-care was explored at an international conference in 2000 and reported in the *Pharmaceutical Journal*.[16] The development of NHS Direct enables any member of the public to get health advice from a professional by a telephone call. This is further explored in Chapter 1.

Information gained over the internet is not restricted to patients, and of course the use of this medium is now almost the first choice for many information queries. The role of evolving technologies for delivering medicines information was described in an article by Shepherd in 2001,[17] and wider initiatives in the use of the internet in a pharmacy department discussed in a linked article by Tugwell.[18] Recognising some of the pressures on information demand and supply the paper *Information for Health*[13] introduced the concept of a National Electronic Library for Health.[19] This went live in November 2000, and gives a central system to access the best information on health matters. It is intended for access by health professionals, managers and patients, and links databases of guidance (e.g. from NICE or National Service Frameworks) with knowledge bases.

Online pharmacy services

A number of pharmacies have established websites offering various facilities, including publicising their services, and, in some cases, medicines information. The Pharmaceutical Group of the European Union (PGEU) has now published guidelines to be used by national authorities to draft national guidelines for internet pharmacy services. These were summarised in a news item in the *Pharmaceutical Journal*, [20] and can be read in full on the PGEU website.[21]

Telemedicine

Telemedicine is a generic term covering the application of a variety of proven electronic and communication techniques to the provision of health care. The range of applications is wide and growing, and the potential benefits for patients are substantial. In essence, it describes a situation where patient and doctor, and sometimes a specialist, can have a remote consultation using information technology. Telemedicine can be delivered anywhere. Depending on what is being provided, it may be in a hospital clinic or surgery or at home, on an oil rig or even in the battlefield. It has been used in Cornwall, for example, for dermatologists to assess a patient who is miles away in the GP surgery. It is not a new clinical procedure, although its effectiveness, safety and acceptability to both clinicians and patients need to be proven in specific cases. Existing clinical procedures link with technology which has usually been developed for non-clinical use, including telephones, data communication links and cameras. By transferring images and other information electronically, travelling time for clinicians and patients should be significantly reduced and waiting time for outpatients or for results could also be cut significantly. The government supports plans for the extension of its use through *Information for Health*,[13] and a website was introduced in 2001 to improve uptake of the process.[22]

Electronic data interchange

Electronic data interchange (EDI) is the technical term for the concept popularly referred to as 'the paperless society'. Many large companies now rely on EDI for much of their operation. Banks transfer money automatically between accounts, including through the Banking Automated Clearing System (BACS) which enables many people (including NHS employees!) to receive their salary, and companies to be paid against invoices. Large retail chains rely on data capture through barcodes to provide management information on sales and stock control, usually through electronic point of sales (EPoS) data capture. The NHS has been slow to introduce such concepts, but the transfer of data will be enabled with the implementation of NHSnet. There will still need, however, to be a common language between systems.

Another reason frequently given by the NHS for not proceeding rapidly with EDI is the additional resource often required to capture data. In the ideal system all data are collected as part of the routine operation rather than as a separate exercise, but this requires specialised equipment. The main method in commerce is by using systems that machine-read the data. Banks use optical character-reading equipment which can read the specially styled print on the bottom of cheques. Trading organisations usually use barcodes which can be read at the point of sale. To ensure that common languages are in use there is an association representing British industry, e-Centre (previously known as the Article Numbering Association) which sets out standards, and works with European associations to agree standard codes, e.g. European Article Numbering (EAN) codes. These EAN codes are in common use today on foods and domestic products; they differ from the American standard codes. Many pharmaceutical suppliers use EAN codes and barcodes, but their slow introduction has inhibited the widespread use of electronic trading. In addition, some wholesalers who were early users of electronic trading systems introduced their own codes, e.g. PIP codes. Ideally, products should be received into the pharmacy, recorded by data capture of EAN, then stock should be controlled and issues recorded by similar means.

Electronic exchange of NHS data is fundamental to the implementation of *Information for Health*.[13] The NHSnet will act as the means of transfer, but there are legal as well as technical issues to be resolved before the system is in common use. A good example of the issues can be gained from a study of electronically transmitted prescriptions, and a useful review article has been published by Middleton.[23] This reviews work undertaken in various countries, including trial work on the use of 'smart cards' for data exchange. These were developed in the 1980s, and act like bank cards, except that information can be accessed or stored on them by any appropriate professional. Patients can therefore carry their own health record with them.

EDI has been discussed in relation to hospital procurement for decades. Its implementation has been slow for a variety of reasons, including that of 'language' and the costs of setting up, but the concept is now gaining credence with the development of the internet in electronic trading; this will be discussed more fully in the next section.

Procurement of medicines

E-commerce

E-commerce is one term, together with e-procurement, used to describe systems for electronic trading. It has been defined as 'the exchange of information across electronic networks, at any stage of the supply chain, whether within an organisation, between businesses, between business and the consumer, or between the public and private sectors'.[24] In this cited article, Fifield draws on the publication of a national e-commerce strategy for the NHS to argue the case for the cost and other benefits of such an approach.

Pharmacists have generally been enthusiastic about the use of e-commerce from its beginnings in EDI, and an interested group of pharmacists and suppliers has met over several years in a group called PharmEDI. A useful article by Wind,[25] on behalf of PharmEDI, describes the various concepts in this area as they affect, in particular, hospital pharmacy. The article includes a helpful table comparing paper systems with EDI, and lists some benefits accruing from paperless trading. A perspective of electronic trading for community pharmacy has been published by Dajani.[26]

Contracting

A contract for supply is a legally enforceable agreement between the purchaser and the supplier. It is crucial therefore to ensure that the details of the agreement are correct. It is usually a supplies officer who acts for the trust as an expert on contract law, and many supplies officers have qualifications related to this, e.g. a law degree, or Associateship of the Chartered Institute of Secretaries. The supplies officer not only acts to ensure that the law is complied with, but also that the terms of the contract are favourable to the trust, and that the trust's own regulations are satisfied. These regulations – SOs and SFIs – are referred to above. They include much detail relating to the whole procurement process – tendering, contracting, ordering, receipt of goods and payment of invoices – with the objective of ensuring that trust resources, e.g. money, are not wasted or abused.

The role of supplies departments

Supply matters are always high-profile because of the volume of NHS spending. In the early 1990s three critical reports on purchasing resulted in major changes, including the formation in 1992 of an NHS Supplies Authority (NHSSA). The National Audit Office (NAO)[27] investigated prices paid for and the organisation of supplies, and found considerable differences in prices. It is interesting to consider that the NAO report specifically excluded drugs from its deliberations, but that subsequently they were subsumed into the arrangements for the NHSSA. The criticisms in the NAO report were mirrored by an Audit Commission report,[28] and both reports acted as the basis for a Public Accounts Committee (PAC) investigation.[29] The PAC is a select committee of the House of Commons which monitors accountability in the use of public funds. It agreed with the NAO and Audit Commission reports that there seemed to be inconsistencies in purchasing which were costing the NHS money, and it was the report of this committee which finally led to the formation of an NHSSA, and set initial targets for its operation. Another review was undertaken in 1999 by the DoH in conjunction with the Treasury,[30] and following that review a new organisation – the Procurement and Supply Agency (PASA) – was formed in 2000. It took over most of the functions of NHS Supplies, which remains a special HA but as a purely wholesaling business and deals with logistics. The Agency's responsibilities are listed in Table 11.7, and there is a useful overview of NHS procurement in *Wellard's NHS Handbook 2000–01*.[31]

PASA obtains pharmaceutical advice in a variety of ways. Apart from local input, and the pharmacists on the Agency staff, a national group of pharmacists – the National Pharmaceutical Supply Group (NPSG) – gives strategic advice to the Agency on the purchase of

Table 11.7 Responsibilities of National Health Service (NHS) Procurement and Supply Agency

To coordinate and guide NHS procurement policy
To develop and improve national purchasing function
To explore the scope for national mandatory contracts
To provide expert advice on procurement
To collate information on procurement for benchmarking
To maintain a market overview of procurement

medicines; acts as a focus for linking professional matters with purchasing, e.g. standardised labelling, and temperature control of distribution; and provides input into any national contracts for medicines.

Generic medicines

Purchasing of generic medicines has historically been more significant in hospital than in community practice. The main reason for this is that, although both sectors use generic medicines now, at the time of writing, only the hospital pharmacist can substitute a generic medicine for one prescribed by its trade name. Community generic supply is regulated by price by the *Drug Tariff*,[32] and until 1999–2000 there were no particular issues regarding supply. At that time, however, severe shortages began to be experienced in community, followed by significant price rises of many items. The government took short-term action to restrict price inflation, and the House of Commons Health Select Committee launched an investigation.[33] As a result, an independent report was commissioned, following which the government published a consultation paper on generics in the summer of 2001.[34]

Shortages and erratic prices had previously been seen in the supply of hospital generics, and a report in 1998 reviewed some of the contributing factors. This report[35] made several recommendations which are being considered for action by the NPSG. An update on this and the whole process of contracting for generics has been published by Stokoe,[36] and the reasons for shortages are explored in an article by Karr.[37] The likelihood is that the response to this consultation will lead to fundamental changes. The use of e-commerce will surely impinge, and this option, together with a consideration of European purchasing, is considered in an article by Matthew Young of the Adam Smith Institute.[38]

Purchasing

The mechanism of purchasing for such a large and complex organisation as the NHS needs considerable control; rules are set out in the SOs and SFIs. There are controls on blank order stationery which is only available to authorised people, and orders are sequentially numbered. Only authorised officers can sign orders, and a copy of all orders is sent to the finance department. Goods should be received by a different officer from the one who placed the order, and details of receipts must be sent to the finance department for payment of invoices. In general, all orders are placed by supplies departments on behalf of requisitioning departments so that extra safeguards against misuse are included.

Pharmacy is the main exception to this arrangement. The operational purchase of most medicines in hospitals is carried out by pharmacists and technicians, within the constraints of SOs and SFIs. The arrangements for pharmaceuticals are unique, and reflect the complexity of buying medicines. Most pharmacists work closely with their supplies colleagues who can give useful support in handling negotiations, on legal matters and in distribution arrangements. Orders for drugs are normally generated within the pharmacy department, signed by a pharmacist, and sent direct to the supplier. The pharmacist's signature is a legal requirement for certain drugs, but it also reflects the urgency of many drug orders, and acknowledges the expertise of the pharmacist in ensuring the correct item. This ordering of a commodity by personnel outside the supplies organisation has been the subject of much discussion, and was originally supported by a report issued in company with a Department of Health and Social Security circular.[39] When pharmacists order non-drug items such as equipment, they have to send a requisition to the supplies officer in the same way as any other hospital officer. Records of purchase and supply must be kept for statutory periods, and are subject to audit inspection.

In addition to local orders, there are frequently consortia of pharmacists from different trusts who work together to obtain the best prices for their hospitals when there is advantage in price or in maintenance of supply by working on this scale. These consortia may be organised on a historic regional basis. Currently there are also arrangements for contracting at this level. A large number of pharmaceutical items are, however, purchased directly from wholesalers who trade at the published hospital price of a medicine, but who often give discounts to regular large customers. Many regions, in addition, utilise a 'short-line' store. This may be independently managed or be within a pharmacy department. The purpose is to purchase bulk quantities of products in order to gain large discounts. Most of these stores keep only a very limited range of items – hence 'short-line' – but these may have a significant turnover and value. Direct purchasing from the manufacturers has the disadvantage of less frequent delivery; increased lead time from placing the order to delivery; and the probability of tying up more cash as stock. The method is therefore only used if significant discounts can be obtained over prices from wholesalers or, as in some cases, if the manufacturer chooses not to distribute through a wholesaler. The proportion of the split quoted above indicates that this is currently quite common, and reflects current pharmaceutical marketing practice. A review of pharmacy procurement issues has been published by Samways *et al.*[40]

When making comparisons of prices, it is important to add additional costs of procurement on to the cost price. These will include overheads in running a store (heat, light, etc.); losses due to capital tied up in stock; and, especially for 'short-line' stores, the distribution costs. The cost of pharmacist and support staff time in the procurement process is often overlooked or not fully accounted for.

Tendering

When a trust wishes to arrange for the supply of goods or services, there are requirements under SOs that it receives competitive tenders for the supply. Invitations to tender are only sent to firms which have been approved both in their financial stability and in the standards of their goods or service. For potential orders of high value there are European rules which must be observed which include advertising the tender in the *Journal of the European Union* to allow open access across Europe. The detailed regulations for tendering are quite rigorous, and are set out in the SOs of each trust. An example is that tenders have to be returned in sealed envelopes, dated upon receipt and only opened after a set date in the presence of approved officers. For high-value items such as major building works these will normally include members of the trust board, but for smaller-value items senior managers may be involved.

It is obviously not practical to invite tenders for every item a trust may require. The procedure is expensive to administer and time-consuming. It would be completely impractical for drugs required in an emergency, for example. Therefore, SOs contain monetary limits within which the formality of tendering may be waived. Goods which are already included in formal contracts are also normally exempted when a purchase is made. In the case of pharmaceutical purchasing, many items are subject to prearranged contracts but, for other items, the pharmaceutical officer is a nominated purchasing officer for drugs and subsequently allowed to initiate the procurement of goods to a certain value.

Management of stock and assets

In common with any large organisation, controls on stock are important in the NHS. Stock control is carried out to monitor the use of a commodity, to control the amount stored, to monitor the efficacy of stock and for its security. For audit purposes, stock is considered by its cash value; many of the controls are set out in SOs and SFIs. Generally, pharmaceutical stores and stock are the responsibility of the trust's senior pharmacy manager. Knowledge of the usage of an item is important for several reasons: it allows efficient purchasing, it may show up abuse or misuse, and finally, the cost may need to be charged to the user, either directly or by cross-accounting, e.g. in management budgeting.

Knowing the amount of an item stored is important not only as an aid to purchasing but also to control the amount of cash tied up in stock. Although superficially this seems more important to a commercial organisation, any cash used for the purchase of stores is money that the health service could otherwise use for direct patient care. The amount stored also relates to the next factor – maintaining the efficacy of stock. This is just as important for other items as it is for pharmaceuticals. Storage conditions must be appropriate with due attention paid to temperature, pest control and security. Stores must be organised so that there is efficient turnover of stock. Particularly important for items with a short shelf-life, it is good practice to ensure that new stock is always behind older stock. Many computerised systems highlight impending time expiry so that steps can be taken to shift the item, possibly by transfer to another trust.

A high level of security is of paramount importance in stores premises, both to prevent theft and to ensure proper documentary control. The degree of physical security will relate to the type of goods within. All stores – not just pharmaceuticals – should have limited access, and be secure from unauthorised entry. Often, burglar alarm systems will be installed. A number of documentary controls are applied to stocks, whether held in store or, in the case of non-consumable items, issued for use. Stock should only be issued against a requisition from an authorised officer. SOs usually require an annual physical stocktake of stores, with reconciliation against book stock. Any discrepancy is investigated by the audit department and reported to the trust board. For disposable items such as syringes, the yearly stocktake must be reconciled with the previous balance, taking account of subsequent issues and receipts. Because of the number of transactions which take place, the legal restrictions on possession and the volume of small items involved, e.g. tablets, drugs have generally been exempted from most of the controls on stocks. It is still necessary to account for them, however. This may be achieved by a physical count at least once each year. Alternatively, auditors may accept a computer valuation if regular, random stock check counts are undertaken throughout the year, and are achieving a result which is typically regularly in excess of 70% accuracy of theoretical stock compared with actual stock. A well-managed pharmacy store, handling unbroken bulk containers, should expect to achieve stock check accuracy values of around 98%.

Asset registers

Assets are the major property of the organisation, i.e. the buildings and fixtures, vehicles, major items of medical and scientific equipment and large installations where the individual components may not have a high value but, taken together, their replacement would require outlay of capital. Examples might be the computer installation or the hot-water and central-heating system. Departmental managers such as the senior manager of the pharmacy will be responsible for the assets listed for their department, and so should make every effort to ensure that the register entries are correct. Trusts and other HAs are now required to maintain registers of assets, like any commercial enterprise. The value of the assets features in the accounts of the trust, and allowance for their depreciation over a period of years, and eventual replacement, has to be included in the financial planning process. New items may be registered by the supplies department as part of the acquisition process; SFIs set out a formal procedure for the disposal of assets and their removal from the register.

References

1. Merry P, ed. *Wellard's NHS Handbook 2001–02*. Wadhurst, East Sussex,: JMH.
2. Department of Health. *Health Authority Revenue Resource Limits 2001/02*. HSC2000/034.
3. News item. New MS patients face restrictions *Pharm J* 2001; 267: 185.

4. Department of Health Consultation Document. *Shifting the Balance of Power within the NHS – Securing Delivery.* London: Department of Health, 2001.

5. Department of Health website (2001). *Private Finance Initiative (PFI)* www.doh.gov.uk/pfi (accessed 19 March 2002).

6. Department of Health and Social Security. *Report of the Resources Allocation Working Party* (1976). London: Her Majesty's Stationery Office, 1976.

7. The NHS and Community Care Act 1990. London: Stationery Office, 1990.

8. NHS Executive. *Directions on Financial Management in England.* HSG(96)12.

9. Department of Health. *Corporate Governance for HAs and Primary Care Groups; Standing Orders, Standing Financial Instructions, Guidance Specific to PCGs and Fraud Policy and Response Plan.* HSC 1999/048.

10. Royal Pharmaceutical Society of Great Britain. *Medicines Ethics and Practice: A Guide for Pharmacists,* published yearly. London: Royal Pharmaceutical Society of Great Britain.

11. Council approves information management strategy for pharmacy. *Pharm J* 1997; 258: 436–443.

12. Bailey L, Jamieson I, Barber N. Hospital pharmacy computing prescription for the 90s? *Pharm J Hosp Suppl* 1991; 246: HS57.

13. NHS Executive. *Information for Health: An Information Strategy for the Modern NHS 1998–2005.* London: Stationery Office, 1998.

14. Whitfield L. Money where the mouth is. *H Serv J* 2001; 111: 18.

15. Department of Health. *Building the Information Core – Implementing the NHS Plan.* London: Stationery Office, 2001.

16. Conference report. The role of the internet in consumer self-care and pharmacy practice. *Pharm J* 2000; 265: 463–464.

17. Shepherd I. The evolving technologies for delivering medicines information. *Hosp Pharm* 2001; 8: 155–157.

18. Tugwell C. Taking pharmacy services to a new level with the intranet. *Hosp Pharm* 2001; 8: 158–162.

19. The National Electronic Library for Health website (2001). www.nelh.nhs.uk (accessed 31 August 2001).

20. News item. European e-pharmacy guidelines published. *Pharm J* 2001; 267: 143.

21. Pharmaceutical Group of the European Union website (2002). www.pgeu.org (accessed 4 January 2002).

22. Telemedicine Information Service website (2001). www.tis.bl.uk (accessed 23 August 2001).

23. Middleton H. Electronically transmitted prescriptions – a good idea? *Pharm J* 2000; 265: 172–176.

24. Fifield J. E-supply chain. *Health Manage* 2001; 5: 12–13.

25. Wind K. Pharmacy procurement: electronic data interchange *Hosp Pharm* 2000; 7: 37–41.

26. Dajani S. IT, e-commerce and pharmac-e! *Pharm J* 2000; 265: 132–133.

27. National Audit Office. *NHS Supplies in England.* London: Her Majesty's Stationery Office, 1991.

28. Audit Commission. *Improving the Supplies Service in the NHS.* Her Majesty's Stationery Office, 1991.

29. Committee of Public Accounts 42nd Report. *NHS Supplies in England*. Her Majesty's Stationery Office, 1991.
30. Department of Health. *Review of NHS Procurement: Implementing the Recommendations*. HSC1999/143.
31. Merry P, ed. *Wellard's NHS Handbook 2000–01*. Wadhurst, East Sussex: JMH.
32. Department of Health and National Assembly for Wales. *Drug Tariff*, published monthly. London: Stationery Office.
33. News article. The House of Commons Health Select Committee's report on generic prices. *Pharm J* 2000; 265: 689–691.
34. News article. Fixed prices or competitive tendering: latest options for generic medicines. *Pharm J* 2001; 267: 109.
35. Mounsey C, Curtis S J. *A Generic Perspective – A Review on Generics Pharmaceuticals within the UK*. London: Unit for Health Services Development, School of Pharmacy, 1998.
36. Stokoe H. Pharmacy procurement: generics contracting in England. *Hosp Pharm* 2001; 7: 42–44.
37. Karr A. Where have all the medicines gone? *Pharm J* 2001; 267: 197–198.
38. Young M. Managing medicines better – smarter purchasing and distribution. *Pharm J* 2001; 267: 235–236.
39. Department of Health and Social Security. *Ordering and Receipt of Pharmaceutical Supplies*. HM(66)33.
40. Samways D, Wind K, Page J. Towards intelligent purchasing. *Hosp Pharm* 2001; 8: 144–146.

Part Three

Health care organisation

12

Health care organisation in the UK

The National Health Service (NHS) is a large organisation which employs nearly one million staff, often said in the days of the Soviet Union to rival the Red Army as the largest employer in Europe. As a pharmacist you will be one of those employees, directly or otherwise, and will be contributing to its success. It is, therefore, important to understand how the NHS is organised.

The NHS is an extremely public organisation, with an anticipated expenditure (raised through general taxation) of over £40 000m in 2000. As befits expenditure of this magnitude, the NHS is accountable to Parliament, and this accountability is exercised through the Secretary of State for Health and supporting ministers. The recent devolution Acts have split some of the control, with, for example, the NHS in Scotland forming about 30% of the budget of the new Scottish Parliament. The structure of the NHS organisation in England is illustrated in Figure 12.1.

Accountability

Parliamentary accountability of the NHS is not just theoretical and has real implications for the practising pharmacist. There are significant areas of practice which are controlled by legislation and where changes need to be debated and passed by Parliament. These will be well-known to students recently concerned with passing law and ethics examinations, but can be further studied in *Medicines, Ethics and Practice*, the guide sent annually to all pharmacists by the Royal Pharmaceutical Society of Great Britain (RPSGB).[1]

More significantly to individual pharmacists, however, is the right of all Members of Parliament to ask parliamentary questions of the Secretary of State on specific issues affecting their constituents. In addition to these occasional questions and enquiries, there are also select committees that monitor the operation of the NHS. The Public Accounts Committee pays particular attention to how the NHS money is spent, and the Health Select Committee looks at more practical or care issues.

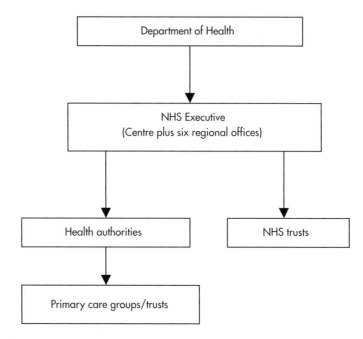

Figure 12.1 Structure of the National Health Service (NHS) in England in 2001.

This central accountability is an ongoing influence in the management of the NHS, and may involve the pharmacist in any area of practice in responding to enquiries. If you are interested and have access to the parliamentary television channel through cable or satellite television, you will be surprised to see the frequency with which health matters are discussed and the occasional specificity of the probing – often related to the care of one specific patient. One relevant matter relates to an enquiry of the Health Select Committee held in 1999 into the market for generics medicines in the NHS and which subsequently initiated a full review of the issue. This has ongoing implications, which are explored in Chapter 11.

Structural change in the NHS

Structural change in the NHS has been continuous since it was nationalised in 1948, and the pace of change has intensified as the expenditure on the service grows and as increasing developments in technology lead governments to look for savings from efficiency before rationing or removing services. Some of the main changes are illustrated in Table 12.1.

Table 12.1 Key reorganisations in the National Health Service (NHS)

1948	Nationalisation
1974	Introduction of area and district health authorities (managed secondary care services)
	Introduction of family practitioner committees
1983	Area health authorities abolished; introduction of general management
1991	Introduction of NHS trusts and internal market
	Family practitioner committees abolished; replaced by health authorities
1995	Abolition of regional health authorities
1999	Introduction of primary care groups
2001	*Shifting the Balance of Power Within the NHS – Securing Delivery*[3]

Government policy documents

The continuing changes in the organisation of the NHS have been reflected recently by three key documents. *The NHS Plan: A Plan for Investment, A Plan for Reform*[2] was published in July 2000. The Health and Social Care Act was passed by Parliament in May 2001, and *Shifting the Balance of Power Within the NHS – Securing Delivery*[3] published in July 2001.

NHS plans for England, Wales and Scotland

In 2000, the government undertook an exceptional consultation process with the public to assess individuals' views on the NHS. As a result of this exercise it produced *The NHS Plan*[2] which introduced some fundamental elements of government thinking. One key element was the creation of two national groups to oversee the NHS changes. These are a Modernisation Board and a Modernisation Agency; the former ensures that the implementation of the plan is being carried out and that patients are at the centre of service reform, while the latter supports the NHS in achieving delivery of the plan. Key elements of the plan are summarised in Table 12.2, and it is usefully reviewed in *Wellard's NHS Handbook 2001–02*.[4]

Amongst some of the radical changes announced in the plan are significant increases in the resources of the NHS. This includes extra beds, more staff – particularly clinical staff – and new hospitals and clinics. It announced clinical priorities which generally follow the National Service Frameworks and the National Cancer Plan, and it announced initiatives around waiting lists for treatment. It also introduced a system for monitoring organisational effectiveness using a

Table 12.2 Key elements of *The NHS Plan*[2]

Provision of a comprehensive range of services for all, based on clinical need, not ability to pay
Services based around the needs and preferences of patients, their families and carers, and to the needs of different populations
Continuous efforts to improve the quality of services and minimise errors
Particular support to and valuing of NHS staff
The objective of keeping people healthy and reducing health inequalities
Respecting the confidentiality of individual patients while providing open access to information about services, treatment and performance

NHS, National Health Service.

red/amber/green listing to indicate closeness to meeting agreed targets. It enabled the creation of care trusts to ensure closer working between social care and primary care.

Similar plans have been announced for Scotland (*Our National Health: A Plan for Action, A Plan for Change*[5]) and Wales *(Improving Health in Wales – A Plan for the NHS with its Partners*[6]*)*.

The Health and Social Care Act 2001

The NHS Plan was soon followed by the Health and Social Care Act 2001, which enabled many of the proposed changes discussed in *The NHS Plan*. Changes are made to funding arrangements, particularly around family practitioner services; arrangements can be made to establish care trusts across primary and community care boundaries; the extension of prescribing rights to other practitioners such as nurses and pharmacists is enabled; and arrangements are put in place to allow the transmission of services using the internet and similar technology. It also allows for the provision of local pharmaceutical services pilots (see below). Much of the change will be implemented by further circulars and reports, and the first significant one was issued in July 2001.

Shifting the Balance of Power Within the NHS – Securing Delivery[3]

The organisational arrangements described in this chapter are those in operation after two decades of significant change. This change is ongoing, and in July 2001 the Department of Health (DoH) issued proposals for yet another structural reorganisation. The discussion document *Shifting the Balance of Power Within the NHS – Securing Delivery*[3] gives details of major changes to be implemented over 2002–04. These include removal of the functions of the NHS regional offices (ROs) and replacing them with four smaller organisations whose prime purpose is to support the DoH and NHS Executive (NHSE) on public health issues. These will be arranged so that they link geographically with the existing regions for local government. The number of health authorities (HAs) in England will be reduced from about 95 to 28, and again their functions will change. Known as strategic health authorities (StHAs), the new bodies came into being in April 2002. The StHAs will take over the performance-monitoring role currently undertaken by the ROs, and will liaise directly with the primary care trusts (PCTs) which, in turn, will gain more independence and accountability. The arrangements described in the following sections will, however, remain during the implementation period, and many of the underlying principles will remain in the new structure.

Current NHS structure and organisation

Government ministers are supported by the DoH (England – see Figure 12.1), the Scottish Office, the National Assembly for Wales, and the Northern Ireland Department of Health and Personal Social Services. These departments all include a pharmacy section with a chief pharmacist responsible for advising on pharmacy issues and for leading on relevant aspects of policy development. The departments work closely with the RPSGB, but have no direct control over professional matters.

The NHS Executive

The DoH in England is very much a strategic organisation that supports the work of ministers. A separate organisation (but within the DoH) – the NHSE – handles the day-to-day running of the NHS. This Executive, whose main office is in Leeds, manages the NHS with the assistance of six ROs across the country. The head of the NHSE is the Chief Executive, who also acts as permanent secretary to the DoH. The Health Ministers also receive advice from a series of standing professional advisory committees, including the Standing Pharmaceutical Advisory Committee (SPAC). These committees are set up with a wide but independent membership from within the profession, and members are chosen by the Secretary of State for their individual expertise rather than any representative position they may hold.

Regional health authorities and regional offices

At the introduction of the NHS in 1948 there were 14 statutory bodies managing the NHS in England – regional health authorities (RHAs). The detailed duties and scale of operation of these authorities changed slightly, but otherwise their role did not change until the 1990 NHS and Community Care Act. This introduced the first major change as part of the introduction of the reforms referred to earlier. At the time, the monitoring of trusts was perceived to cause problems because, as they were accountable directly to the NHSE, RHAs no longer had any role in monitoring the services they provided; there was a lack of detailed service monitoring, coordination and development of trusts. In October 1993, therefore, the Secretary of State made an announcement of further changes to the management of the NHS, resulting in the creation of regional outposts of the NHSE. This was by setting up separate organisations known as 'regional outposts/offices'. There are currently six of these, and their title reflects the fact that they are not statutory bodies like the RHAs, but operated as outposts of the NHS Management Executive. Set up as part of the central management organisation, their task was to monitor NHS trusts on behalf of the Secretary of State, mainly dealing with financial issues. They are small organisations, with staffing of only 10–20 people, and generally have kept to their financial remit.

The main task of the ROs is to monitor the performance of HAs and trusts in meeting their targets as set by the government. The RO agrees an annual contract with each HA and monitors this through an annual review, and also monitors the financial control of trusts. This performance management currently includes a significant interest in the use of medicines. Each RO has a pharmacist appointed to contribute to this process. The six pharmacists in the ROs meet regularly with the Chief Pharmacist of the DoH and with colleagues in Scotland, Wales and Northern Ireland to discuss common issues and policy. All pharmacists should at least know the name and geography of their own RO and its pharmaceutical adviser so that they can follow developments affecting their locality.

NHS management

The day-to-day management of the NHS in England and Wales is currently carried out at two levels – that of the HAs and of the NHS trusts. In Scotland, Wales and Northern Ireland there are some

Table 12.3 Main roles of a health authority

Assessing needs for health care for the population of the district
Preparation of Health Improvement Programmes (HImPs)
Administration of delegated aspects of management of primary care groups/trusts
  and of contractors
Discharging statutory objectives (such as maintaining services within budget)

differences in detail (e.g. the HA is called the health board) but the functions are broadly similar. However, the introduction of primary care groups (PCGs) and their development into PCTs is fundamentally changing these arrangements.

Health authorities and boards

Until April 2002, there were about 100 HAs in England, each responsible for a population of about 500 000. HAs were statutory bodies as set up in the NHS Act 1977 and amended by the NHS and Community Care Act 1990. The authorities comprised a board chaired by an appointee of the Secretary of State, with an equal number of executive and non-executive members. The non-executive members act substantially in a voluntary capacity. HAs had a legal status similar to that of a limited company. Any decision of the authority was thus binding on its members and employees. The same management principles will apply to their successors, the StHAs and PCTs. In order to conduct the business in an efficient manner within the law, such authorities have a set of rules, called 'standing orders'. These include standing financial instructions which, as their name indicates, give details on handling matters such as bank accounts, cheque signatories and accounting for cash. These are discussed in more detail in Chapter 11.

The main roles of HAs are summarised as in Table 12.3.[7] Their role has been primarily strategic and they must assess the health needs of their population, formulate a strategy to meet these needs, plan for the provision of services for their residents and, most recently and importantly, support the development of PCGs and PCTs. The link between health needs and organisational achievement has been enhanced recently, as all HAs in conjunction with local primary care organisations and local authorities, and in collaboration with local health care providers such as NHS trusts, have had to produce a Health Improvement Programme (HImP). The HImP outlines a 3-year strategy for a HA to improve health in its locality, and ensures that the HA has to work on

Table 12.4 Examples of special health authorities

Commission for Health Improvement
Health Development Agency (previously Health Education Authority)
Medical Devices Agency
National Institute for Clinical Excellence
NHS Purchasing and Supply Agency
National Clinical Assessment Authority
National Blood Authority
Prescription Pricing Authority

NHS, National Health Service.

these issues with its constituent PCG/PCTs. (See also Chapter 10.) The HA also has a public health role in matters such as outbreaks of infectious disease, and it manages the contracts for independent practitioners such as general practitioners (GPs) and pharmacists.

Special health authorities

In addition to HAs there are a number of special health authorities (SHAs). These are responsible directly to the Secretary of State for the provision of their services. Within the NHS, the SHAs cover a range of services of a highly specialised or critical nature that require direct accountability. At one stage, some of the London postgraduate teaching hospitals were included, but these are now managed as NHS trusts. Current examples of SHAs are included in Table 12.4.

These HAs are set up with a chair and board comparable with other authorities, and are subject to similar financial and statutory controls. Their finance comes directly from the DoH.

NHS trusts

The 1990 NHS and Community Care Act introduced completely new arrangements for the organisation of health care within the NHS. In place of the previously fairly rigid line management structure, it introduced a system based on an internal market (see below). The main consideration in this was that hospitals were encouraged to become more independent by applying for NHS trust status. The Act gave powers to the Secretary of State to establish bodies known as NHS trusts to assume responsibility for the management of hospitals or other establishments previously managed by regional, district or SHAs for the purpose of providing hospitals or other facilities. Trusts are statutory bodies with a board of directors consisting of a chair appointed by the Secretary of State, and executive and non-executive directors. A review of the role of trusts was published by Brookes.[8]

Within the NHS, the purpose of establishing trusts was to give them as much freedom to manage as possible. They are therefore accountable directly to the Secretary of State through the ROs of the DoH, and are not managed by HAs. Their detailed powers were set out in the Act and regulations made under it. They can, for example, borrow and invest money (forbidden to the rest of the NHS), and can use non-Whitley Council terms of service (including pay) for employment of staff. They are, however, bound to comply with directions from the Secretary of State, including circulars specifically directed to them. They are required to submit annual accounts to the Secretary of State. They obtain income by contracting to provide services to purchasing organisations, e.g. HAs, PCGs.

There are about 400 NHS trusts in the UK and these are responsible for the management of hospital services, community health services and supporting services such as ambulances. The trust structure was established in 1991, as described above, and although there have been changes to their operation, they are still the foundation of hospital management. They are independent bodies accountable to the Secretary of State, but their performance – particularly regarding financial targets – is monitored by ROs. They will be increasingly monitored with the introduction of clinical governance to improve quality in the NHS. Many trusts are based on acute hospitals, but some include community services or are based on mental health services. Each trust will have a pharmacy service, often on-site, and the chief pharmacist has an important role in the control of medicines within the organisation. As in primary care, this will include an element of cost control.

It is important that trust chief pharmacists and their supporting staff work closely with their colleagues in community pharmacy and at the HA/board. Each has specific skills and knowledge, which can be harnessed to improve patient care and control expenditure. The wider role of pharmacy is not particular to a single area of practice and is enhanced by cooperation and joint working.

Primary care groups and primary care trusts

PCGs were established in England in 1999 as the latest step in ongoing reforms to ensure that GPs play their full part in the management of a primary care-led NHS. They are paralleled in Scotland by local health care cooperatives and in Wales by local health groups. There are differences in the detailed composition and the level of power in each example, and some issues are still to be confirmed by the appropriate devolved parliament/assembly. English PCGs are formally committees of the HA and have certain functions delegated to them. These include improvement of the health of their community, development of primary and community health services and commissioning of secondary care services.

Over time PCGs will become free-standing bodies called PCTs. The first 14 of these became operational in April 2000, with successive waves operational from October 2000 onwards. Many PCTs have been formed from groups of PCGs and cover a larger geographical area. PCTs will take over the management of the services for their patients from the HA. This diminution in their role will lead to the widespread merging of HAs, discussed above.

In England, nearly 500 PCGs were established, and each is managed by a board comprising four to seven GPs, two nurses, one social services representative, one lay member, one HA representative and the chief executive. There was some controversy at the time of establishment that there was no statutory place for a pharmacist. Some of these concerns have been reduced over time, as a few PCGs appointed a pharmacist to the board, and most have appointed at least one pharmacist as adviser.

Some pharmacists have been appointed as chief executive of a PCG. These contributions by pharmacists reflect the importance of medicines at this level of health care. It also gives an important indication of the difference between a board-level post and an adviser. As a board member the individual has to make decisions on a corporate basis, including dealing with statutory matters referred to the PCG. In other words, there is not great freedom to act on behalf on the individual's profession. An adviser – this can be a senior post – has this freedom.

PCG pharmaceutical advisers have functions similar to those described for the HA, but obviously deal with a smaller population base. Their role is no less important, however, because it is at GP practice level that the introduction of a cash-limited unified budget has most effect. (See also Chapter 3.) In addition, the PCG is different from earlier models of management, such as GP fundholding, in that there is no element of choice of membership by GPs. All GPs are members of a PCG and must support the management process, including maintaining expenditure within budget.

Because of the local nature of PCGs it is essential that community pharmacists know the detailed arrangements of PCGs/PCTs in their area. This will include understanding the boundaries, knowing which GP is in which organisation and knowing which GPs are leaders in the organisation. Working with local medical leaders is likely to enhance the pharmacists' contribution to health care. In addition it is necessary to have positive communication with the PCG pharmacist adviser. Many of these are being appointed with a community pharmacy background and will be in an ideal position to develop pharmacy services within the PCG. As PCGs become trusts, there is an unrivalled opportunity for pharmacy to take its full role as part of the primary health care team.

Patient involvement

The Secretary of State is accountable to Parliament for the provision of health services; this means that there has to be public accountability for the way in which the NHS is run. The 1974 reorganisation sought to improve links with the public by the introduction of community health councils (CHCs). They are statutory bodies; there is usually one for each HA. Their main functions are to represent consumer views to HAs, e.g. by participating in the formulation of the HImP (see above), and to provide the public with information about local health services.

The government announced its intention to strengthen patient/public involvement with the publication of a report *Patient and Public Involvement in the New NHS* in September 1999.[9] This set out a whole series of measures to make partnership working a reality and these are summarised well in an article by Covey.[10] *The NHS Plan*,[2] published in 2000, made wider proposals for the involvement of the public and patient groups in service design and provision. The proposals included the abolition of CHCs and their replacement by local patients' forums and patients' advocacy and liaison services. In addition, the Modernisation Board set up following *the NHS Plan* would have up to a third patient interest membership.

Contracting for health care

A main purpose of the NHS and Community Care Act 1990 was to introduce an 'internal market' to the provision of health care. In parallel with the formation of trusts, health service bodies, including the then district health authorities (DHAs: now HAs) were given the power to place contracts with providers for the provision of goods and services required for their function; GP fundholders (GPFHs) were established with similar powers. They are both therefore referred to as 'purchasers' of health care. A review of the initial position of purchasers and providers has been published by Gilbey.[11]

This internal market caused considerable disruption to the historic pattern of service provision. The rising cost of health care imposed pressures on purchasers to obtain minimum costs for treatments in order to maintain the numbers of cases they could afford to treat. In many cases this led to a reduction in work going to specific hospitals, with resultant closures of wards or even, potentially, complete hospitals. In August 1993 the press was full of reports indicating such problems, with mergers of trusts being proposed to overcome deficits,[12] and HAs indicating major changes to their pattern of spending. Around London and other large conurbations, local hospitals were sometimes gaining at the expense of city-centre teaching institutions because of both cost and convenience. As a result, subsequent government policy documents removed the competitive element of the internal market. Competition is now encouraged for efficiency, but competition on cost is not permitted.

Family health services in primary and community care

Since the beginning of the NHS, those services provided by GPs, pharmacists and dentists in the community have been referred to as family health (or practitioner) services. Initially these had evolved from local-authority-run services, and the 1948 Act put them into the NHS for the first time, but run by separate organisations known as executive councils. The 1974 reorganisation brought them under mainstream NHS control, and they were managed by the then area HAs. After a short period when they existed separately again, first as family practitioner committees and then as Family Health Services Authorities (FHSAs), they were linked in with the then DHAs in 1995; the DHAs were superseded by HAs.

The prime functions which have been undertaken are listed in Table 12.5. A key one for pharmacy was the control of prescribing, and the role of prescribing advisers (see also Chapter 3) has evolved from this.

With the introduction of PCGs and PCTs, the latter organisations will gradually take over the management of primary care contractors. It is anticipated that legislation will come into force in October 2002 to enable this and remove one of the last operational tasks residing with the HA.

Table 12.5 Primary care contractors: the current role of health authorities

Paying practitioners according to their contracts

Planning for local service development in primary health care

Managing the contracts of general practitioners (GPs) and other professionals, including pharmacists

Financial management, including prescribing and allocation of funds for GP practice development

Provision of information to the public and dealing with complaints from them

The majority of professionals working within primary care are independent contractors. They work, therefore, from their own premises, and employ their own staff. The number of staff managed directly by the HA or PCT is quite small. Professionals, i.e. GPs, pharmacists, dentists and opticians, are in contract to provide services to the population of that authority, and must comply with the terms and conditions of this contract to be able to undertake NHS work. For example, a community pharmacy cannot dispense NHS prescriptions unless it has a contract with the HA. The various contracts are different for each profession.

An important change for all groups of primary care contractors was introduced in December 2001 under provisions of the Health and Social Care Act. The new regulations gave HAs disciplinary powers over their contractors, and for the first time will enable them to suspend or remove existing contractors as a disciplinary measure on grounds of inefficiency, fraud or unsuitability. This supersedes the previous arrangement where suspension or removal could only result as an outcome of an NHS Tribunal hearing. Appeals against HA decisions will be referred to the Family Health Services Appeals Authority (FHSAA). While HA decisions will only apply to their own list, FHSAA rulings can apply throughout England and Wales.[13,14] It is not yet clear how these changes will be implemented when the operational role of HAs ceases when the StHAs take over.

General practitioners' terms and conditions of service

GPs are paid a basic practice allowance, and then various additional fees – a capitation fee for each patient registered (higher for elderly patients), out-of-hours allowance, maternity and contraceptive services, etc. They can also claim payment for certain 'items of service', maternity medical services and attending temporary residents. A new feature of the 1992 General Medical Services regulations is that, in order to achieve full payment for childhood immunisations and cervical smears, targets set nationally as norms for the number of patients on the doctor's list must be achieved by each GP.

Certain GPs offer additional facilities, such as maternity medical services or family planning advice. The 1992 regulations for the first time offered payment to GPs for performing certain specified minor surgical procedures. Others may have beds available in local hospitals to which they can admit patients directly under their own care, i.e. without prior referral to a hospital consultant; these are usually for medical or maternity cases. These patients usually receive their medicines from the hospital pharmacy during their stay. Some hospital diagnostic and treatment services may also be open to the GP ('open access'); this invariably includes laboratory facilities for blood tests and microbiological tests, and at some hospitals may be extended to X-rays, ultrasound scans and physiotherapy. Some GPs hold part-time hospital appointments as clinical assistants, usually assisting consultants in outpatient clinics; any drugs they prescribe during these sessions will be dispensed either by the hospital pharmacy or by a community pharmacy upon receipt of a hospital-type form FP10(HP).

All permanent UK residents are entitled to register with a GP who, by accepting them on to his/her list (which he/she is not obliged to do), undertakes to provide medical care in accordance with the terms of service. HAs publish a local directory of doctors, including details of qualifications and sex, range of services offered and practice hours, the number of assistants and trainee GPs, and whether any languages are spoken in addition to English. Practices are now required to furnish each patient with a practice leaflet, updated annually, detailing the services on offer. GPs' lists usually number between 2000 and 4000 patients.

Doctors are required to supply drugs or appliances included in the *Drug Tariff*[15] needed for immediate treatment before a supply can be obtained. These should be purchased in advance from a pharmacy by the doctor. Further supplies are prescribed on form FP10 and, to quote from the regulations: [16]

> The prescription shall not refer to a previous prescription. The doctor shall himself sign the prescription form, in ink with his initials, or forenames, and surname in his own handwriting and not by means of a stamp, and shall so sign only after particulars of the order have been inserted in the prescription form. A separate form shall be used for each patient except where a doctor is prescribing in bulk for a school or institution . . .

(A 'bulk' prescription is an order, written on form FP10, for several patients in an institution or school; see *Drug Tariff* Part VIII DTA/26. Such prescriptions are exempt from prescription charges.)

Local medical committees

The local medical committee (LMC) is analogous in function to the local pharmaceutical committee (LPC). Its members, elected from among the GPs in the area, advise the HA about matters affecting local GPs, and liaise with hospital medical staff on matters of common interest. If, for example, the local trust hospitals wanted input from GPs to their drug and therapeutics committee, a nominee could be sought from the LMC. This committee would also probably nominate the doctors serving on the committee which the HA has to convene to investigate complaints against doctors by patients.

Dental services

General dental practitioners are, like doctors and pharmacists, in contract with the HA to provide services under the NHS. Many dentists have decided that NHS remuneration is insufficient to cover their costs, and have therefore withdrawn from a contract with the NHS. This has led to problems in some areas where it is difficult to find a dentist to give NHS treatment. The HA has an obligation to find a dentist who will provide treatment, and so should be contacted in this instance. (See also Chapter 1.)

Pharmaceutical services

In order to be able to dispense NHS prescriptions from a registered pharmacy, the pharmacist must hold a contract with the local HA. The HA has to publish a list of persons providing pharmaceutical services; the list also includes surgical appliance contractors and oxygen concentrator contractors. The terms of the NHS contract are defined by the NHS Act 1977, as subsequently amended. The details of the contract divide into two main areas: the opening of a pharmacy and the conditions of service required.

Opening a pharmacy

In 1992, the NHS Regulations were amended, resulting in changes to the way in which entry to the Pharmaceutical List was controlled.[16] Under these regulations, in consultation with the LPC, the HA determines whether or not to grant a new dispensing contract or to permit a minor relocation. The HA grants a contract if it considers that a new pharmacy in that location is both necessary and desirable, e.g. in a new premises or perhaps in-store in a supermarket. If the pharmacy does not meet either of the criteria, the application will be refused. An alternative method for a new pharmacy to acquire a contract to dispense may be to purchase the NHS contract from an existing pharmacy in the neighbourhood, in which case the HA may permit a minor relocation; this is also the method by which an existing contractor may be able to move, e.g. to larger premises nearby. The 1992 Regulations also changed the mechanism for dealing with appeals against decisions, and now any appeals are referred to the FHSAA, an SHA.

The arrangements for providing pharmaceutical services described are those in force at present, but changes are planned. In *Pharmacy in the Future*[17] the government sets out a number of proposals, including piloting local pharmaceutical services schemes (see below) and gives notice that the control of entry arrangements for community pharmacy will be changed if they block the development of better services for patients, or if they are clearly inappropriate. The Office of Fair Trading is currently reviewing the market for pharmaceutical services, and is due to report its findings during 2002.

Rural areas

Regulations were introduced in 1983 to control dispensing in rural areas.[18] These arose from the earlier Clothier Report, which considered the relationship of dispensing doctors and pharmacists. Under the 1983 regulations, a pharmacist wishing to open a new pharmacy in a rural area has to make the case direct to the HA. Appeals against decisions are dealt with as described in the previous paragraph. The existing controls led to considerable ill will between doctors and pharmacists in rural areas and new regulations are to be drafted by the government following 3 years of negotiations between the Pharmaceutical Services Negotiating Committee and representatives of dispensing doctors.[19] The new regulations will prevent doctors from establishing dispensaries in surgeries in locations that are already adequately provided with pharmaceutical services, and will discourage new pharmacies in areas where they may not be viable. HAs are not to be allowed to authorise new contracts to dispense in rural areas unless they are satisfied that they will not prejudice existing medical or pharmaceutical services in that area.

Guidance on the organisation of collection and delivery services in rural areas in England and Wales will be found in the *Medicines, Ethics and Practice* guide.[1]

Terms of service

Being accepted by an HA on to the Pharmaceutical List under the above regulations means that the pharmacy is under contract to the NHS to provide a dispensing service. The detailed regulations for this are set out in the NHS Act 1977 as amended, but useful summaries can be found in *Dale and Appelbe's Pharmacy Law and Ethics*[20] and in the *Chemist and Druggist Directory*.[21] The main provisions of the contract, apart from remuneration, cover hours of service, supply of dispensed items, quality of service through sampling and action taken in alleged breach of contract conditions.

Pharmacists in contract with the HA to provide NHS dispensing services are paid by a complex formula which is negotiated nationally. Some aspects of this, together with the regulations governing the entry into a contract with the NHS, will be explored below.

Remuneration of contractors for their NHS contract is determined by the Secretary of State after negotiation with the Pharmaceutical Services Negotiating Committee (PSNC). The arrangements are then published in the *Drug Tariff*,[15] which is sent to all contractors. In essence, the global sum paid to contractors is determined net of costs such as stockholding, and this global sum is increased annually by negotiation (in effect, the contractors' 'pay rise'). The costs of the service are taken from a sample of contractors who are monitored for the full costs of dispensing. There is often considerable debate, about both the cost figures which have been used, and also the detailed arrangements for the settlement.

For many years the arrangements for the payment of contractors were based almost exclusively on two concepts: the cost of a prescription, by adding an on-cost, and the number of prescriptions, by a fee. The on-cost had been removed prior to 1993, and in imposing the 1993 settlement, the Secretary of State announced the wish of government to move towards a professional fee to reflect the desire to develop the role of pharmacists in the health team. This concept is only recently being effected with the introduction of local pharmaceutical services pilots (see below).

Having a contract with the NHS is not essential to carry out a retail pharmacy business. The regulations for registration with the RPSGB allow an almost automatic grant of entry to the Register. This allows the pharmacy to undertake all duties except NHS dispensing, including the sale of Pharmacy medicines, and dispensing private prescriptions. This fact has been used by some contractors at non-contracted premises who receive NHS prescriptions, which are then dispensed at a nearby pharmacy which has a contract. In effect this bypasses the regulations which limit the entry of contractors to the list. Considerable debate has ensued, and in Scotland the process has been banned.

Hours of opening

The hours of opening are controlled by the HA within guidelines set out in the contract. In general, these hours are 9.00 a.m. to 6.00 p.m. (or 5.30 p.m. if that is normal local practice) for 6 days, with a maximum 1 hour for lunch and the normal local half-day closing from 1.00 p.m. In addition, the HA has to determine what service is needed to cover Sundays, bank holidays and urgently required prescriptions, and must organise and pay for pharmacies to participate in a rota which covers these extended times.[22] These services are known as additional pharmacist access services (formerly rota services). If a pharmacy chooses to open longer hours, it may do so, but must accept any prescription presented.

Supply of dispensed items

Supply must be made with 'reasonable promptness' to any prescription presented. Thus, a pharmacist cannot choose not to accept any particularly difficult prescription, and must endeavour to fulfil it as quickly as possible. Failure to comply with this requirement is a breach of contract, which can lead to a service case (see below). It is also part of the terms of service that the prescription is dispensed as written unless the prescriber has agreed to a change, or there are professional reasons why not to dispense, e.g. an error which cannot be rectified as the prescriber cannot be contacted. It is also a requirement that the pharmacist provides any ancillary service needed to fulfil the prescription, e.g. the supply of a 5-ml spoon, and for provision to measure for, and fit, appliances.

Drug Testing Scheme

Compliance with the conditions of service is monitored by a testing scheme for prescriptions set up by the local HA in accordance with national guidelines. Inspectors of the RPSGB, acting as agents of the HA, visit premises and take for analysis a prescription which has been dispensed and is awaiting collection. In summary, the prescription is

Table 12.6 Key sections of the *Drug Tariff*[15]

Arrangements for the payment of fees and allowances for contractors
Detail on the sums payable for imbursement for individual drugs
Approved lists of appliances, surgical dressings and other items prescribable on the NHS using form FP(10)
Arrangements for the supply of domiciliary oxygen
Details relating to prescription charges
Drugs and other substances not prescribable on the NHS ('Black List')

NHS, National Health Service.

weighed or counted as appropriate, and then divided into three approximately equal parts into containers provided by the pharmacist. These are sealed, and the inspector takes two containers, and one is left with the pharmacist. The inspector sends one sample to the Medicines Testing Laboratory in Edinburgh for testing, and the other is retained by the HA. Should the test results be unsatisfactory, the pharmacist is informed so that he/she may send his/her sample to an independent laboratory for testing. Should the two test results differ, the HA will send the results, together with the remaining sample, to the laboratory of the government chemist for further study.

Drug Tariff

The *Drug Tariff*[15] is prepared and published by the Secretary of State. It is published monthly and circulated to all contractors. It is full of essential information for contractors set out in 18 main sections. The important ones are listed in Table 12.6. (Further details about collecting prescription charges and checking exemptions will be found in Chapter 5.)

Prescription Pricing Authority (PPA)

The PPA is an SHA, and is thus directly responsible to the Secretary of State. It is responsible for the pricing of all NHS prescriptions in England; similar bodies operate in Wales and Scotland. Contractors are required to sort their NHS prescription forms as directed by the PPA. In summary, this means sorting forms into those for which prescription charges have been collected and those exempted, and within each category sorting the forms into doctor order. Forms other than the normal FP10s/GP10s used by GPs are treated as a separate category. The

PPA prices the forms and notifies the HA, which pays the contractors on a monthly basis. The scale of fees payable is set out in the *Drug Tariff*.[15]

Local pharmaceutical services pilots

The government in its *NHS Plan*[2] is committed to redesigning services around patients. Its interpretation of this in the context of pharmaceutical services is set out in *Pharmacy in the Future*:[17]

- pilot local pharmaceutical services (LPS) schemes will demonstrate new ways in which to organise and pay for community pharmacy, to deliver a wider range of services than under the current national contract, enabling local needs to be met more effectively;
- the national contract for community pharmacists will be developed to reward high-quality services at the expense of those prepared only to provide the basic minimum;
- pharmacy services
- will be designed around the needs of patients, not organisations;
  - — will be integrated with other services;
  - — make best use of all staff and their skills;
  - — take advantage of modern technologies;
  - — and will operate within more flexible contractual arrangements which promote and reward high quality, convenient access and good service, while tackling poor quality.

In 2001, the first step towards establishing pilot LPS schemes was taken when the DoH issued a briefing document.[23] From this, it appears that there is no fixed model proposed, but it is expected that successful bids, expected to start operating in 2002, will:

- contain good ideas on linking rewards for pharmacists to measures and outcomes other than prescription numbers, as in the present contract;
- increase the clinical input of community pharmacists in medicines management;
- integrate pharmacists into the primary health care team;
- use the accessibility of pharmacies in public health and neighbourhood renewal schemes;
- NHS prescriptions will be dispensed, but unlike the present contract, these could be limited to certain groups of patients or specific circumstances, e.g. out-of-hours services. PCTs or NHS trusts could be involved in pilot schemes, e.g. by establishing posts involving joint working between hospital and community pharmacies.

Advice on making successful bids was given in an article by Belling-ham,[24] and this would be a useful starting point for anyone planning to formulate a proposal.

Although some extra funding will be given to HAs to enable them to get started on the development of pilot schemes, it appears that for new services not covered by the existing contract, funding will have to be found locally. The threat to existing contractors implicit in this arrangement has led to considerable opposition to the new proposals from within the profession. Schemes analogous to LPS have already been initiated for doctors and dentists. Russell and Craig[25] reviewed the lessons to be learned by pharmacists from these pilots; they concluded that 'early winners may be those who do less well from the current contract such as those with a low dispensing volume'.

Hospital organisation and administration

Trust organisation and administration

As discussed above, most operational units within the NHS exist as NHS trusts. These can be acute trusts, running large hospitals and related services, or primary/community care trusts, which run services in these areas, including non-acute hospitals. Trusts are managed independently and acquire their work by obtaining contracts with purchasers, currently HAs and soon PCTs. Management arrangements for each unit, for matters not covered by statutory regulations, are made by local decision, and this means that there is no nationwide model. This section will there-fore describe typical arrangements.

The NHS and Community Care Act 1990 established NHS trusts to provide and manage the services to hospitals or other health care estab-lishments and facilities. Each trust has a board of directors consisting of a chair appointed by the Secretary of State, and executive directors and non-executive directors, i.e. not employed by the trust. One of the execu-tive members of the board will be the chief executive who manages the operation of the trust. Chief executives have been appointed from a variety of backgrounds, with the majority having an administrative back-ground, but with several being professionals, e.g. doctors, nurses and a few pharmacists. Some have been appointed from outside the NHS.

The chief executive is supported by a management board of vari-able membership. Typically there will be a director of finance, a medical director, a director of operations, a business manager (who might also be contracts manager) and one or more clinical directors. There is no

Table 12.7 Principal recommendations of the *Noel Hall Report*[26]

Hospital pharmaceutical services should be organised on a scale large enough to ensure that pharmacists and supporting staff are fully occupied on relevant professional and managerial activities, and that conditions create an adequate career structure
The unit of organisation will normally include 4000–6000 beds
Pharmacists should be supported by adequate technical and other staff
Training needs should be kept under review, and attendance at courses for further education should be encouraged

common pattern, as trusts are all trying to bring in new management styles, and are generally steering away from traditional hierarchies to much more devolved structures.

Pharmacy organisation at trust level

The Noel Hall Report

Prior to 1970, hospital pharmacy services were provided solely to each hospital in isolation. This led to problems, which were acknowledged in a report by Sir Noel Hall, published in 1970,[26] and commended to the NHS by a Department of Health and Social Security circular.[27] For many years, this report formed the basis of hospital pharmacy organisation, and its proposals are summarised in Table 12.7.

Since the implementation of the report there have been many management changes in the NHS, described above. Many of these changes have reduced or eliminated the management structures introduced by the report, but substantial elements of the concepts are maintained in other areas. Even with the introduction of the internal market and the formation of NHS trusts, many benefits have been maintained by informal cooperation. Managers have found professional and economic advantages arising from cooperation and networking and in most parts of the country groups of pharmacy managers still meet regularly for this purpose.

Pharmacy management within a trust

Pharmacy services within a trust are normally managed by a senior pharmacist whose job title will vary: sometimes chief pharmacist, sometimes director of pharmacy; these posts are generically known as senior pharmacy managers (SPMs). Such pharmacy managers are occasionally on the boards of their trusts, but more commonly are accountable to a board member. Many pharmacy managers also have a wider responsibility than pharmacy, commonly managing the central sterile supply department, medical supplies such as dressings, and/or other clinical or non-clinical departments. The logic for this is that the skills required to manage a diverse pharmacy department can easily be applied to similar services.

Pharmacists' grading structure

Although NHS trusts have the authority to pay staff according to locally agreed pay scales, to date most have decided substantially to follow nationally agreed rates. These are negotiated by Whitley Councils. Introduced at the beginning of the health service, the Whitley structure was set up to negotiate pay and conditions of service for all staff. In outline, there is a General Whitley Council, which deals with conditions of service applicable to all staff, e.g. travelling expenses, removal expenses, and there are several functional councils dealing with specific staff groups. Hospital pharmacists' conditions are dealt with by a committee within the Scientific and Professional Council. Each committee comprises a management side (which includes representatives from the DoH as well as NHS employers) and a staff side. Most of the representatives on the staff side are nominated by the Guild of Healthcare Pharmacists.

Conditions of service for all staff on Whitley conditions can be studied by reference to the relevant circulars or handbooks. These are often available from the senior pharmacist, but if not, can be consulted in the local personnel office. Changes which occur during a year, such as pay awards, are usually issued in a circular of notification, of which an example might be AL(PH)2/2001.[28] This reference number indicates that it is an Advance Letter, i.e. early warning of change; in this case it relates to PH or pharmacists, and it is the second letter of 2001.

The national agreement for pharmacists results in a grading scale rising from Grade A for newly qualified pharmacists to Grade H for the most senior pharmacy managers in charge of large (normally teaching) units and includes a grade for preregistration pharmaceutical students. The grading structure definitions were originally based on the increasing management complexity of the posts as they ascend the scale, and were not related to the experience or age of the post-holders. Thus, post-holders in the higher grades, i.e. E, F, G and H, will undertake an increasing proportion of management, and a decreasing proportion of practical pharmacy. Increasingly, however, clinical and technical expertise is being taken into account in grading. In addition, because of the trend for some SPMs to take on additional responsibilities outside pharmacy, a few are graded on general management scales, which in effect extends the range of salaries available. These latter scales often have an element of performance-related pay.

Pharmacy support staff

One of the more significant changes in pharmacy staffing in recent years has been the more effective use of supporting staff. There are two main categories – qualified pharmacy technicians and assistant technical officers (ATOs or pharmacy assistants).

Pharmacy technicians

Pharmacy technicians are recognised as having qualified by a variety of routes. Many will have successfully completed a 2- or 3-year part-time college course for a Business and Technicians' Education Council (BTEC) certificate. New technicians, however, qualify by undertaking study leading to the award of a National Vocational Qualification (NVQ). They are normally employed within the hospital service while attending the college course on a day-release basis, and will undertake a programme of job-based training in parallel with the college work. NVQs are being introduced for all technical staff to replace classic teaching methods, and are based on the requirement for students to achieve competence in undertaking tasks appropriate to their qualification. There are nationally five levels of NVQ relating to the level of interpretation, or working on one's own initiative involved in the job, and they are intended to give a commonality of competence across all technical areas. An introduction to the subject can be found in a book by Fletcher,[29] and the development of NVQs in pharmacy was detailed in a series of articles in the *Pharmaceutical Journal* in 1996.[30] The majority of pharmacy technicians are awarded a level three certificate, but it is also possible that certificates may be awarded in pharmacy in due course for achievement of competencies at levels two and four, and discussions are underway to use level two for pharmacy assistants. As a comparison, it is considered that level five equates roughly with a degree award.

Pharmacy technicians have a grading structure introduced by the Professional and Technical Whitley Council. This allows up to five grades of qualified medical technical officer (MTO) for technicians, and two grades for unqualified ATOs. As with pharmacists, grades are dependent on the complexity of the post rather than the experience of the post-holder.

Pharmacy technicians have an education in basic pharmacology and pharmaceutics, and support pharmacists both in dispensing and in support services. In addition, they often have management roles which may place them in charge of junior pharmacists, e.g. in dispensary management or in a technical service such as aseptic dispensing.

Pharmacy assistants

Pharmacy assistants or ATOs support pharmacists and technicians by carrying out routine tasks under supervision. They are generally unqualified, although with the introduction of NVQs, it is possible that a level one or two certificate may be introduced for this grade of staff. The two job titles as described indicate a historic anomaly, in that these staff were originally covered, as pharmacy assistants, by the Ancillary Staffs Whitley Council. The regrading of pharmacy technicians on to MTO grades allowed for the assistants to be reclassified as ATOs, but in some places this has not been done because of differences in conditions of employment, e.g. hours of work per week differ. Some ATOs have taken on supervisory roles for junior staff, and they can then be graded as senior ATO (SATO). Included in the duties that some ATOs and SATOs carry out are stock control and distribution of stocks. Some larger hospitals employ specific storekeeper clerks (an administrative and clerical grade) for these tasks.

Administrative staff

In addition to the operational staff described above, most pharmacies are also supported by clerical staff who undertake a range of duties from typing to financial duties such as checking invoices. These staff are normally paid under the Administrative and Clerical Whitley Council.

Specialist pharmacy services

The emphasis above has rightly been on pharmacy staff within a unit. In the new NHS, this is where operational matters should be decided. Over many years, however, since the implementation of the Noel Hall Report,[26] there has been a range of specialist pharmacy services organised on a larger scale – normally at the level of the former regions. They have been organised this way for two main reasons: they can be managed by an expert with scarce skills and knowledge who can contribute such expertise to a wide range of units, and they help economise on scale both through the centralisation of staff and of specialised expensive resources such as equipment or subscriptions. Such regional units are often supported by local units which deal with operational matters, e.g. a local medicines information unit may deal directly with enquirers and answer all queries, while a regional centre maintains a specialist literature base, prepares evaluated information and acts as a centre of expertise for the training of local staff (see Chapter 7).

The organisation of regional specialities has always varied across the country, and the recent management reorganisations have led to difficulties in maintaining these services. Generally, however, most regional specialities have been maintained in a variety of models. Some have been funded by an RO, while others have been funded on a cooperative basis by a group of hospitals, often in a regional or similar grouping.

Medical staff grading structure

Consultants

The most senior doctor in the hospital service is the consultant, who takes professional responsibility for the clinical care of all the patients referred to him/her. To be eligible for appointment as an NHS consultant, a doctor has to complete an extended professional training and be accredited in his/her speciality. Some consultant posts entail work at two or more hospitals, not necessarily within the same NHS trust. Many consultants are allocated a specific number of beds in the hospital, but others work in specialities that do not admit patients to their direct care, e.g. radiology and pathology. Most consultants head a team of junior doctors. These junior staff are responsible for their own professional decisions, but the amount of freedom that they have to do more specialised work, e.g. operations, is determined by their consultant. In hospitals, most of the day-to-day medical care of inpatients, including diagnostic procedures and minor operations, is carried out by junior doctors under the supervision of their consultant or registrar. There are various grades of increasing seniority and responsibility. Not every consultant's team (traditionally spoken of as a 'firm') will include all of the following grades, but a typical structure is as follows.

Senior registrars

This is the final 'junior' post that a doctor undertakes before becoming a consultant. It is normally held for 4 years, and is designed to give the final experience and specialised training required for professional accreditation. These posts often rotate between a teaching hospital and a district general hospital. A senior registrar may have responsibilities beyond his/her immediate team, e.g. a senior surgical registrar may be available to support junior staff in all surgical specialities at night and at weekends.

Registrars

The next most senior doctor in the hierarchy is the registrar – again a fixed-term post running for 1 or 2 years. By this stage, the doctor will have decided to pursue a career in the hospital service in the chosen speciality, and will be studying for or have obtained a higher qualification.

Senior house officers

After registration, doctors work for several further periods of 6 months or a year as senior house officers. The posts are usually designated as suitable for training for further professional qualifications, covering a variety of specialities, including gynaecology, paediatrics and casualty. These are sometimes combined in a structured rotational programme, including general practice trainee attachments as part of the vocational training: all intending GPs must undergo this.

Preregistration house officers

These are provisionally registered postgraduate doctors who are working for full registration with the General Medical Council. Two posts are held for 6 months each, in general medicine and general surgery; these are usually arranged by the doctor's medical school. To facilitate the training scheme, all such posts nationally are synchronised to change on 1 February and 1 August each year. There are usually two to a consultant's team, one for the male ward and one for the female, changing places after 3 months; they cover for each other's off-duty, and sometimes for the off-duty of other doctors in related specialities, known as 'baby-sitting'.

Medical staff training

Undergraduate training of doctors is organised by the medical schools of universities. It is based on success in degree examinations of the university, but also has a practice component. After students have successfully completed the first section of theoretical examinations, the clinical part of their training consists of attending ward rounds and clinics, and participating in the work of the wards under supervision. This experience is divided between the wards of the university hospital ('teaching hospital') and those of district general hospitals. In their final year, selected students may work for short periods assisting a house officer whose opposite number is on leave – a so-called medical student assistantship. The amount of authority they are given is set out in an NHS Executive circular.[31] (See also Chapter 6.) They are not permitted to initiate treatment or to write prescriptions for Controlled Drugs or Prescription Only Medicines.

Postregistration training for doctors is largely based on qualification for membership of one of the medical Royal Colleges. These colleges set standards of practice within their speciality, and membership of the appropriate college is essential for career progression. Many of the junior doctor grades, and the conditions attaching to them, link with the training programmes for qualifications for the college examinations. The first level of higher qualification in medicine is Membership of the Royal College of Physicians (MRCP): fellowship is awarded to distinguished members by election. The equivalent first-level qualification for surgeons is, somewhat confusingly, Fellow of the Royal College of Surgeons (FRCS). This is because there is an undergraduate diploma designated MRCS. It is on award of their FRCS that surgeons revert in title from 'Dr' to 'Mr/Mrs/Miss'. Some surgeons also obtain a postgraduate degree, Master of Surgery (MS).

Medical staff organisation

In most NHS trusts individually consultant-led teams of similar specialities are formed for managerial purposes into organisational units known variously as service groups, directorates or divisions. An example might be a medical division, which could include gastroenterology, renal medicine, rheumatology, cardiology, dermatology and sexual health. One of the consultants will be designated as the clinical director, possibly on a rotational basis, and he/she will have some managerial responsibilities on behalf of the group, although each consultant retains clinical autonomy. Each directorate is a self-contained unit of management, with responsibility for its own staffing, operational management and control of budgets. The clinical director works closely with the service manager, who will head up an organisation including management accountants as well as nursing managers. Together they will have to make decisions about the allocation of resources, and will contribute to service planning as well as making bids for capital and revenue for the service.

Medical directors

Using the same model as commercial companies with their boards of directors, the activities of NHS trusts are directed by a board headed by a chief executive; one of the consultants will be appointed as a medical director, with a seat on the trust board. Usually this doctor will divide his/her time between clinical responsibilities as a consultant, and managerial responsibilities. Typically the appointment would be for a 5-year period, and at the end of this time another consultant would take over. A British Medical Association working party issued guidance about the role of medical directors. They considered, *inter alia*, that:

- They should have overall responsibility for medical staffing, including consultant appointments, contracts and job plans.
- They should play an important part in disciplinary procedures for medical staff.
- They should be the source of medical advice to the board, and convey the views of the clinical directors.
- They should have board-level responsibility for medical audit and postgraduate education.
- They should also play an important role in the reporting and managing of untoward incidents and medical complaints.

It should be noted that they do *not* manage the other consultants.

Nursing staff organisation

Nursing staff management structures are largely determined locally and there is no universally accepted model. Until recently, the only career pathway upwards meant that ambitious nurses had to move away from patient care into administration or teaching. It has now been recognised that this did not improve patient care, and new grades have been introduced which enable clinical nurses designated as consultants to be financially rewarded. Such posts must involve working directly with patients, clients or communities for at least 50% of the time. The circular[32] introducing this change defined the core functions that could lead to a post being designated:

- an expert practice function;
- a professional leadership and consultancy function;
- an education, training and development function;
- a practice and service development, research and evaluation function.

Senior sisters/charge nurses: modern matrons

As part of the implementation of the government's NHS plan, a new grade of senior sister/charge nurse (female/male respectively) has been introduced.[33] With the emphasis on a high profile on the wards, and a job description that should give the post-holder real authority to implement change, it is intended that these post-holders will raise both the standards of clinical nursing practice and public awareness of the government's ongoing quality initiative. According to the circular, 'matrons will be accountable for a group of wards. They will be easily identifiable to patients, highly visible, accessible and authoritative figures to whom patients and their families can turn to for assistance, advice and support and upon whom they can rely to ensure that the fundamentals of care are right'. Many units already have nurse managers that equate to senior sisters, so the concept is not entirely new. In addition, many district general hospitals have a senior nurse on duty at night, with hospital-wide responsibilities, to whom the night sisters/charge nurses report.

Ward and departmental managers

Each conventional ward or unit directly involved in patient care, such as day surgery, outpatients' department or accident and emergency department, has a senior nurse manager, who will report to the senior sister/charge nurse, discussed above. The ward manager has overall responsibility for the day-to-day running of the ward, organising staff rotas and ensuring that stocks of consumables are ordered and that equipment is present and maintained. Pharmacists should already be familiar with the fact that the ward manager is responsible for Controlled Drug stocks on the ward, although routine ordering and checking activities may be delegated.

During the evening and night, night sisters/charge nurses are responsible for groups of wards, which they visit as necessary to supervise the night ward team. When Controlled Drugs are administered, they are taken from the ward's stock, under the supervision of night sisters/charge nurses, who have no stocks of their own.

The ward team

Several qualified nurses will work on the ward; they are known as staff nurses and are managed by the ward manager. The team will include some who permanently work at night. In addition, the ward will have student nurses assigned to it on rotation. They are supernumerary to the ward team. While on the ward, their work will be supervised by the qualified nurses, sometimes supplemented by visiting nursing school staff. The students have to participate fully in the rota, and may work at night. Also reporting to the ward manager are nursing assistants, who undertake most of the routine tasks such as patient toilet procedures and bedmaking. Many wards have a ward clerk who probably answers the telephone and who handles the myriad clerical duties required, e.g. making follow-up outpatient appointments for patients being discharged and filing reports in case notes. In addition, funding is being made available over the next 3 years to introduce by 2004 ward housekeepers to manage the hotel services on the ward – food service, cleaning and linen provision.

Nurse practitioners

Nurse practitioners are specialists in a particular field who have extra responsibilities and, according to their area of expertise, have patients referred to them and may hold clinics. They do not usually form part of a ward team, although they may visit wards to advise on specialist treatment. Some examples of nurse practitioner roles are listed in Table 12.8. Such nurses are likely to achieve nurse consultant status, as discussed above.

Nurse practitioners currently may prescribe or issue medicines within the hospital under the authority of patient group directions (see Chapter 1), and also appliances and surgical equipment such as syringes. They are likely to extend their prescribing rights in the future. The government has recently recommended that appropriately trained nurses working in accident and emergency departments should be given extended powers, including ordering X-rays, diagnostic tests and the interpretation of results, and give medication and discharge patients.[34]

Table 12.8 Examples of nurse practitioner

Breast care and mastectomy advice	Family planning
Chemotherapy specialist	Minor injuries clinic
Continence adviser	Stoma care
Control of infection	Wound management and tissue viability
Diabetic specialist	

Nurse training

On 1 April 2002, the Nursing and Midwifery Council replaced the UK Central Council, formerly responsible for maintaining a register of all qualified nurses and midwives. This new statutory body has taken over the registration of nurses and midwives, and sets and monitors education and professional standards for entry to the register. It also investigates allegations of misconduct and incompetence, and is able to order removal from the register.

Since 1989, a new college or university-based system of nurse education has been introduced. Students now study for a Diploma of Higher Education in Nursing or a degree in nursing, both of which lead to registration as a nurse in the chosen branch of nursing. In both cases, the course lasts for a minimum of 3 years, combining theoretical studies with practical experience in hospital and community settings. The first year is a common foundation programme, but thereafter the student has to choose between adult nursing, mental health nursing, children's nursing and learning-disability nursing. During the course, which lasts for 3 years altogether, the student has full student status, and instead of a salary, receives a bursary. Midwifery is now regarded as a separate profession, and it is possible to take a 3-year Diploma of Higher Education in Midwifery, without previously qualifying as a registered nurse; registered nurses in adult nursing can also qualify by taking further training in midwifery.[35]

In most care settings, whether in hospitals or in residential and nursing homes, many practical nursing tasks are undertaken by nursing or care assistants, who may work independently or under the supervision of qualified nurses. There are many unstructured training programmes to impart the skills needed, but in addition, there is a move towards the more structured approach afforded by the NVQ scheme. Teaching and assessment for NVQs are task-oriented and practice-based, and NVQs gained in one area of work may be used to progress towards higher qualifications in other technical fields.

Table 12.9 Professions registered with the Health Professions Council

Chiropodists	Physiotherapists
Dieticians (or nutritionists)	Radiographers
Medical laboratory scientific officers	Orthoptists
Occupational therapists	Speech and language therapists

Other staff groups

The NHS is not only an employer of large numbers of staff, but because of the range of expertise needed, these staff represent over 100 special interests. Doctors, nurses and pharmacists have already been discussed, but it is worthwhile mentioning at least some of the other groups.

Health Professions Council

Several groups of health professional are linked through their membership of the Health Professions Council (HPC), a new statutory body that has replaced the Council for the Professions Supplementary to Medicine. Registration with the Council is mandatory for workers within the NHS, although it is not necessarily required for entry to the profession. The main professions that pharmacists are likely to encounter are listed in Table 12.9.

Dentists

Dentists have a similar education to doctors, and those who choose to stay in the hospital service can progress to consultant status. The main subspeciality is oral surgery (where senior practitioners are sometimes medically qualified as well), but there are also posts in orthodontics and restorative dentistry.

The majority of dentists work in the community, in private practice, NHS general practice under contract to the HA, or in the community dental service. The latter service is managed by a community dental officer, who also liaises with dentists in general practice. The community dental service is provided to schools and to handicapped adults, as well as advising on policy matters such as fluoridation.

Management and administration

To support the large numbers of health professionals in the NHS, many managers are employed by the NHS. They are appointed from a variety

Table 12.10 Patient services: main functions

Manage Patient Administration System (PAS)	Master index of patients
	Allocates hospital (unit) numbers
	Outpatient appointments
	Tracks patient attendances, admissions, transfers and deaths
	Waiting lists
	Hospital performance statistics
	Purchaser/provider information
Medical records department	Files and retrieves case notes 24 hours a day
	Files reports, letters and prescription sheets
Medical secretariat	Consultant and ward/departmental secretaries
	Write referral letters and discharge summaries
Death registration department	Organises medical certificates of death, cremation certificates
	Liaises with bereaved families
	Liaises with undertakers, coroners' officers
	Stores and issues deceased patients' effects

of backgrounds, but most career managers are members of the Institute of Health Services Management. Membership is by examination after taking an appropriate course of study. This studying is normally carried out part-time while working in junior grades of the NHS. Increasingly, managers are appointed with relevant qualifications such as business, management or law degrees, which exempts them from some of the Institute's examinations. Much of the work of managerial staff is outside the scope of this book, but it is relevant to mention their role in patient services in more depth.

Patient services department

The main roles of the patient services department (PSD) are listed in Table 12.10.

Perhaps the commonest reason for a pharmacist to interact with the PSD is the need to locate a patient's case notes. Pharmacists must be aware of, and follow, hospital procedures designed to restrict access to confidential patient information. In 1997, the Caldicott Committee, set up by the Chief Medical Officer, published a report[36] that recommended that NHS organisations should be held accountable through clinical governance procedures for continuously improving confidentiality and security procedures governing access to and storage of personal

Table 12.11 Retention of hospital patient individual case records

Children and young people	Until 25th birthday, or 26th if person was 17 at conclusion of treatment, or 8 years after death if death occurred before 18th birthday
All obstetric and midwifery records, including drug prescription and administration records	25 years
Mentally disordered persons (within the meaning of Mental Health Act 1983)	20 years after no treatment considered necessary, or 8 years after death if patient died while receiving treatment
Patients involved in clinical trials	15 years after conclusion of treatment
General (not covered above)	8 years

information. There is now a Controls Assurance Standard for record management, which enables practice to be audited.[37]

Case records and the Public Records Act

Hospital records have legal significance not only for the patient, but also because they form part of NHS records generally, which are treated by law as public records.[38] The case records or notes should form a consecutive account of every clinic visit, medical examination and consultation. Also included are the results of diagnostic tests and X-ray reports, prescription sheets and copies of correspondence, mainly with the referring doctor. Public records are subject to regulations concerning their preservation and destruction, which are set out in a Health Circular.[39] The guidance is intended to retain the confidentiality of the patient's medical records while allowing access to other types of information, e.g. financial records. The periods of time for the retention of hospital patient individual case records are set out in Table 12.11.

As public records, however, if there is some inclusion of national importance, this may warrant retention for a longer period. The magnitude of the storage problem which this presents is potentially huge, as there could be a set of notes in store for every member of the population. This possibility is reduced by the time limit, but conversely increased by the fact that an individual may have sets of notes at several different hospitals. (See Chapter 8 for confidentiality and laws relating to disclosure of medical records.)

Table 12.12 Retention of non-medical records

Delivery notes	1.5 years
Establishment records – major (personal files, letters of appointment, related correspondence)	6 years after person leaves or until 70th birthday, whichever is later (summary only need be retained until 70th birthday)
Attendance records Annual leave records Timesheets	2 years
Job applications Job descriptions	3 years after termination of employment
Job advertisements	1 year
Pharmacy records	Local decisions should be made with regard to the permanent preservation of these records, in consultation with relevant health professionals and places of deposit.
Product records	11 years (Consumer Protection Act)
Quality assurance records	12 years
Stock control reports	1.5 years
Record of custody and transfer of keys	1.5 years
Inspection reports (boilers, lifts, etc.)	Lifetime of installation

Retention of non-medical records

In addition to medical records, several other records generated within the pharmacy are classified as public records, as discussed above, and are subject to regulations about their retention and disposal set out in the same circular. The main examples affecting pharmacy practice are set out in Table 12.12.

References

1. Royal Pharmaceutical Society of Great Britain. *Medicines, Ethics and Practice: A Guide for Pharmacists.* published yearly, London: Royal Pharmaceutical Society of Great Britain.
2. Department of Health. *The NHS Plan: A Plan for Investment, A Plan for Reform* (Cm 4818–1). London: Stationery Office, 2000.
3. Department of Health. *Shifting the Balance of Power Within the NHS – Securing Delivery.* London: Stationery Office, 2001.

4. Merry P, ed. *Wellard's NHS Handbook 2001–02*. Wadhurst, East Sussex: JMH.
5. Scottish Department of Health. *Our National Health: A Plan for Action, A Plan for Change*. London: Stationery Office, December 2000.
6. National Assembly for Wales. *Improving Health in Wales – A Plan for the NHS with its Partners*. Cardiff: National Assembly for Wales, 2001.
7. Department of Health. *Leadership for Health: The Health Authority Role*. HSC 1999/192.
8. Brookes W T. Self-governing trusts. *Pharm J* 1991; 246: 47.
9. Department of Health. *Patient and Public Involvement in the New NHS*. London: Stationery Office, 1999.
10. Covey D. *Patients and the NHS. Wellard's NHS Handbook 2000–01*: Wadhurst, East Sussex: JMH: 246–253.
11. Gilbey J. The changing NHS – purchaser and provider. *Pharm J* 1991; 246: 76.
12. News item. DoH rethinks GP freedoms as two-tier service emerges. *H Serv J* 1993; 103: 3.
13. News item. Health authorities gain new power over contractors from next week. *Pharm J* 2001; 267: 737.
14. News item. What will new disciplinary and control powers for health authorities mean? *Pharm J* 2002; 267: 774.
15. Department of Health and National Assembly for Wales. *Drug Tariff*. Published monthly. London: Stationery Office.
16. National Health Service (Pharmaceutical Services) Regulations 1992. SI 1992 no. 662.
17. Department of Health. *Pharmacy in the Future – Implementing the NHS Plan*. London: Stationery Office, 2000.
18. Report. Clothier Regulations to take effect on April 1st. *Pharm J* 1993; 230: 312.
19. News item. New rural dispensing settlement agreed. *Pharm J* 2001; 266: 342.
20. Appelbe G E, Wingfield J. *Dale and Appelbe's Pharmacy Law and Ethics*, 7th edn. London: Pharmaceutical Press, 2001.
21. *Chemist and Druggist Directory*, published annually. Tonbridge, Kent: United Business Media Information Services.
22. NHS Executive. *Additional Pharmaceutical Services: Arrangements for Locally Managed Pharmaceutical Services for 1999/2000*. HSC 1999/076.
23. News item. First wave of local pilots in 2002. *Pharm J* 2001; 266: 270.
24. Bellingham C. How to win bids and influence future pharmacy services in your locality. *Pharm J* 2001; 267: 81–82.
25. Russell R, Craig G. Local pharmaceutical services – what can we learn from doctors and dentists? *Pharm J* 2001; 267: 865–866.
26. Department of Health and Social Security. *Report of the Working Party on the Hospital Pharmaceutical Service*. London: Her Majesty's Stationery Office, 1970.
27. Department of Health and Social Security. *Hospital Pharmaceutical Service*. HM(71)70.
28. Department of Health. *Health Care Pharmacists: Increases to National Salary Scales for 2001/02*. AL(PH)2/2001.
29. Fletcher S. *Designing Competence Based Training*. London: Kogan Page, 1992.

30. Mansfield R, Benson A, Morgan L. National Vocational Qualifications. *Pharm J* 1996; 257: 602–605.
31. NHS Executive (1991). *Medical Students in Hospitals: A Guide to their Access to Patients and Clinical Work.*
32. NHS Executive. *Nurse, Midwife and Health Visitor Consultants.* HSC 1999/217.
33. NHS Executive. *Implementing the NHS Plan – Modern Matrons.* HSC 2001/010.
34. News item. Extended role for A and E nurses. *Pharm J* 2000; 264: 357.
35. NHS Careers. *Nursing and Midwifery in the New NHS.* London: Stationery Office, 2000.
36. Caldicott Committee. *Review of Patient Identifiable Information.* London: Stationery Office, 1997.
37. NHS Executive. *Controls Assurance Standard: Records Management.* London: Stationery Office, 1999.
38. Public Records Act 1958 s.3(1)–(2).
39. NHS Executive. *For the Record: Managing Records in NHS Trusts and Health Authorities.* HSC 1999/53.

Index

A & E, *see* accident and emergency departments
ABPI, *see* Association of the British Pharmaceutical Industry
Access to Health Records Act 1990, 220
accident and emergency departments, 18
accounting in community pharmacies, 91
accreditation, 270–273
  British Standards Institute, 271–272
  Investors In People, 272–273
ADROIT, *see* adverse drug reactions, On-Line Information Tracking
adverse drug reactions
  On-Line Information Tracking, 43
  reporting scheme for, 43–44
advisers, pharmaceutical, 314–315
agencies, medical
  Care Standards Act, 60
  independent, regulation of, 60
Aitken Report, and midwifery, 147
'alternative' medicines, 82–83
antibodies, monoclonal, 199
asset
  management, 298–299
  registers, 299
assistant technical officers, 329
assistants
  clinical, 318
  nursing, 335
Association of the British Pharmaceutical Industry, 23, 35
  Code of Practice, 23, 34–35
ATOs, *see* assistant technical officers
audit
  clinical, 258
  computer, 286

financial, 284–286
internal, 284–285
professional, 273–274
Audit Commission, **258–259**
  NHS trust accounts, 285
  procurement, 294

BASICS *see* British Association for Immediate Care
Borderline Substances, 33–34
Breckenridge Report, 154, 195
British Association for Immediate Care, 167
British Standard
  ISO 9000, 202
  pharmaceutical containers, 112–114
  quality management, 271–272

cardiopulmonary resuscitation kits, 169
Care Council for Wales, 60
care homes
  administration and control of medicines, 62, **63–64**
  'homely remedies', 64
  monitored-dose systems, 63–64
  pharmaceutical services, 63–65
  training for work in, 64–65
Care Standards Act 2000, 58–61
centralised intravenous additive service, 154–155, **195–200**
  guidelines for, 196
  National Group, 196
Centre for Pharmacy Postgraduate Education, 74, 251
Charter
  NHS, 261–262
  Patients', 261–262
CHC, *see* community health council
chemotherapy
  dispensing, 198–200

chemotherapy *(continued)*
  prescriptions, 100–101
CHI, *see* Commission for Health
      Improvement
CIVAS, *see* centralised intravenous
      additives service
clinical governance, **263–265**
  Hospital Pharmacists' Group
      policy, 265
  role of CHI, 267
  RPSGB policy, 264–265
clinical indicators, 267–268
clinical pharmacists
  advisory role, 173–175
  control of infection committee, 174
  drug and therapeutics committee,
      174
clinical pharmacy, **169–172**
  intervention monitoring, 172
  intervention recording, 171
clinical trials
  certificates, 40
  Doctors' and Dentists' Exemption
      Scheme, 44
  of established drugs, 44
  European Directive on, 40
  exemption certificates, 40
  planning for, 40–41
  postmarketing surveillance
      guidelines, 37
  role of the pharmacy, 40–42
  running of, 41–42
clinical waste
  categories, 226
  disposal, 225–227
  licensed waste contractors,
      226–227
  procedures, 227
  waste disposal carriers, 226
clinics, independent, regulation, 59
Clothier Report (on contaminated IV
      fluids), 28
code of practice
  Association of the British
      Pharmaceutical Industry, 23,
      34–35
  medical gas cylinders, 129, 206
  Proprietary Association of Great
      Britain, 23
cold chain
  audit of, 206

  maintaining in clinics, 165–166
  quality assurance of, 206
College of Pharmacy Practice,
      251–252
  Faculty of Prescribing and
      Medicines Management, 252
Commission for Health
      Improvement, 261, **266–267**
Committee
  Caldicott, 338–339
  NHS Pharmaceutical Quality
      Control, 202
  Standing Pharmaceutical Advisory,
      309
committees
  control of infection, 174
  drug and therapeutics, 174
  local medical, 319
  local research and ethics, 41
  select, role of, 305–306
communication, 118–119
community
  care, 3
  community clinics, **164–165**
    childhood immunisation
        programme, 165–166
    cold chain, 165–166
    patient group directions, 164
    refrigerators, 165–166
  family health services in, **316–325**
  health councils, 315
  health services, access to, 3
  midwives, 148
  pharmaceutical services, **319–325**
    control of entry, 319–320
    dispensing contract, 319
    pharmaceutical list, 319–320
    rural areas, 321
community pharmacies
  accounting, 91
  administration, 85–91
  computer technology, 85–86
  contraception and sexual health,
      80–81
  design of premises, 83–85
  diagnostic services, 80
  Disability Discrimination Act,
      84–85
  ear piercing, 82
  emergency hormonal
      contraception, 80–81

financial controls, 90–91
goods returned for credit, 89–90
health promotion, 77–80
opening, 83–84
organisation, 83–85
patient areas, 85
protocols, 75
purchasing for, 87–89
purchasing via wholesalers, 88–89
receipt of goods, 89
response to symptoms, 75–76
security, 85
services provided by, 74–83
smoking cessation, 79
stock control, 86–87
supply and control of medicines,
    86–90
supply of 'alternative' medicines,
    82–83
supply of complementary therapies,
    82–83
supply of veterinary medicines, 83
surgical appliances, 76–77
wound management products,
    76–77
community pharmacists
extended role, 69–70
prescribing by, 74–76
complaints
procedure, NHS, 19–20
review panel, 20
complementary therapies, 82–83
compliance, **114–119**
aids, 116–118
aids, nurses and, 118
see also concordance
computers
audit, 286
Common Basic Specification,
    287–288
in community pharmacy, 85–86
in pharmacy, 286–288
concordance, **114–119**
pharmacist's role in, 115–116
see also compliance
confidentiality, 219–220
continuing professional development,
    252–253
contraception and sexual health,
    80–81
contracts, tendering for, 297–298

Control of Substances Hazardous to
    Health Regulations, 239–240
Controlled Drugs in hospitals,
    142–144
destruction, 144–145
monitoring, 147
storing, 143–144
supplying, 143
unwanted, 144
Controls Assurance Documents,
    National, **270**
decontamination of medical
    devices, 224
emergency preparedness, 270
medical devices management, 270
medicines management, safe and
    secure handling, 138
record management, 270, 339
waste management, 226, 270
COSHH, see Control of Substances
    Hazardous to Health
    Regulations
CPD, see continuing professional
    development
CPP, see College of Pharmacy
    Practice
CPPE, see Centre for Pharmacy
    Postgraduate Education
CPR see cardiopulmonary
    resuscitation kits
Crown Report, 11
CTX, see clinical trials, exemption
    certificates
cytotoxics, dispensing, 198–200

Data Protection Act, 1998, 220
Data Protection Commissioner, 220
DDX, see clinical trials, Doctors'
    and Dentists' Exemption
    Scheme
defective products, reporting,
    222–223
dentists, **9–10**
dental service, community, 10, 319,
    337
prescribing, 9
Devonport incident, 28
diagnostic services in community
    pharmacies, 80
DIAL, see Drug Information
    Advisory Line

directors
  clinical, 332
  medical, 333
Disability Discrimination Act, 84–85
dispensaries
  layout and house keeping, 108
  safe system of work, 105–108
  standard operating procedures,
    105–106
dispensing
  cytotoxics, 198–200
  errors, 108–110
  extemporaneous preparations,
    110–114
    documentation of, 201
    formulation, 201
    hazards, 112
    standards, 111–112
  infants and children, 121–124
  labels, 107
  near-patient, 152
  non-sterile specials, 200–201
  older people, 119–121
  packaging, 112–114
  quality assurance of, 205
  records of 'specials', 112
  specialised services, 26
  training assistants, 105–106
doctors
  dispensing, 7, 320
  limited registration, 215
  provisionally registered, 215
  registration, 215
  visiting EU practitioner, 215
domiciliary visits, 17
drug addicts
  clinical management guidelines for,
    125
  needle and syringe exchange
    schemes, 126–127
  prescribing for, 125–126
  services for, 124–127
Drug Alerts, 223
  classification of, 224
Drug Information Advisory Line,
  121–122
drug information centres, *see*
  medicines information centres
Drug Information Manual, 182
Drug Tariff
  bulk prescribing, 318

key sections for contractors, 323
medical gases, 128, 130
outpatients, 161
prescribing and, 31
wound management products,
  127
Drug Testing Scheme, 322–323
drug usage review, 187–188
drugs, new, 37–44
Drugs Squad, 217–218
DUMP campaigns, 227–228
Duthie Guidelines, 270
  patients' own medicines, 225

ear piercing, 82
EDI, *see* electronic, data interchange
education
  Centre for Pharmacy Postgraduate,
    251
  continuing, 250–253
    role of the RPSGB, 250–251
  education and training, **249–253**
EHC, *see* emergency hormonal
    contraception
EHR, *see* electronic, health records
electronic
  data interchange, 292–293
  health records, 290
  information, 290–291
  patient record, 290
  see also computers
EMEA, *see* European Medicines
    Evaluation Agency
emergency hormonal contraception,
  80–81
emergency
  cupboards, 168
  procedures, 166–169
employment
  appointing staff, 236
  contracts, 236
  discrimination in, 235–236
  dismissal of staff, 236–238
  equal opportunities in, 235–236
  law, 235–242
Environmental Protection Act 1990,
  225–226
EPACT Net, 50
EPR, *see* electronic, patient record
European Medicines Evaluation
    Agency, 38

evidence-based medicine, 188–189
excise officers, 218–219
stills and, 219

Family Health Services Appeals
    Authority, 317
FHSAA, *see* Family Health Services
    Appeals Authority
financial controls
    cash flow, 91
    invoices, 90–91
financial management
    audit, 284–286
    budget statements, 284
    budgets, 283–284
    internal audit, 284–285
flammables, storage, 200
formularies, 189–190
    management of, 190
FP10 (HP) prescription form,
    157–159
    abuse of, 158–159
funding, NHS, **279–283**
    capital and revenue, 281
    cash limits, 280
    NHS cash allocation, 279–280
        distribution of allocation,
            281–282
    private finance, 281

general practice
    deputising services, 8
    out-of-hours
        co-operatives, 9
        services, 8–9
general practitioners, **5–9**
    group practices, 6–7
    health centres, 7
    private practice, 6
    training and education, 5–6
General Social Care Council, 60
generic medicines,
    manufacture and marketing, 25–26
    prescribing, 31–32
    procurement, 295
    substitution in hospitals, 150
GPs, *see* general practitioners
guidelines
    centralised intravenous additives
        services, 196
    Duthie, 144

postmarketing surveillance, 37
    SAMM, 42–43
    TPN for children, 198

HASAWA, *see* Health and Safety at
    Work etc. Act
Hazard Notices, 223
HDA, *see* Health Development
    Agency
Health and Safety at Work etc. Act,
    238–239
Health and Safety Executive, role of,
    238
Health and Social Care Act 2001,
    308
    disciplinary powers over
        contractors, 317
health authorities, **311–312**
    family health services, 316
    regional, 310
    special, 312
health boards, 311–312
health care
    contracting for, 315–316
    co-operatives, local, 314
    organisation, 305–306
    providers, private, **58–61**
        pharmaceutical requirements,
            61–63
        regulation and standards, 58–61
health centres, 7
Health Development Agency, 78
Health Education Council, 78
health groups, local, 314
Health Improvement Programmes,
    260, 269
    role of HAs, 311
Health Professions Council, 337
health
    promotion, 77–80
    services, family, 316–325
The Health of the Nation, 73
Health Technical Memorandum
    2010, 194
    2022, 129, **207**
Health Technology Appraisals, 266
Health Technology Assessments, 188
High Level Performance Indicators,
    267–269
HIMPs, *see* Health Improvement
    Programmes

HLPIs, *see* High Level Performance
Indicators
home care teams, 163
hospices, 64
hospital
admission, 17–18
at home, 163
inpatients
administration of medicines,
150–152
dispensing for, 152–156
patients' own drugs, 152
self-medication, 151–152
organisation and administration,
325–326
outpatients
dispensing for, 156–162
FP10 (HP), 157–159
non-*Drug Tariff* items, 161
prescription charges, 159–160
prescription receipts, 160
prescription sheets for, 157–158
prescriptions owing, 161
pharmaceutical service
on-call schemes, 168
out of hours, 167–169
pharmacokinetics service,
172–173
production, 190–201
residency schemes, 167–168
ward and department stock
drugs, 138–142
staff as patients, 162
hospitals, independent
Care Standards Act, 59
HTA *see* Health Technology
Assessments
HTM, *see* Health Technical
Memorandum

incidents, major **166–167**
mobile teams, 167
industrial tribunals, 237–238
infants and children
calculating dosage, 122
'off-label' prescribing, 121
presentation of drugs, 122–123
Information for Health, 263, 288
electronic health records, 290
information technology, 286–288
insurance

professional indemnity, 213–214
public liability, 214
intermediate care, **163–164**
Care Standards Act, 59
providers, regulation of, 59
internal market, 315–316
International Organisation for
Standardisation, 271
intravenous fluids
additives, 154
total parenteral nutrition, 154–156
Investors in People UK, 272–273
IPPR *see* Itemised Prescription
Payment Report
ISO 9001 (2000), 271–272
ISO, *see* International Organisation
for Standardisation
Itemised Prescription Payment
Report, 50

kits
anaphylactic shock, 169
cardiopulmonary resuscitation, 169

management
authority in, 254
communication, 253–254
delegation, 254–255
departmental, 253–256
NHS, 310–311
planning, 255–256
managers, ward and departmental,
334–335
manufacturers, special-order, 111
Manual of Cancer Services Standards,
198
marketing authorisation
mutual recognition procedure, 38
stages leading to, 38–40
maternity pay and leave, 241–242
MDA, *see* medical devices, agency
medical devices
agency, and defective products, 222
Controls Assurance Standard for
decontamination, 224
decontamination of, 223–224
medical directors, 333
medical gases, **128–132**
cylinders, *Code of Practice*, 129,
206
domiciliary oxygen, 130

Health Technical Memorandum No 2022, 129, 207
liquid, 131–132
oxygen concentrators, 130
quality assurance of, 206–207
medical practitioners, general, *see* general practitioners
medicinal products
marketing authorisation
application for, 37–40
new, 37–44
registration of, 37–40
medicine measures, British Standards for, 113
Medicines Act 1968, 191
Medicines Control Agency
Defect Reporting Centre, 223
defective products, 222
Medicines for Older People, 119–120
medicines
collection for charity, 228
generic, 25–26
marketing
commercial sponsorship, 36
promotional activities, 36–37
standards of conduct, 34–35
not prescribable on the NHS, 32–33
over-the-counter, 25
patient's own, 225
postlicensing evaluation, 34
postmarketing
safety assessment, 42–43
studies, 42–44
prescribing on form FP 10, 318
procurement, 293–295
purchasing, 296–297
reuse, 225
in schools, 123–124
take-home, 17–18
unlicensed indications, 44
unwanted, 224–225, 227–228
disposal, 228
WHO guidelines for donations, 228
medicines information
centres, local, 183–184
centres, regional, 182–183
and clinical audit, 187–188
drug usage review, 187–188
evidence-based medicine, 188–189
formularies, 189–190
information sources, 186–187
proactive, 185–186
quality, 184–185
records, 184
service **179–180**
new products assessments, 180–181
organisation, 180
standards for enquiry answering, 185
Medicines Information, UK
Pharmacists Group, 180–182
medicines management, **71–74**
Collaborative National Medicines
Management Services
Programme, 52–53
performance management
framework, 263
see also pharmaceutical care
mercury spillage, 228
midwifery
Aitken Report, 147
'flying squad', 148
services, **147–148**
midwives, registration, 336
Modernisation Agency, 307
Modernisation Board, 307
monitored-dosage systems, 116–118
Moving Forwards, 58, 60

National Care Standards
Commission, **58–60**, 61
National Horizon Scanning Centre, 181
National Institute for Clinical
Excellence, 261, **265–266**
National Patient Safety Agency, 109
National Performance Assessment
Framework, **267–269**
clinical indicators, 267–268
High Level Performance Indicators, 267–269
National Pharmaceutical Association
and insurance, 213–214
National Pharmaceutical Supply
Group, 294–295
National Prescribing Centre, **51–52**
new products assessments, 181
Prescribing Nurse Bulletins, 15
National Service Frameworks, 262–263

National Vocational Qualification
  Scheme, 248
  ATOs, 329
  care assistants, 336
NCSC, *see* National Care Standards
  Commission
nebuliser therapy, 130–131
needle and syringe exchange schemes,
  126–127
The New NHS: Modern,
  Dependable, 260–261, 262,
  264
NHS
  complaints procedure, 19–20
  local pharmaceutical services
    pilots, 324
  management and administration,
    337–340
  networks, 289–290
  The NHS Plan, 307–308
  stores, centralised pharmaceutical,
    141–142
  structure and organisation,
    309–315
  treatment, eligibility for, 162
NHS and Community Care Act 1990,
  4
  contracting for health care, 315
  internal market, 282
NHS Centre for Review and
  Dissemination, 188
NHS Direct, 10
NHS Executive, 309
  regional offices, 310
    and NHS trusts, 313
NHS Information
  Authority, 288
  Strategy, 288–289
NHS Litigation Authority, 214
NHS trusts, **312–313**
  organisation and administration,
    325–326
  pharmacy organisation, 326–327
  primary care
NHSE, *see* NHS Executive
NHSSA, *see* NHS Supplies Authority
NICE, *see* National Institute for
  Clinical Excellence
Noel Hall Report, 326
NPA, *see* National Pharmaceutical
  Association

NPC *see* National Prescribing Centre
NSFs, *see* National Service
  Frameworks
nurse practitioners, **335–336**
  A & E, 18
nurse prescribers, **14–15**
  Formulary, 14
  prescription forms for, 14
  supplementary prescribing, 14
  training, 15
nurses
  community, 217
  consultants, 333–334
  Macmillan, 11
  modern matrons, 334
  organisation of, 333–336
  palliative care, 11, 14
  student, 217
  training, 336
  ward and departmental managers,
    334–335
Nursing and Midwifery Council,
  336
nursing homes, 58
NVQ, *see* National Vocational
  Qualification Scheme

'off-label' prescribing, 103
  for infants and children, 121
Ombudsman, *see* Parliamentary and
  Health Service Commissioner
orders, standing, 311
'orphan drugs', 27
out-of-hours services
  dentists, 9
  general practice, 8–9
  GP co-operatives, 9
  procuring drugs, 168–169
outpatient clinics
  form FP10 (HP), 16
  NHS consultant, 16–17
oxygen
  concentrators, 130
  cylinders, supply on FP10, 130
  domiciliary, 130

PACT, *see* Prescribing Analysis and
  Cost
PAGB, *see* Proprietary Association of
  Great Britain
parallel importing, **29**

Parliamentary and Health Service
    Commissioner, 20–21
Partnership in Action, 263
PASA, *see* Procurement and Supply
    Agency
patient
    focused care, 152
    group directions, **11–14**
        A and E nurses, 18
    information leaflets, 107
    information, use of, 219–220
    medication records, 221
        and counter prescribing, 221
        Data Protection Act, 220
    services department, 338
patients'
    own drugs, 152
    rights, 19–21
PCCLG *see* Pharmacy Community
    Care Liaison Group
PDGs, *see* pharmacy, development
    groups
PFI, *see* Private Finance Initiative
PGDs, *see* patient, group directions
pharmaceutical advisers, 54–55
pharmaceutical care, 71–74
    Minnesota Project, 72
    see also medicines management
pharmaceutical containers, British
    Standards for, 112–114
Pharmaceutical Industry
    Competitiveness Task Force,
    30–31
Pharmaceutical Price Regulation
    Scheme, 30
pharmaceutical services, local pilots,
    324
    specialist, organisation of, 329–330
Pharmaceutical Services Negotiating
    Committee, 321
pharmaceuticals
    branded products, 24–25
        labelling, 24
    government control, 27–34
    manufacture, 23–27
    marketing, 24–27, 34–37
        standards of conduct, 34–35
    'specials', 26
    storage on wards, 144–145
    suppliers, 24–27
        control of, 27–31

pharmacists
    primary care, 55–57
        core competency framework, 55
    hospital, grading, 327–328
pharmacokinetics service, 172–173
pharmacy
    assistants, 329
    development groups, 70–71
    managers, senior, 327
    services, online, 291
    technicians, 328–329
Pharmacy Community Care Liaison
    Group, 53–54
    and carers, 118
Pharmacy in a New Age, **69–70**
    clinical governance policy,
    264–265
Pharmacy in the Future
    community pharmaceutical
        services, 320
    local pharmaceutical services
        pilots, 324
PharmEDI, 293
Pharm-line, 182
PIANA, *see* Pharmacy in a New Age
PICTF, *see* Pharmaceutical Industry
    Competitiveness Task Force
PILS, *see* patient, information leaflets
planned preventative maintenance,
    204
PMCPA, *see* Prescription Medicines
    Code of Practice Authority
poisoning, **229–230**
    identification of poisons, 229–230
    treatment of, 230
police officers, **217–218**
    chemist inspection officers, 218
    confidentiality, 218
policy, disciplinary, 237–238
PPA *see* Prescription, Pricing
    Authority
PPM, *see* planned preventative
    maintenance
PPP, *see* Public Private Partnership
PPRS, *see* Pharmaceutical Price
    Regulation Scheme
Prescribing Analysis and Cost, 50
prescribing
    'Black List', 32–33
    borderline substances, 33–34
    bulk prescriptions, 318

prescribing *(continued)*
  by community pharmacists, 74–76
  by dentists, 9
  Drug Tariff, 31
  generics, 31–32
  government controls, 31–34
  in hospitals
    electronic, 149–150
    generic substitution, 150
    inpatients, 148–150
    medical students, 150
  nurse, 14–15
    Formulary, 14
  'off-label', for infants and children, 121
  support
    practice level, 56–57
    primary care, 49–51
    training for, 57
  'White List', 32
Prescription
  Medicines Code of Practice Authority, 34
  Pricing Authority, **323–324**
    FP10 (HP)s, 159
    Fraud Investigation Unit, 96
    retention of FP 10s, 216
prescriptions
  abbreviations in, 100
  charges
    evasion, 96–97
    exemption, 96–97
  checking procedure, 153–154
  chemotherapy, 100–101
  contraindications, 104
  data, anonymised, 220
  dispensing, 96–105
  extemporaneously dispensed, 104–105
  forged, 214–215
  fraud, 96–97
  hospital inpatients, 152–156
  hospital outpatients, 159–160
  incorrect, 102
  interactions, 104
  non-NHS, 97–98
  'off-label', 103
  private, 97–98
  problem, 98–102
  queries, 216
  reading and checking, 98
  receiving, 96–97
  repeat, 102–103
  'specials', 104–105
  'take-home', 154
  unlicensed products, 103
  urgent, 218
  weekend leave, 154
primary care, 3
  dental services in, 9–10
  family health services in, 316–325
  groups, 51, 313–315
  medical services in, 5–9
  NHS trusts, 313–315
  nurses in, 10–15
  pharmacists, 55–57
  prescribing support, 49–51
  trusts, 51
Private Finance Initiative, 281
procedures
  running clinical trials, 41–42
  standard operating, in dispensary, 105–106
procurement
  contracting, 293–295
  e-commerce, 293
  medicines, 293–295
    generic, 295
  supplies departments, 294–295
Procurement and Supply Agency, 294–295
production, pharmaceutical, 190–201
  Medicines Act 1968
    Section 10 exemptions, 191
    Section 55 exemptions, 191
  terminally sterilised products, 194
  training manual, 192
  Orange Guide, 191, **192–193**
  unlicensed units, standards, 191
Proprietary Association of Great Britain, 23
protocols
  group, 11–14
  medicines counter assistants, 75
  shared care, 16
PSNC, *see* Pharmaceutical Services Negotiating Committee
Public Private Partnerships, 281
Public Records Act 1958
  case records, 339
  hospital prescriptions, 158

purchasing
  controls on, 296
  drug orders, 296
  medicines, 296–297
  pharmacy consortia, 296
  requisitions, 296
  'short-line' stores, 296–297

quality
  circles, 274–275
  standards, imposed by government,
    258–269
  suggestion schemes, 275
quality assurance
  cold chain, 206
  dispensing, 205
  documentation, 203–204
  environmental monitoring, 204
  good laboratory practice, , 207
  hospital manufacture, 202–205
  in hospitals, 201–207
  master documents, 203
  medical gases, 206–207
    Permit to Work, 207
  personnel and training, 202–203
  planned preventative maintenance,
    204
  premises and equipment, 204
  process and materials, 204–205
  quarantine storage, 204–205
  storage, 205–206
  transportation, 205–206
Quality Control, NHS Pharmaceutical
  Committee, 202

radiopharmacy, **194–195**
  regulations governing, 195
  UK Radiopharmacy Group, 195
RAWP, *see* Resource Allocation
    Working Party
reagents, 128
receptionists, 8
  prescribing, 8
records
  case, retention of, 339–340
  non-medical, retention of, 340
refrigerators
  community clinics, 165–166
  drug, on wards, 146
Registered Homes Act 1984, 58
Registered Homes Tribunal, 60

repackaging, 193–194
Reporting of Injuries, Diseases and
    Dangerous Occurrences
    Regulations, 240
representatives, medical, 35
  samples, 35
residential homes, 58
Resource Allocation Working Party,
    281–282
response to symptoms, 75–76
RIDDOR, *see* Reporting of Injuries,
    Diseases and Dangerous
    Occurrences Regulations
Rosenheim Report, 28
RPSGB, National Syllabus for
    Continuing Education, 250
rural areas
  dispensing, 321
  prescription collection and delivery
    services, 320

safe system of work, 105–108
SAMM Guidelines, 42–43
schools, medicines in, 123–124
SCOPE, *see* Standing Committee for
    Pharmacy Postgraduate
    Education
Scottish Centre for Post Qualification
    Pharmaceutical Education, 74
Scottish Social Services Council, 60
secondary referral, 15–17
service, additional pharmacist access,
    322
service-level agreements, 283
service, rota, *see* service, additional
    pharmacist access
SFIs, *see* standing financial
    instructions
SHA, *see* health authorities, special
*Shifting the Balance of Power within
    the NHS – Securing Delivery*,
    307, 308–309
smoking cessation, 79
SOs, *see* standing orders
SOPs, *see* standard operating
    procedures
SPAC, *see* Committee, Standing
    Pharmaceutical Advisory
'specials'
  manufacturers, 26
  ordering, 111

'specials' *(continued)*
  prescriptions for, 104–105
SSP, *see* Statutory Sick Pay
staff
  appointing, 236
  appraisal, 246–247
  competencies, 247–248
  development, 246–249
  dismissal, 237–238
  identification of training needs,
    248–249
  job descriptions, 242
  maternity pay and leave, 241–242
  medical
    grading structure, 330–331
    organisation, 332–333
    training, 332
  performance review, 247
  person specifications, 243
  recruitment, 242–246
  selection, 244–245
standard operating procedures, in
    dispensary, 105–106
Standing Committee for Pharmacy
    Postgraduate Education, 251
standing financial instructions, **285,**
    311
  drug promotion, 35
  procurement, 294
  stock management, 298
standing orders, **285**
  procurement, 294
  stock management, 298
Statutory Sick Pay, 240–241
stills, 219
stock
  checks, 299
  management, 298–299
  security, 298–299
stores
  centralised NHS pharmaceutical,
    141–142
  'short-line', 296–297
students, medical, 332
  prescribing by, 150
supplies departments, 294–295
surgical appliances, 127–128
  community pharmacies, 76–77
surgical equipment, 127–128

TDM *see* therapeutic drug monitoring

technician top-up, 140
technicians, checking, 106
Technology Appraisal Guidances, 266
telemedicine, 291
terms of service
  community pharmacists, 321–324
  general practitioners, 317–318
  pharmacy contractors'
    remuneration, 321
  pharmacy opening hours, 322
  supply of dispensed items, 322
therapeutic drug monitoring,
    172–173
total parenteral nutrition, **197–198**
  and specialised dispensing services,
    26
  cold chain in, 198
  guidelines for children, 198
TPN *see* total parenteral nutrition
training, staff, 249–253
  preregistration students, technical
    services, 192
treatment, private
  consultations, 18–19
  NHS hospitals, 162–163
trusts, NHS, 312–313

UK Central Council, 336
UK Medicines Information
    Pharmacists Group, 180–182
UKMIPG, *see* UK Medicines
    Information Pharmacists
    Group

veterinary medicines, 83

walk-in centres, 10–11
ward pharmacy, **169–172**
ward visit, 170–172
  stock orders
    creating, 140–141
    lists, control of, 139–140
    processing, 141–142
  stock, top-up service, 140
  stocks, monitoring, 145–147
Whitley Council
  Administrative and Clerical, 329
  Ancillary Staffs, 329
  conditions of service, 327
  General, 327
  Professional and Technical, 328–329

Scientific and Professional, 327
wholesalers
   control of, 28–29
   use by community pharmacies,
      88–89
Woods Report, 101
Working for Patients, 257–258, 259

Working Together, 263
wound management products, 127
   in community pharmacies, 76–77

'Yellow Card' Scheme, *see* adverse
      drug reactions, reporting
      scheme for